Schizophrenia

Guest Editor

PETER F. BUCKLEY, MD

PSYCHIATRIC CLINICS OF NORTH AMERICA

www.psych.theclinics.com

September 2012 • Volume 35 • Number 3

SAUNDERS an imprint of ELSEVIER, Inc.

W.B. SAUNDERS COMPANY
A Division of Elsevier Inc.

1600 John F. Kennedy Boulevard ● Suite 1800 ● Philadelphia, PA 19103-2899

http://www.theclinics.com

PSYCHIATRIC CLINICS OF NORTH AMERICA Volume 35, Number 3
September 2012 ISSN 0193-953X, ISBN-13: 978-1-4557-4928-7

Editor: Joanne Husovski
Developmental Editor: Donald Mumford

Psychiatric Clinics of North America (ISSN 0193-953X) is published quarterly by Elsevier Inc., 360 Park Avenue South, New York, NY 10010-1710. Months of issue are March, June, September, and December. Business and Editorial Offices: 1600 John F. Kennedy Blvd., Suite 1800, Philadelphia, PA 19103-2899. Periodicals postage paid at New York, NY and additional mailing offices. Subscription prices are $265.00 per year (US individuals), $473.00 per year (US institutions), $131.00 per year (US students/residents), $321.00 per year (Canadian individuals), $589.00 per year (Canadian Institutions), $399.00 per year (foreign individuals), $589.00 per year (foreign institutions), and $194.00 per year (international & Canadian students/residents). Foreign air speed delivery is included in all *Clinics*' subscription prices. All prices are subject to change without notice. **POSTMASTER:** Send address changes to *Psychiatric Clinics of North America*, Elsevier Health Sciences Division, Subscription Customer Service, 3251 Riverport Lane, Maryland Heights, MO 63043. Customer Service: 1-800-654-2452 (US). From outside the United States, call 1-314-447-8871. Fax: 1-314-447-8029. E-mail: journalscustomerservice-usa@elsevier.com (for print support) and journalsonlinesupport-usa@elsevier.com (for online support).

Reprints. For copies of 100 or more, of articles in this publication, please contact the Commercial Reprints Department, Elsevier Inc., 360 Park Avenue South, New York, New York 10010-1710. Tel.: (212) 633-3813, Fax: (212) 462-1935, E-mail: reprints@elsevier.com.

Psychiatric Clinics of North America is covered in *MEDLINE/PubMed (Index Medicus)*, *Current Contents/Social and Behavioral Sciences, Social Science Citation Index, Embase/Excerpta Medica,* and PsycINFO.

Printed and bound by CPI Group (UK) Ltd, Croydon, CR0 4YY

Transferred to digital print 2012

Contributors

GUEST EDITOR

PETER F. BUCKLEY, MD
Dean and Professor of Psychiatry, Medical College of Georgia, Georgia Health Sciences University, Augusta, Georgia

AUTHORS

MARIO ÁLVAREZ-JIMÉNEZ, PhD, DClinPsy, MAResearchMeth
Orygen Youth Health Research Centre, Melbourne, Australia; Centre for Youth Mental Health, The University of Melbourne, Melbourne, Victoria, Australia

ANTHONY O. AHMED, PhD
Department of Psychiatry and Health Behavior, Georgia Health Sciences University, Augusta, Georgia

SARAH BENDALL, PhD, MClinPsych
Orygen Youth Health Research Centre, Melbourne, Victoria, Australia; Centre for Youth Mental Health, The University of Melbourne, Melbourne, Victoria, Australia

MONICA BENEYTO, PhD
Department of Anatomy and Neurobiology, University of Vermont, Burlington, Vermont

DENIS BIRGENHEIR, MS
Department of Psychiatry and Health Behavior, Georgia Health Sciences University, Augusta, Georgia

CHRISTOPHER R. BOWIE, PhD
Associate Professor of Psychology and Psychiatry, Queens University, Ontario, Canada

JOHN BUCKLEY
Senior Student, Davidson Fine Arts High School, Augusta, Georgia

PETER F. BUCKLEY, MD
Dean, School of Medicine, Medical College of Georgia; Department of Psychiatry and Health Behavior, Georgia Health Sciences University, Augusta, Georgia

THOMAS H.J. BURNE, PhD
Queensland Brain Institute, University of Queensland, St Lucia; Queensland Centre for Mental Health Research, The Park Centre for Mental Health, Wacol, Queensland, Australia

MARY CANNON, PhD, MRCPsych
Department of Psychiatry, Royal College of Surgeons in Ireland, Education and Research Centre, Beaumont Hospital, Dublin, Ireland

MAURICE CLANCY, MB, MRCPsych
Department of Psychiatry, Royal College of Surgeons in Ireland, Education and Research Centre, Beaumont Hospital, Dublin, Ireland

MARY C. CLARKE, PhD
Department of Psychiatry, Royal College of Surgeons in Ireland, Education and Research Centre, Beaumont Hospital; Department of Psychology, Division of Population Health Sciences, Beaux Lane House, Dublin, Ireland

CHRISTOPH U. CORRELL, MD
Division of Psychiatry Research, The Zucker Hillside Hospital, North Shore-LIJ Health System, Glen Oaks, New York; Hofstra North Shore-LIJ School of Medicine, Hempstead, New York; Albert Einstein College of Medicine, Bronx, New York; The Feinstein Institute for Medical Research, Manhasset, New York

NANCY J. DOANE, PhD
Department of Psychiatry and Health Behavior, Georgia Health Sciences University, Augusta, Georgia

DARRYL W. EYLES, PhD
Queensland Brain Institute, University of Queensland, St Lucia; Queensland Centre for Mental Health Research, The Park Centre for Mental Health, Wacol, Queensland, Australia

ADRIANA FOSTER, MD
Associate Professor of Psychiatry, Department of Psychiatry and Health Behavior, Medical College of Georgia, Georgia Health Sciences University, Augusta, Georgia

JAMES GABLE, PharmD
Senior Medical Student, Medical College of Georgia, Georgia Health Sciences University, Augusta, Georgia

JUAN A. GALLEGO, MD, MS
Psychiatry Research, The Zucker Hillside Hospital, North Shore-Long Island Jewish Health System, Glen Oaks, New York; The Feinstein Institute for Medical Research, Manhasset, New York

JOHN F. GLEESON, PhD, MClinPsych
Department of Psychology, Australian Catholic University, Melbourne, Victoria, Australia

NADA M. GOODRUM, BS
Department of Psychiatry and Health Behavior, Georgia Health Sciences University, Augusta, Georgia

PHILIP D. HARVEY, PhD
Professor, Department of Psychiatry and Behavioral Sciences, University of Miami Miller School of Medicine, Miami, Florida

IAN KELLEHER, PhD
Department of Psychiatry, Royal College of Surgeons in Ireland, Education and Research Centre, Beaumont Hospital, Dublin, Ireland

JOHN G. KERNS, PhD
Associate Professor, Psychological Sciences Department, University of Missouri, Columbia, Missouri

MATCHERI S. KESHAVAN, MD
Stanley Cobb Professor and Vice Chair for Public Psychiatry, Department of Psychiatry, Beth Israel Deaconess Medical Center and Massachusetts Mental Health Center, Harvard Medical School, Boston, Massachusetts

E. KILLACKEY, DClinPsy
Orygen Youth Health Research Centre, Melbourne, Victoria, Australia; Centre for Youth Mental Health, The University of Melbourne, Melbourne, Victoria, Australia

JOHN LAURIELLO, MD
Professor, Department of Psychiatry, University of Missouri, Columbia, Missouri

R. LEDERMAN, PhD
The Department of Computing and Information Systems, The University of Melbourne, Melbourne, Victoria, Australia

DAVID A. LEWIS, MD
Department of Psychiatry, University of Pittsburgh, Pittsburgh, Pennsylvania

P. ALEX MABE, PhD
Department of Psychiatry and Health Behavior, Georgia Health Sciences University, Augusta, Georgia

PATRICK D. McGORRY, PhD, MD
Orygen Youth Health Research Centre, Melbourne, Victoria, Australia; Centre for Youth Mental Health, The University of Melbourne, Melbourne, Victoria, Australia

JOHN J. McGRATH, MD, PhD
Professor, Queensland Brain Institute, University of Queensland, St Lucia; Queensland Centre for Mental Health Research, The Park Centre for Mental Health, Wacol, Queensland, Australia

ANILKUMAR PILLAI, PhD
Associate Professor of Psychiatry, Department of Psychiatry and Health Behavior, Medical College of Georgia, Georgia Health Sciences University, Augusta, Georgia

MICHAEL PIPER, PhD
School of Biomedical Science, Queensland Brain Institute, University of Queensland, St Lucia, Queensland, Australia

JAI SHAH, MD
Resident in Psychiatry and Dupont-Warren Research Fellow, Harvard Longwood Psychiatry Residency Training Program, Department of Psychiatry, Harvard Medical School, Boston, Massachusetts

VINOD H. SRIHARI, MD
Associate Professor, Department of Psychiatry, Yale University; Director, Clinic for Specialized Treatment Early in Psychosis (STEP), Connecticut Mental Health Center, New Haven, Connecticut

RAJIV TANDON, MD
Professor of Psychiatry, University of Florida, Gainesville, Florida

G. WADLEY, PhD
The Department of Computing and Information Systems, The University of Melbourne, Melbourne, Victoria, Australia

Contents

Although dementia praecox or schizophrenia has been considered a unique disease entity for more than a century, definitions and boundaries have changed and its precise cause and pathophysiology remain elusive. Despite uncertain validity, the construct of schizophrenia conveys useful clinical and etiopathophysiologic information. Revisions of the Diagnostic and Statistical Manual of Mental Disorders and the International Classification of Diseases seek to incorporate new information about schizophrenia and include elimination of subtypes, addition of psychopathological dimensions, elimination of special treatment of Schneiderian "first-rank" symptoms, better delineation of schizoaffective disorder, and addition of a new category of "attenuated psychosis syndrome".

The neurodevelopmental hypothesis of schizophrenia suggests that the disruption of early brain development increases the risk of later developing schizophrenia. This hypothesis focuses attention on critical periods of early brain development. From an epidemiologic perspective, various prenatal and perinatal risk factors have been linked to schizophrenia, including exposures related to infection, nutrition, and obstetric complications. From a genetic perspective, candidate genes have also been linked to altered brain development. In recent decades evidence from neuropathology has provided support for the neurodevelopmental hypothesis. Animal models involving early life exposures have been linked to changes in these same brain systems, providing convergent evidence for this long-standing hypothesis.

This article gives an overview of genetic and environmental risk factors for schizophrenia. The presence of certain molecular, biological, and psychosocial factors at certain points in the life span, has been linked to later development of schizophrenia. All need to be considered in the context of schizophrenia as a lifelong brain disorder. Research interest in schizophrenia is shifting to late childhood/early adolescence for screening and preventative measures. This article discusses those environmental risk factors for schizophrenia for which there is the largest evidence base.

combination and discontinuation trials are necessary to determine the effectiveness, safety, and role of APP in the management of severely ill patients with insufficient response to antipsychotic monotherapy.

This article discusses the measurement of cognition in schizophrenia, its role as a determinant of disability, and treatment efforts to date, including pharmacological and behavioral interventions as well as effective treatments that lead to improved outcomes. The measurement of functioning when patients with schizophrenia receive treatment in the office is addressed. The review focuses on new developments in the creation and adoption of a consensus method for the assessment of cognitive functioning in treatment studies, on the increased appreciation for assessment of functional skills in the prediction of everyday outcomes, and on developments in the basic neuroscience of cognition.

This article provides a snapshot of the nature, guiding philosophy, and empiric status of interventions for people with schizophrenia that go beyond traditional psychopharmacological and psychosocial treatments to include peer-led interventions. The authors discuss the nature and principles of peer-led interventions for people with schizophrenia and the types of peer-led interventions along with evidence of their effectiveness in fostering the recovery of people with schizophrenia and other severe mental illnesses. Focus is on 3 types of peer-led interventions: (1) mutual support/self-help, (2) consumer-operated services, and (3) peer support services.

The impact of mental illness, comorbid substance abuse, and medication nonadherence, coupled with disjointed psychiatric and social services, conspires to a disproportionately high rate of psychiatric disorders among people who are homeless in the United States. This article reviews the prevalence of homeless among the mentally ill as well as the prevalence of mental illness among the homeless and details barriers in access to care and the solutions that have been attempted. The need and solutions to introduce a new generation of physicians and allied health care workers to the unique health care needs of the homeless population are highlighted.

The Internet and mobile technologies are becoming ubiquitous. However, the potential of these technologies to support people with psychosis has been unexplored and the development of innovative e-based interventions is overdue. Research suggests the acceptability and effectiveness of such interventions in psychosis. Internet-based technologies have the potential to transform psychosis treatment by enhancing the accessibility of evidence-based interventions, fostering engagement with mental health services, and maintaining treatment benefits over the long term. This article reviews the current evidence on Internet-based interventions for psychosis, including potential benefits, risks, and future challenges. Recommendations are proposed for developing future online interventions for psychosis.

PSYCHIATRIC CLINICS OF NORTH AMERICA

FORTHCOMING ISSUES

Forensic Psychiatry
Charles Scott, MD, *Guest Editor*

Integrative Therapies in Psychiatry
Philip Muskin, MD, Robert Brown, MD,
and Patricia Gerbarg, MD, *Guest Editors*

Disaster Psychiatry
Craig Katz, MD, and Anand Pandya, MD,
Guest Editors

RECENT ISSUES

June 2012
Addiction
Itai Danovitch, MD, and
John J. Mariani, MD, *Guest Editors*

March 2012
Depression
David L. Mintz, MD, *Guest Editor*

December 2011
**Obesity and Associated Eating
Disorders: A Guide for Mental Health
Professionals**
Thomas A. Wadden, PhD,
G. Terence Wilson, PhD,
Albert J. Stunkard, MD, and
Robert I. Berkowitz, MD,
Guest Editors

DOWNLOAD
Free App!

Review Articles
THE CLINICS

NOW AVAILABLE FOR YOUR iPhone and iPad

Preface

Early Diagnosis and Intervention in Schizophrenia

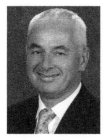

Peter F. Buckley, MD
Guest Editor

Schizophrenia remains a poorly understood and yet a profoundly serious condition among all the major medical illnesses. We have witnessed a major shift in the past 5 years with the belief now that diagnosing and intervening early may have a positive influence on the outcome of schizophrenia. This shift has led to a search for key diagnostic clusters to enhance early diagnosis as well as to concerted efforts to find biomarkers of disease and disease progression. To that end, this issue of the *Psychiatric Clinics of North America* is dedicated to these contemporary issues that promote "early intervention" in schizophrenia. Distinguished academic clinicians and neuroscientists provide comprehensive overviews of the present state of knowledge on the epidemiology, early clinical characteristics and diagnostic changes, proposed pathogenesis, neurobiology, and treatment requirements for this disorder.

The optimism and excitement for real progress in schizophrenia research treatment are incorporated into this text. The current state of knowledge is substantial, academically credible, and scientifically based, although it is true that we remain a ways off from robust biomarkers to primary and secondary prevention efforts. I am most grateful to our outstanding group of contributors for their expert reviews that provide the most current "state of play" about schizophrenia.

Peter F. Buckley, MD
Medical College of Georgia
Georgia Health Sciences University
1120 15th Street, AA-1002
Augusta, GA 30912, USA

E-mail address:
pbuckley@georgiahealth.edu

Psychiatr Clin N Am 35 (2012) xiii
doi:10.1016/j.psc.2012.06.012
0193-953X/12/$ – see front matter © 2012 Elsevier Inc. All rights reserved.

The Nosology of Schizophrenia
Toward *DSM-5* and *ICD-11*

Rajiv Tandon, MD

KEYWORDS

• Schizophrenia • *DSM-5* • *ICD-11* • Nosology • Classification • Psychosis

KEY POINTS

- Based on the absence of clear boundaries around schizophrenia, the multiplicity of implicated etiologic factors, and pathophysiologic mechanisms, schizophrenia is likely a conglomerate of multiple disorders.
- Dissection of schizophrenia's heterogeneity is proving difficult, with the dimensions/endophenotypes approach coupled with illness staging currently the most promising approach toward resolving this disease admixture.
- An etiopathophysiologic nosology of schizophrenia and related psychotic disorders is currently elusive, so the hope is that the *Diagnostic and Statistical Manual of Mental Disorders* (Fifth Edition) (*DSM-5*) and the *International Classification of Disease, Eleventh Revision* (*ICD-11*) will provide a more useful platform than the current *DSM-IV* and *ICD-10* in integrating emerging genetic and other neurobiologic information about these conditions that ultimately may serve as a bridge between the clinically useful psychopathologic nosology of today and an etiopathophysiologic classification of tomorrow.
- Proposed changes in DSM-5 include elimination of the classic subtypes, addition of unique psychopathological dimensions, elimination of special treatment of "Schneiderian" first-rank symptoms, better delineation of schizoaffective disorder, and addition of a new category of "attenuated psychosis syndrome" for further study.

OVERVIEW

The present nosologic system (ie, system of classification of disease) for psychiatric disorders originated in efforts during the late nineteenth and early to mid-twentieth century, culminating in a section related to mental disorders (section V) in the *ICD-6*[1] in 1949 and the first edition of the *DSM-1*[2] in the United States in1952. Schizophrenia and related psychotic disorders comprised one of the major sections in both manuals. In subsequent revisions (*ICD-7, ICD-8, ICD-9, ICD-10, DSM-II, DSM-III*, and *DSM-IV*), changes have been made in specific diagnostic criteria, but the basic

Disclosure statement: Rajiv Tandon is a member of the *DSM-5* Work Group on Schizophrenia and Related Disorders and the World Psychiatric Association Pharmacopsychiatry Section. The opinions expressed in the article are those of the author alone and do not purport to represent any of the organizations that the author belongs to.
Department of Psychiatry, University of Florida, PO Box 103424, Gainesville, FL 32610-3424, USA
E-mail address: tandon@ufl.edu

Psychiatr Clin N Am 35 (2012) 557–569
http://dx.doi.org/10.1016/j.psc.2012.06.001
0193-953X/12/$ – see front matter Published by Elsevier Inc.

structure has been retained. Differences in criteria between the *DSM* and *ICD* systems have narrowed with considerable similarity between *DSM-IV*[3] and section V of *ICD-10*.[4] The process of revising both *DSM-IV* and *ICD-10* is under way, with *DSM-5* likely released in 2013 and *ICD-11* expected to be finalized by 2016. Current versions of both *ICD-10* and *DSM-IV* are marked by considerable complexity, variable validity, and limitations in clinical and research utility; the revisions under way seek to address these limitations.

Schizophrenia has been studied as a specific disease entity for the past century with the assumption that it is caused by a distinct pathologic process whose nature continues to be unknown. Its precise core definition, boundaries, pathogenesis, and cause remain undefined.[5,6] Since its demarcation as dementia praecox by Kraepelin and Robertson[7] and schizophrenia by Bleuler and Zinkin,[8] its definitions have varied and its boundaries have expanded and receded. Thus, it is instructive to examine its origins and varying definitions over the past 150 years (**Fig. 1**).

Concept of Schizophrenia from the Nineteenth Century to DSM-IV and ICD-10

Although there are descriptions of insanity from ancient times, the concept of schizophrenia is of relatively recent origin. In the mid to late nineteenth century, European psychiatrists began describing a range of mental disorders affecting young adults that were associated with deterioration and chronicity. Morel termed them, *démence precoce*,[9] Clouston called them *adolescent insanity*,[10] Kahlbaum described *katatonia*,[11] and Hecker described *hebephrenia*.[12] The current construct of schizophrenia derives from Kraepelin's formulation of dementia praecox in the late nineteenth century and his elaboration of this concept in the early part of the twentieth century.[7,13] Until that time, there were two broad prevailing views about the nature of major psychiatric illness. Based on his study of persons with mental disorders in large psychiatric hospitals, Griesinger postulated that there was only one basic form of psychosis with diverse manifestations attributable to endogenous and environmental factors (einheitspsychose).[14] In contrast to this concept of a unitary psychosis, others suggested that there were several distinct disorders (catatonia, hebephrenia, folie circulaire, dementia paranoides, and melancholia, among other disorders). Kraepelin's genius was in identifying two distinct patterns of illness course around which the many different conditions could be grouped. He was influenced by the then-recent success in defining the etiopathophysiology of general paresis of insanity (neurosyphilis or tertiary syphilis) — its distinctive course and outcome among patients in psychiatric hospitals led to its delineation, identification of the causative spirochete, and the diagnostic Wassermann test and later to definitive treatment with penicillin. Kraepelin, therefore, believed that course and outcome could similarly best distinguish other psychiatric disease entities. Based on a study of several hundred cases of hospitalized patients,[15] Kraepelin delineated two distinct disorders: (1) dementia praecox, combining catatonia, hebephrenia, and paranoid states, and (2) manic-depressive insanity, combining folie circulaire and melancholia. Kraepelin[7,13] identified schizophrenia on the basis of its onset (in adolescence or early adulthood), course (deteriorating), and outcome (démence or mental dullness). He distinguished dementia praecox from manic-depressive insanity on the basis of the chronicity and poor outcome of the former contrasted with the episodicity and good outcome of the latter. Kraepelin acknowledged the enormous diversity of clinical expression subsumed under the rubric of dementia praecox but surmised some shared etiopathogenetic process. Bleuler[8] renamed this condition "the group of schizophrenias" because he believed it was comprised of several diseases with the splitting of different psychic functions the common defining characteristic. They identified a set of basic or

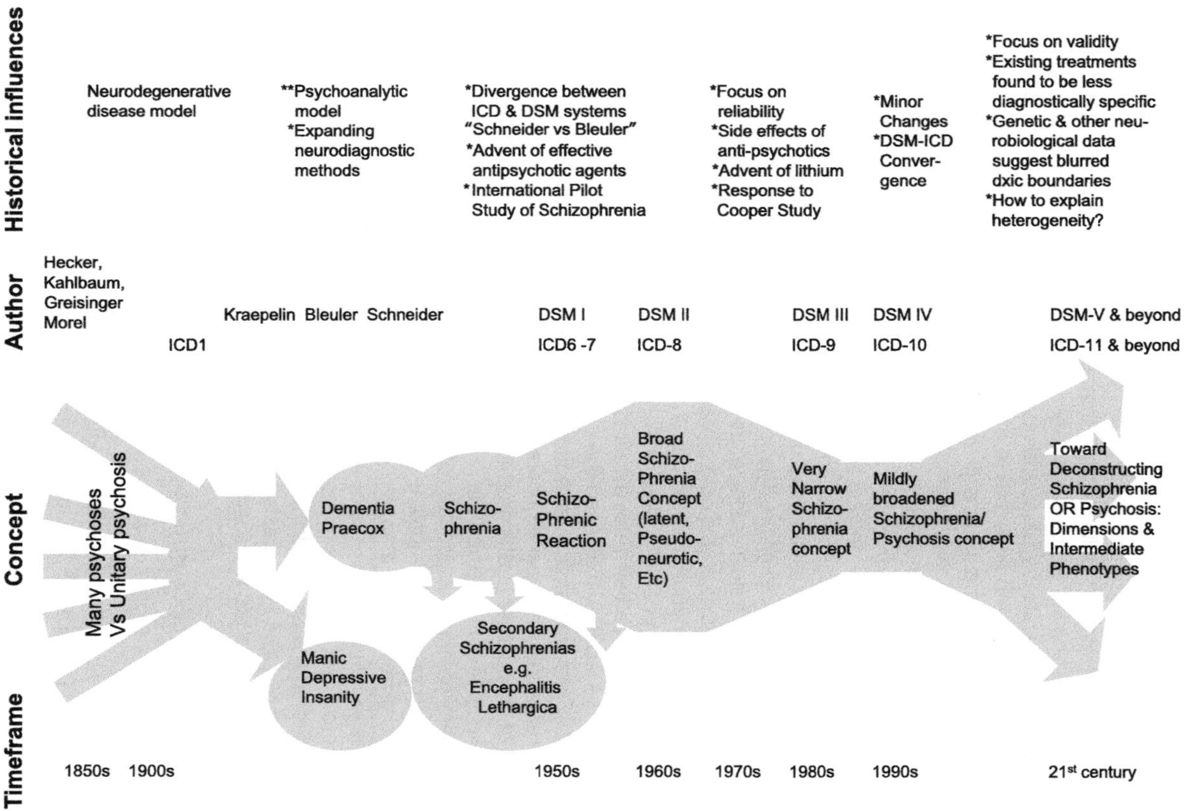

Fig. 1. Evolution of the concept of schizophrenia. (*From* Tandon R, Nasrallah HA, Keshavan MS. Schizophrenia, "just the facts." 4: Clinical features and conceptualization. Schizophr Res 2009;110:1–23; with permission.)

fundamental symptoms—4 A's: ambivalence, affective incongruity, autistic thinking, and associative disturbances—which were unique to schizophrenia and always present in those with the condition, whereas they considered the course and outcome variable.[8,13] Influenced by the work of Sigmund Freud, Bleuler considered accessory symptoms (eg, such as delusions and hallucinations) psychogenically determined, variable, and nonspecific. They further believed that many mild cases existed and considerably broadened the scope of the disease entity of schizophrenia, including latent and simple forms as part of this entity.

Schneider and Hamilton[16] believed that impairment of empathic communication was the fundamental defect in schizophrenia and considered "un-understandability" of the personal experience as pathognomonic. Based on this premise, Schneider defined 11 first-rank symptoms (a range of "bizarre" delusions and hallucinations), which they considered diagnostic of schizophrenia.[13,16] Incorporated into the Present State Examination,[17] these positive symptoms have been prominent in *ICD-8, ICD-9, and ICD-10)* and in *DSM-III and DSM-IV* definitions of schizophrenia. Schizophrenia has increasingly been defined on the basis of positive symptoms because these were considered more reliably defined and measured than negative symptoms.

Current definitions of schizophrenia (including *ICD-10* and *DSM-IV*) all incorporate kraepelinian chronicity, bleulerian negative symptoms, and schneiderian positive symptoms as part of their definition. The relative emphasis paid to these three roots has, however, varied over time. Looking at the *DSM* system, the bleulerian perspective (emphasis on negative symptoms and broad definition of the schizophrenias, including latent, pseudoneurotic, pseudopsychopathic, and residual subtypes) is reflected most strongly in *DSM-I*[2] and *DSM-II*.[18] This overly broad definition led to a marked discrepancy between the diagnosis of schizophrenia in the United States and the rest of the world, which used the *ICD* system and emphasized kraepelinian chronicity (*ICD-7*) as well as schneiderian positive symptoms (*ICD-8*).[19] In reaction to these discrepancies, the operationalized criteria of *DSM-III*[20] provided the narrowest definition of schizophrenia with an emphasis on kraepelinian chronicity and schneiderian positive (first-rank) symptoms. From *DSM-III* to *DSM-IV*,[3] there has been a modest expansion of the boundaries of schizophrenia, with some greater consideration of bleulerian negative symptoms but a continued emphasis on positive symptoms. All versions continue to emphasize kraepelinian chronicity.

Looking ahead, what are the major limitations in the current construct of schizophrenia in the context of new information about the disorder accumulated over the past 2 decades and what are the current *DSM-5*[21] efforts to address these challenges? Outlines of *ICD-11* proposals are not available at the time of writing this article, although they are expected to be similar to the *DSM-5* recommendations.

Limitations in the Present Construct of Schizophrenia

It is increasingly evident that schizophrenia is unlikely a single disease.

1. Many etiologic factors and pathophysiologic processes seem relevant to what is considered schizophrenia[22,23] and it is almost certain that this construct encompasses several diseases.
2. The boundaries of the disorder are not clearly demarcated (**Fig. 2**); in particular, the boundary between schizophrenia and schizoaffective disorder is imprecisely defined and a significant proportion of individuals with schizophrenia and mood symptoms may inappropriately receive a diagnosis of schizoaffective disorder. This is compounded by the poor reliability and low diagnostic stability of the diagnosis of schizoaffective disorder.[5,24]

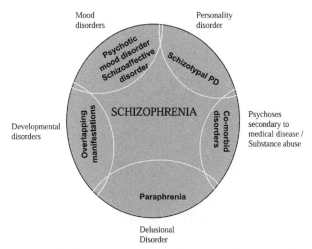

Fig. 2. The boundaries of schizophrenic disorders. (*From* Tandon R, Nasrallah HA, Keshavan MS. Schizophrenia, "just the facts." 4: Clinical features and conceptualization. Schizophr Res 2009;110:1–23; with permission.)

3. The current classic subtypes of schizophrenia provide a poor description of its heterogeneity, longitudinal subtype stability is low, and only the paranoid and undifferentiated subtypes being used with some frequency.[25,26]
4. The prominence that continues to be given to schneiderian first-rank symptoms ("bizarre" delusions or "special" hallucinations) seems misplaced.[27,28]
5. The current construct of schizophrenia is inadequate in describing the major psychopathologic dimensions of the condition[26] or stages in its evolution (**Figs. 3 and 4**).[29]
6. The clinical construct as currently defined does not match neurobiologic markers[23] and genetic findings[22,30] or specific pharmacologic treatment provided.[31]

CURRENT *DSM-5* PROPOSAL FOR DEFINITION OF SCHIZOPHRENIA

The currently proposed *DSM-5* definition of schizophrenia[21] advocates several changes to the *DSM-IV* description to address some of these limitations. These changes and their rationale are briefly described.

Schizophrenia Syndrome

Changes proposed in the diagnostic criteria of schizophrenia are modest and continuity with *DSM-IV* is broadly maintained. Three modest changes are proposed in criterion A (active-phase symptoms):

1. Elimination of special treatment of bizarre delusions and other schneiderian first-rank symptoms. In *DSM-IV* (as in *ICD-10*), only 1 criterion A is required if it is a bizarre delusion or hallucination. Schneiderian first-rank symptoms have not been found specific for schizophrenia, however, and the distinction between bizarre versus nonbizarre delusions has poor reliability. Consequently it seems appropriate that schneiderian first-rank symptoms be treated like any other positive symptom with regard to their diagnostic implication. This change should have little impact on the observed prevalence of the disorder because fewer than 5% of individuals receive a diagnosis of schizophrenia based on a single bizarre delusion or hallucination.

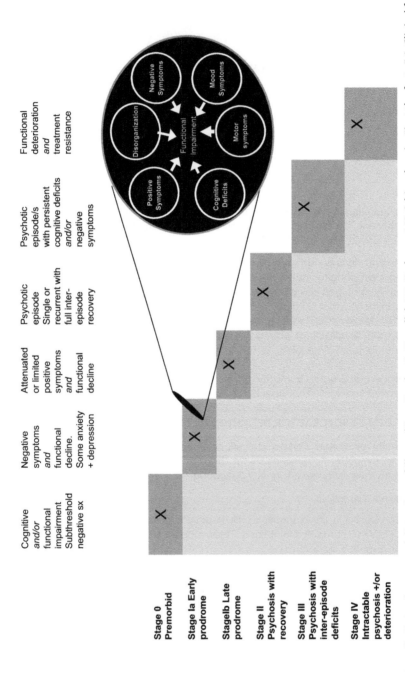

Fig. 3. New findings of stages and dimensions of illness. (*From* Tandon R, Nasrallah HA, Keshavan MS. Schizophrenia, "just the facts." 4: Clinical features and conceptualization. Schizophr Res 2009;110:1–23; with permission.)

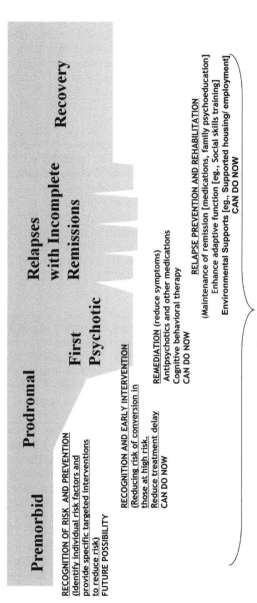

Premorbid   Prodromal   First Psychotic   Relapses with Incomplete Remissions   Recovery

RECOGNITION OF RISK AND PREVENTION
(Identify individual risk factors and provide specific targeted interventions to reduce risk)
FUTURE POSSIBILITY

RECOGNITION AND EARLY INTERVENTION
(Reducing risk of conversion in those at high risk.
Reduce treatment delay
CAN DO NOW

REMEDIATION (reduce symptoms)
Antipsychotics and other medications
Cognitive behavioral therapy
CAN DO NOW

RELAPSE PREVENTION AND REHABILITATION
(Maintenance of remission [medications, family psychoeducation]
Enhance adaptive function [eg., Social skills training]
Environmental Supports [eg., Supported housing/ employment]
CAN DO NOW

Primary, Secondary, and Tertiary Prevention

Reduce Likelihood of developing disease, Reduce manifestations of illness once it develops,
Reduce negative impact of illness once it develops. On mortality, productivity, and quality of life

Fig. 4. Stages of schizophrenic illness and opportunities for intervention.

2. Clarification of types of negative symptoms that are considered active-phase symptoms. It is proposed that the *DSM-5* consider diminished emotional expression and avolition as the 2 domains of negative symptoms, which count toward the A criteria because they better describe distinguishable aspects of negative symptoms; there is no change in the criteria itself.
3. Addition of a requirement that at least 1 of 2 required symptoms to meet criterion A be delusions, hallucinations, or disorganized thinking. These are core positive symptoms diagnosed with high reliability and might reasonably be considered necessary for a reliable diagnosis of schizophrenia. This should not affect caseness because one of these symptoms is present in all cases of *DSM-IV* schizophrenia across different datasets.

Schizophrenia Subtypes

The current *DSM-5* proposal for describing schizophrenia advocates that the *DSM-IV* subtypes of schizophrenia be eliminated. These subtypes have limited diagnostic stability, low reliability, poor validity, and little clinical utility. They do not exhibit distinctive patterns of treatment response or longitudinal course and are not heritable. Furthermore, except for the paranoid and undifferentiated subtypes, the other subtypes are rarely used in most mental health care systems across the world. For example, in a large sample of 19,000 psychiatric patients in a hospital in China with a diagnosis of schizophrenia over a 10-year period, the catatonic subtype was diagnosed in 0.2% of patients and the disorganized type in 1.0% of patients, with 91% receiving a diagnosis of undifferentiated schizophrenia.[32]

Schizoaffective Disorder

Many patients with schizophrenia exhibit prominent mood symptoms at some stage of their illness. Conversely, mania and severe depressive states are frequently marked by psychotic symptoms. Characterization of patients with both psychotic and mood symptoms either concurrently or at different points during their illness has always been a source of controversy. In *DSM-I* and *DSM-II*, a diagnosis of schizophrenia was generally recommended with schizophrenia, schizoaffective subtype, used for conditions with prominent mood symptoms. In *DSM-III*, this approach was reversed and the strong mood disorder bias led to the recommendation that schizophrenia be diagnosed only in the absence of prominent mood symptoms. Furthermore, in *DSM-III*, a diagnosis of schizoaffective disorder was strongly discouraged and schizoaffective disorder was the only condition in *DSM-III* without operational criteria. Schizoaffective disorder saw a revival in *DSM-III-R* that continued into the *DSM-IV*. Almost a third of patients with psychotic symptoms currently receive a diagnosis of schizoaffective disorder in many mental health care systems. One of the insidious changes in the definition of schizoaffective disorder from *DSM-III-R* to *DSM-IV* is that it moved from a lifetime diagnosis to a cross-sectional diagnosis (ie, in *DSM-IV*, the relative severity and temporal relationship of mood and psychotic symptoms only in the current episode are considered whereas the longitudinal course of these symptoms in an individual's life history are ignored). In the current *DSM-5* proposal, an effort is made to improve reliability of this condition by providing more specific criteria and schizoaffective disorder is reconceptualized as a longitudinal and not a cross-sectional diagnosis. Toward this end, the most significant change is proposed in criterion C, requiring that a major mood episode be present for greater than 50% of the total duration of the illness for a diagnosis of schizoaffective disorder in contrast to schizophrenia with mood symptoms.

Psychopathologic Dimensions of Schizophrenia

It is clear that schizophrenia is characterized by several psychopathologic domains (see **Fig. 3**), each with distinctive courses, patterns of treatment response, and prognostic implications. The relative severity of these symptom dimensions varies across patients as well as within patients at different stages of their illness. Measuring the relative severity of these symptom dimensions through the course of illness in the context of treatment can provide useful information to clinicians about the nature of an illness in a particular patient and in assessing the specific impact of treatment on different aspects of a patient's illness (analogous to measuring pulse, temperature, blood pressure, respiratory rate, and so forth). As a simple rating scale (akin to a thermometer or a sphygmomanometer), it should encourage clinicians to explicitly assess and track changes in the severity of these dimensions and to use this information to guide treatment. Although 9 different psychopathologic dimensions were evaluated in *DSM-5* field trials, the question of how many dimensions are useful, necessary, and practicable remains open. Furthermore, the reliability of measuring these dimensions is being assessed in the field trials and results will guide selection of the schizophrenia dimensions to be included in *DSM-5*. In addition to their clinical utility, dimensional measurement should prove useful from a research perspective and thereby permit studies on cause and pathogenesis that cut across current diagnostic categories. Such approaches would be consistent with recent findings in genetics and neuroscience and the recent research domain criteria project initiated by the National Institute of Mental Health.[33]

Attenuated Psychosis Syndrome

It is believed that the still unsatisfactory outcome of schizophrenia in a significant proportion of individuals with the disorder is because the illness is identified and treatment initiated late in the course of an illness after a substantial amount of damage has already occurred. The introduction of attenuated psychosis syndrome will support the efforts of clinicians in recognizing and monitoring psychotic symptoms early in the course of their evolution, and, if necessary, intervene in these crucial early stages. Early recognition and intervention are important in other branches of medicine and these changes in *DSM-5* should stimulate the development of a similar practice in psychiatry. The proposal is controversial[34–36] and it is unclear if this category will finally appear in *DSM-5* and, if it does, whether it will be in the main text or in the appendix.[37]

Current Status of Schizophrenia in DSM-5

Three of the proposed changes in the *DSM-5* definition of schizophrenia have been field-tested. These include evaluating

1. The impact of the change in the concept and criteria for schizoaffective disorder: reliability, feasibility, impact on prevalence, and so forth
2. The addition of a series of psychopathology dimensions: feasibility, utility, reliability, and so forth
3. The impact of adding attenuated psychosis syndrome as a new class: reliability, feasibility, and so forth

The field trials have been completed and their results are being evaluated. Based on their results and other emerging data and discussions, some additional changes in the current *DSM-5* proposals may be expected. The final proposals regarding *DSM-5* definition of schizophrenia, schizoaffective disorder, and attenuated psychosis syndrome are expected by the end of 2012. The *DSM-5* manual with the final set of diagnostic criteria is expected to be published in 2013.

ICD-11 DEFINITION OF SCHIZOPHRENIA

Although the gap between the *DSM* and *ICD* definitions of schizophrenia has narrowed from *ICD-8/DSM-II* to the current *ICD-10/DSM-IV*, there remain some significant differences. Whereas *DSM-IV* mandates a total duration of a minimum of 6 months, *ICD-10* requires a minimum duration of 1 month. In contrast to the *DSM-IV* requirement for social/occupational dysfunction, *ICD-10* has no such requisite. Although both systems provide special treatment to schneiderian first-rank symptoms, *ICD-10* places a greater emphasis on them than *DSM-IV*. Finally, *ICD-10* explicitly acknowledges schizophrenia as a group of disorders whereas *DSM-IV* implicitly treats it as a unitary condition.

The World Health Organization Psychosis Work Group has recently begun discussions about the definition of schizophrenia and other psychotic disorders in *ICD-11*. Some revisions being considered include an increase in the duration criterion for diagnosing schizophrenia (from the current 1 month to possibly 6 months as in *DSM*), deconstruction of *ICD-10* category of acute and transient psychotic disorders and introduction of a category of schizophreniform disorder (as in *DSM*), and consolidation of various delusional disorders (as in *DSM-5*). Although *ICD-11* deliberations are in their early stages, a better concordance between *ICD-11* and *DSM-5* definitions of schizophrenia and other psychotic disorders is expected.

SUMMARY

Although the shortcomings of the current diagnostic approach to schizophrenia are currently easy to enumerate, it is more difficult to come up with something that is more valid, more clinically useful, and more reliable all at the same time. Starting with *DSM-III*, both *DSM* and *ICD* systems have promoted better diagnostic agreement (reliability), thereby improved diagnostic communication and consistency of health statistics reporting across the world. The validity of the construct of schizophrenia has, however, been increasingly drawn into question.[38–40] The *DSM-5* workgroup on schizophrenia and related disorders reviewed the group of schizophrenia and related psychotic disorders against a range of validating criteria, including shared genetic risk factors and familiality, environmental risk factors, gene-environment interactions, neural substrates, biomarkers, temperamental antecedents, cognitive and emotional processing abnormalities, comorbidity, illness course, and treatment response.[41] They concluded that there was insufficient evidence of cause and pathophysiology to base group membership on causality, and that it was unclear if the other validating criteria would support a clustering of schizophrenia and related psychotic disorders. Based on the absence of clear boundaries around the condition, the multiplicity of implicated etiologic factors and pathophysiologic mechanisms, schizophrenia is likely a conglomerate of multiple disorders. Dissection of its heterogeneity is proving difficult, however, and the dimensions/endophenotypes approach coupled with illness staging is currently the most promising approach toward resolving this disease admixture.[26,33,42,43]

Although maintaining high reliability and improving validity are important considerations, the principal objective of the *DSM* system is clinical utility.[44,45] Any proposed changes must primarily facilitate clinical assessment and treatment, must be implementable in routine clinical settings, and must provide meaningful distinctions

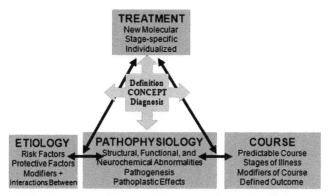

Fig. 5. Defining disorder, generating new information about disorder based on definition, redefining disorder, and so on—an iterative process. (*From* Tandon R, Keshavan MS, Nasrallah HA. Schizophrenia, "just the facts": what we know in 2008. Part 1: overview. Schizophr Res 2008;100:4–19; with permission.)

between different kinds of mental illness. Additionally, the *DSM* system is designed to facilitate research aimed at better understanding cause and pathogenesis. Hopefully, the revisions in *DSM-5* and *ICD-11* criteria for schizophrenia and related disorders will make them more useful to patients, clinicians, researchers, and society at large.

Although an etiopathophysiologic nosology of schizophrenia and related psychotic disorders is currently elusive, *DSM-5* and *ICD-11* will hopefully provide a more useful platform than the current *DSM-IV* and *ICD-10* in integrating emerging genetic and other neurobiologic information about these conditions (**Fig. 5**). They may serve as a bridge between the clinically useful psychopathologic nosology of today to an etio-pathophysiologic classification of tomorrow. Likely iterative changes in *DSM-5* and *ICD-11* might serve as the launching platform for a future paradigm shift to a classification of distinct psychotic disorders based on cause and pathophysiology.[46]

REFERENCES

1. World Health Organization. Manual of the International Statistical classification of diseases, injuries and causes of death, sixth revision (ICD-6). Geneva: World Health Organization; 1949.
2. American Psychiatric Association. Diagnostic and statistical manual of mental disorders: DSM-I. 1st edition. Washington, DC: American Psychiatric Association; 1952.
3. American Psychiatric Association. Diagnostic and statistical manual of mental disorders (DSM-IV). 4th edition. Washington, DC: American Psychiatric Association; 1994.
4. World Health Organization. The ICD-10 classification of mental and behavioral disorders: clinical descriptions and diagnostic guidelines (CDDG). Geneva (Switzerland): World Health Organization; 1992.
5. Tandon R, Maj M. Nosological status and definition of schizophrenia. Some considerations for DSM-V and ICD-11. Asian J Psychiatr 2008;1:22–7.
6. Tandon R, Keshavan MS, Nasrallah HA. Schizophrenia, "just the facts": what we know in 2008. Part 1: overview. Schizophr Res 2008;100:4–19.
7. Kraepelin E. Dementia praecox and paraphrenia. New York: Krieger; 1971. [Robertson GM, Trans; original work published 1919.]

8. Bleuler E. Dementia praecox, or the group of Schizophrenias. New York: International University Press; 1950. [Zinkin J, Trans; original work published 1911.]

9. Morel B. Traite des maladies mentales. Paris: Masson; 1860.

10. Clouston TS. Clinical lectures on mental disorders. 6th edition. London: Churchill; 1904.

11. Kahlbaum KL. Clinische abhandlungen einige psychische krankheiten. I. Katatonia oder das spannungsirresein. Berlin: Springer; 1874.

12. Hecker E. Die hebephrenie. Arch Pathol Anat Physiol Clin Med 1871;52:394–429.

13. Hoenig J. The concept of schizophrenia. Kraepelin-Bleuler-Schneider. Br J Psychiatry 1983;142:547–56.

14. Berrios GE, Beer M. The notion of unitary psychosis: a conceptual history. Hist Psychiatry 1994;5:13–36.

15. Jablensky A, Hugler H, von Cranach M, et al. Kraepelin revisited: a reassessment and statistical analysis of dementia praecox and manic-depressive insanity in 1908. Psychol Med 1993;23:843–58.

16. Schneider K. Clinical psychopathology. New York: Grune and Stratton; 1959. [Hamilton MW, Trans; original work published 1950.]

17. Wing JK, Cooper JE, Sartorius N. The measurement and classification of psychiatric symptoms. Cambridge (United Kingdom): Cambridge University Press; 1974.

18. American Psychiatric Association. Diagnostic and statistical manual of mental disorders-(DSM-II). 2nd edition. Washington, DC: American Psychiatric Association; 1968.

19. Cooper JE, Kendell RE, Gurland BJ, et al. Psychiatric diagnosis in New York and London. Maudsley monograph # 20. London: Oxford University Press; 1972.

20. American Psychiatric Association. Diagnostic and statistical manual of mental disorders-(DSM-III). 3rd edition. Washington, DC: American Psychiatric Association; 1980.

21. Tandon R, Carpenter WT. DSM-5 status of psychotic disorders: 1 year prepublication. Schizophr Bull 2012;38:369–70.

22. Tandon R, Keshavan MS, Nasrallah HA. Schizophrenia, "just the facts": what we know in 2008. 2. Epidemiology and etiology. Schizophr Res 2008;102:1–18.

23. Keshavan MS, Tandon R, Boutros N, et al. Schizophrenia, "just the facts": what we know in 2008. Part 3: neurobiology. Schizophr Res 2008;106:89–107.

24. Jager M, Haack S, Becker T, et al. Schizoaffective disorder—an ongoing challenge for psychiatric nosology. Eur Psychiatry 2011;26:159–65.

25. Helmes E, Landmark J. Subtypes of schizophrenia: a cluster analytic approach. Can J Psychiatry 2003;48:702–8.

26. Tandon R, Nasrallah HA, Keshavan MS. Schizophrenia, "just the facts." 4: Clinical features and conceptualization. Schizophr Res 2009;110:1–23.

27. Carpenter WT, Strauss JS, Muleh S. Are there pathognomonic symptoms in schizophrenia. An empiric investigation of Schneider's first-rank symptoms. Arch Gen Psychiatry 1973;28:847–52.

28. Nordgard J, Arnfred SM, Handest P, et al. The diagnostic status of first-rank symptoms. Schizophr Bull 2008;34:137–54.

29. McGorry PD. Risk syndromes, clinical staging, and DSM V: new diagnostic infrastructure for early intervention in psychiatry. Schizophr Res 2010;120:49–53.

30. Insel TR. Rethinking schizophrenia. Nature 2010;468:187–93.

31. Tandon R, Keshavan MS, Nasrallah HA. Schizophrenia, "just the facts." 5: Treatment and prevention. Schizophr Res 2010;122:1–23.

32. Xu TY. The subtypes of schizophrenia. Shanghai Arch Psychiatry 2011;23:106–8.

33. Insel T, Cuthbert B, Garvey M, et al. Research domain criteria (RDoC): toward a new classification framework for research on mental disorders. Am J Psychiatry 2010;167:748–51.
34. Woods SW, Walsh BC, Saksa JR, et al. The case for including attenuated psychotic symptoms syndrome in DSM-5 as a psychosis risk syndrome. Schizophr Res 2010;123:199–207.
35. Yung AR, Nelson B, Thompson AD, et al. Should a "Risk Syndrome for Psychosis" be included in the DSMV? Schizophr Res 2010;120:7–15.
36. Carpenter WT, van Os J. Should attenuated psychosis syndrome be a DSM-5 diagnosis? Am J Psychiatry 2011;168:460–3.
37. Tandon N, Shah J, Keshavan MS, et al. Attenuated psychosis and the schizophrenia prodrome: current status of risk identification and psychosis prevention. Neuropsychiatry 2012;2(4):1–10.
38. Robins E, Guze SB. Establishment of diagnostic validity in psychiatric illness: its application to schizophrenia. Am J Psychiatry 1970;126:983–7.
39. Cuesta MJ, Basterra V, Sanchez-Torres A, et al. Controversies surrounding the diagnosis of schizophrenia and other psychoses. Expert Rev Neurother 2009;9: 1475–86.
40. Jablensky A. The diagnostic concept of schizophrenia: its history, evolution, and future prospects. Dialogues Clin Neurosci 2010;12:271–87.
41. Carpenter WT, Bustillo JR, Thaker GK, et al. The psychoses: cluster 3 of the proposed meta-structure for DSM-V and ICD-11. Psychol Med 2009;39:2025–42.
42. Hyman SE. The diagnosis of mental disorders: the problem of reification. Annu Rev Clin Psychol 2010;6:155–79.
43. Kupfer DJ, Regier DA. Neuroscience, clinical evidence, and the future of psychiatric classification in DSM-5. Am J Psychiatry 2011;168:672–4.
44. Kendell RE, Jablensky A. Distinguishing between the validity and utility of psychiatric diagnoses. Am J Psychiatry 2003;160:4–12.
45. Tandon R. Getting ready for DSM-5. The process, challenges, and introduction to series. Curr Psychiatr 2012;11:33–7.
46. Kendler KS, First MB. Alternative futures for the DSM revision process: iteration versus paradigm shift. Br J Psychiatry 2010;197:263–6.

The Neurodevelopmental Hypothesis of Schizophrenia
Convergent Clues from Epidemiology and Neuropathology

Michael Piper, PhD[a,b], Monica Beneyto, PhD[c],
Thomas H.J. Burne, PhD[b,d], Darryl W. Eyles, PhD[b,d],
David A. Lewis, MD[e], John J. McGrath, MD, PhD[b,d],*

KEYWORDS

- Schizophrenia • Epidemiology • Neuropathology

KEY POINTS

- MRI evidence indicates that schizophrenia is associated with changes in brain volume that predate the onset of the clinical syndrome and continue to change after onset.
- It is feasible that early disruption of brain development can alter the trajectory of brain growth and involution across the lifespan.
- At the cellular level, there is evidence to suggest that schizophrenia is associated with subtle abnormalities in cytoarchitecture of different brain regions.
- The best research returns will come from linking schizophrenia epidemiology with molecular, cellular, and behavioral neuroscience, as research inspired by epidemiologic clues is likely to lead to the identification of informative pathways. Cross-disciplinary projects related to candidate genetic or nongenetic risk factors can address the biologic plausibility of these factors, and can also provide a road to new discoveries in neuroscience.

Conflicts of interest: Michael Piper, Monica Beneyto, Darryl Eyles, and Thomas Burne report no competing interests. David A. Lewis currently receives investigator-initiated research support from Bristol-Myers Squibb, Curridium Ltd, and Pfizer and in 2009–2011 served as a consultant in the areas of target identification and validation and new compound development to BioLine RX, Bristol-Myers Squibb, Merck, and SK Life Science. Monica Beneyto reports no competing interests. John J. McGrath has received conference travel support from Janssen and Eli Lilly.

[a] School of Biomedical Science, University of Queensland, St Lucia, Queensland 4072, Australia; [b] Queensland Brain Institute, University of Queensland, St Lucia, Queensland 4072, Australia; [c] Department of Anatomy and Neurobiology, University of Vermont, Burlington, VT 05405, USA; [d] Queensland Centre for Mental Health Research, The Park Centre for Mental Health, Wacol, Queensland 4076, Australia; [e] Department of Psychiatry, University of Pittsburgh, Pittsburgh, PA 15213, USA
* Corresponding author. Queensland Brain Institute, University of Queensland, St Lucia, Queensland 4072, Australia.
E-mail address: john_mcgrath@qcmhr.uq.edu.au

Psychiatr Clin N Am 35 (2012) 571–584
http://dx.doi.org/10.1016/j.psc.2012.06.002
0193-953X/12/$ – see front matter © 2012 Elsevier Inc. All rights reserved.

INTRODUCTION

In schizophrenia research, it is unusual to find a theory, such as the neurodevelopmental hypothesis, that has grown stronger during the past two to three decades. This hypothesis, presented in its current formulation nearly a quarter of a century ago, proposes that genetic or environmental factors during critical early periods of brain development adversely impact on adult mental health.[1,2] Early formulations of this hypothesis proposed that after the developmental insult, the "lesion" was clinically dormant (silent) until after puberty, after which maturational events (or other environmental factors, such as cannabis use) were postulated to lead to the emergence of the characteristic psychotic features of schizophrenia. Whether such early exposures produce static (allostasis) or dynamic alterations in brain ontogeny remains an important research question.[3]

The neurodevelopmental hypothesis provided a degree of coherence to a wide range of findings associated with schizophrenia. Several epidemiologic clues had implicated early life exposures (eg, season of birth, obstetric complications). People with schizophrenia have more minor physical anomalies, suggestive of prenatal disruptions,[4–6] and subtle changes in cognitive and psychological function in early childhood, predating the onset of schizophrenia.[7]

In some respects, the initial formulation of the neurodevelopmental hypothesis was an unsatisfactory guide for research; it lacked a precise form that predicted a particular causal factor or even a particular category of risk factors (eg, genetic vs nongenetic). Nevertheless, it did provide guidance as to the timing of key events; it proposed that disruptive events during early brain development (eg, prenatal or perinatal period, or during the first few years of life) contribute to the risk architecture of schizophrenia. The use of the label "neurodevelopmental" has led to some debate about static versus progressive encephalopathies.[3,8,9] This issue has come into sharper focus in recent years as the MRI evidence has accumulated indicating that schizophrenia is associated with changes in brain volume that predate the onset of the clinical syndrome and continue to change after onset.[10,11] It is feasible that early disruption of brain development can alter the trajectory of brain growth and involution across the lifespan.

Clearly, genetic factors are also implicated in the neurodevelopmental hypothesis[12]; major advances have occurred in this field in recent years. In particular, it is now clear that common single nucleotide polymorphisms and rarer structural variants are associated with an unexpectedly wide range of neuropsychiatric disorders.[13] For example, a large study recently implicated MIR137, a short, noncoding RNA molecule known to regulated dendritic development and the maturation of neurons.[14] In this article we examine evidence for the neurodevelopmental hypothesis from two perspectives: modifiable risk factors from observational epidemiology, and recent developments from neuropathology at the molecular and cellular levels.

MODIFIABLE RISK FACTORS FOR SCHIZOPHRENIA THAT IMPACT DURING EARLY LIFE
Nutrition

Catastrophic prenatal famine has been linked to an increased risk of schizophrenia. Individuals who were in utero during the Dutch famine during World War II showed an increased risk of schizophrenia and schizophrenia-spectrum personality disorders.[15] The finding has been replicated in studies based on a catastrophic famine in China during the Cultural Revolution (**Box 1**).[16–18]

With respect to the association between risk of schizophrenia and specific maternal micronutrients, elevated homocysteine (a marker of impaired folate metabolism) from maternal third-trimester sera has been linked to an increased risk of schizophrenia.[19]

Box 1
Clues from epidemiology that implicate the neurodevelopmental hypothesis

Excess risk of schizophrenia associated with exposures and proxy markers that could impact on early brain development:

- Winter-spring birth
- Born or raised in urban areas
- Prenatal infection
- Prenatal famine
- Prenatal micronutrient deficiency (eg, vitamin D, iron, folate)
- Pregnancy and birth complications
- Early life motor and cognitive antecedents in cohort studies
- Increased prevalence of minor physical anomalies

Based on clues from season of birth, low prenatal vitamin D has also been proposed as a risk factor for schizophrenia.[20] A recent case-control study lends weight to this candidate.[21] There is now robust evidence from rodent models demonstrating that transient prenatal vitamin D deficiency results in persistent changes in adult brain structure, neurochemistry, and behavior.[22–27] Maternal iron deficiency has also been linked to an increased risk of schizophrenia.[28] Even if altered prenatal nutrition contributes to only a small fraction of those with schizophrenia, the potential to use safe and inexpensive interventions in at-risk groups makes these candidate exposures attractive from a public health perspective.[29]

Infection

Evidence linking prenatal infection with an increased risk of schizophrenia has accumulated over recent decades.[30] The association was initially mostly based on ecologic studies (eg, examining the rate of schizophrenia in cohorts who were in utero during influenza epidemics[31]). More recent studies have been able to access biobanks to test these hypotheses in stronger, analytic settings. To date, some evidence suggests that the risk of schizophrenia is elevated in those with prenatal exposure to influenza,[32] rubella,[33] or *Toxoplasmosis gondii*,[34,35] with mixed evidence for herpes simplex virus type 2.[36,37] Evidence from animal models suggests that the prenatal infection may impact on brain development by features of the maternal immune response rather than the direct impact of infectious agents.[38]

Pregnancy and Birth Complications

Two meta-analyses have examined the association between pregnancy and birth complications and the risk of schizophrenia.[39,40] Both have found that a diverse range of pregnancy and birth complications are associated with a significant but modest increased risk of later schizophrenia. Based on prospective population-based studies, Cannon and colleagues[40] reported that the following specific exposures were associated with increased risk of schizophrenia: antepartum hemorrhage, gestational diabetes, rhesus incompatibility, preeclampsia, low birth weight, congenital malformations, reduced head circumference, uterine atony, asphyxia, and emergency caesarean section. Animal models based on these exposures have been informative for schizophrenia research.[41,42]

Advanced Paternal Age

The offspring of older fathers have an increased risk of a range of neurodevelopmental disorders, including schizophrenia,[43–45] autism,[46] and epilepsy.[47] The offspring of older fathers have slightly impaired neurocognitive development during early childhood.[48,49] With respect to schizophrenia, a meta-analysis[50] reported that the offspring of fathers aged 30 years or older had a significantly increased risk of schizophrenia compared with fathers aged 29 years or younger. The greatest increased risk was found in fathers who were 50 years or older. These findings raise the possibility that an age-related accumulation of de novo mutations in paternal sperm contributes to the risk of schizophrenia. A recent animal model based on advanced paternal age confirmed that the offspring of older male mice had a significantly increased risk of de novo copy number variants.[51] Although paternal age may impact on health outcomes by genetic factors, this risk factor is potentially modifiable with public health education (much as has happened with the risks associated with advanced maternal age).

Other Risk Factors that May Impact on Early Brain Development

There is now robust evidence showing that migrant groups in some countries have an increased risk of schizophrenia.[52,53] Meta-analysis of the primary studies shows that first- and second-generation migrants have an increased risk of developing schizophrenia, and that the effect is most pronounced in dark-skinned migrants.[53] Veling and colleagues[54] have recently examined age-at-migration and risk of schizophrenia in first-generation migrants. They found that migrants who arrive as babies or infants had the highest risk of schizophrenia, with risk decreasing with age at migration thereafter, such that those who migrated aged 29 years or older had no greater risk of psychotic disorder than the indigenous population. They conclude that the critical window of exposure is during early life.

There is also evidence linking an increased risk of schizophrenia in those who are born and grow up in urban, more densely populated settings (eg, in population-based studies from Holland[55] and Denmark[56]). The evidence suggests that urbanicity of place of birth is a proxy marker for a yet-to-be-identified risk-modifying variable operating at or before birth.[57] However, because most people who are born in a city are also brought up there, it is difficult to disentangle prenatal and perinatal effects from those operating later in childhood. Early life stress has also been proposed as a risk factor for schizophrenia.[58,59]

Although this review focuses on early life exposures, it should be noted that puberty is also a critical time for brain development and maturation, and exposures during this period have also been linked to risk of schizophrenia. In particular, cannabis use during early teenage years increased the risk of psychotic-related outcomes.[60,61] There is also evidence linking exposure to trauma and an increased risk of psychotic-related outcomes.[62–64]

NEUROPATHOLOGIC CORRELATES OF SCHIZOPHRENIA: CLUES RELATED TO THE NEURODEVELOPMENTAL HYPOTHESIS

Findings from morphologic and molecular postmortem studies support the hypothesis that schizophrenia is a consequence of a developmental process, and not a degenerative process, affecting the cellular connectivity and network plasticity of the cerebral cortex. Macroscopic morphologic studies of postmortem tissue show a reduction in the normal brain asymmetry (torque)[65] in subjects with schizophrenia that, because brain asymmetries are first apparent prenatally, is consistent with a neurodevelopmental disruption in brain development.[66] The absence of prominent gliotic or other neurodegenerative changes in schizophrenia makes adult-onset brain insults unlikely (eg, as would be expected from the neuropathology associated with adult-onset infection or autoimmune or other degenerative processes).[67]

At the cellular level, there is evidence to suggest that schizophrenia is associated with subtle abnormalities in cytoarchitecture of different brain regions; for example, certain populations of cortical neurons are smaller and the density of white matter neurons just below the cortex is greater in schizophrenia.[68] Recent studies have demonstrated that schizophrenia pathology is not only characterized by macroscopic or cytoarchitectural alterations, but also by molecular disturbances in circuits that are substantially remodeled during developmental periods critical for the cognitive functions that are impaired in schizophrenia. When examined at the level of individual types of neurons, molecular alterations in schizophrenia can be quite robust (**Box 2**).[69]

Disturbances in certain cognitive processes, such as attention, context representation, and working memory, seem to form part of the core clinical landscape of schizophrenia.[1,70] These cognitive deficits seem to correlate with abnormal activation of the dorsolateral prefrontal cortex (DLPFC) in patients with schizophrenia.[71–73] At the cellular level, working memory performance requires the precise timing and coordination of activity in subsets of pyramidal neurons in the DLPFC.[74] This "tuning" of pyramidal cells is accomplished by inhibitory inputs from γ-aminobutyric acid (GABA) interneurons.[75,76]

Developmental refinements in the connectivity between GABA neurons and pyramidal cells are thought to provide the neural substrate for age-related improvement in working memory performance.[77–79] Recent findings suggest that working memory impairments in schizophrenia might reflect disturbances in the developmental trajectories of DLPFC synaptic circuitry.[80] Given the protracted nature of these circuitry refinements, several different environmental risk factors, acting at different stages of development, could converge on a common pathology. Such alterations, even if minor initially, could become progressively more detrimental as they lead to a diversion from the normal developmental trajectory. In addition, inflection points in these trajectories may delineate periods of increased risk for specific components of cortical circuits.

The Ontogeny of Cortical GABA Interneurons

Interneurons comprise a suite of neurons that display a diverse range of cellular mophologies, laminar distributions, patterns of connectivity, and electrophysiologic properties. Within the cortex, interneurons contribute approximately 20% of the total neuronal complement. Cortical GABAergic interneurons are born in the ganglionic eminence, migrate tangentially into the cortical plate following well-defined

---

Box 2
Clues from neuropathology that implicate the neurodevelopmental hypothesis

Schizophrenia is associated with findings suggestive of altered early brain development:

- Loss of normal cerebral asymmetry
- Lack of prominent gliosis or related markers of adult-onset neuropathology
- Subtle alterations in cytoarchitecture
  - Smaller neurons
  - Shorter dendrites
  - Increased density of neurons in the subcortical white matter
- Altered expression of markers of genes/proteins implicated in brain development

pathways,[81–85] and then vertically into specific cortical layers.[86,87] In recent years, much work has focused on defining the signaling systems that may influence the migration of these cells; these include such well-known agents as Slit/Robo, Neuregulin/Erb4, semaphorin/neuropilin, and BDNF and NT4 by TrkB receptors. Microarray experiments have also discovered specific genes that are differentially expressed in these cells during migration.[88] Curiously, several of the genes expressed by these cells during migration are of broad interest to schizophrenia. These include ErbB4[89]; Pcdhh8; Nr4a1 (also known as Nur77); Rora; and several genes involved in calcium channels.

Inhibitory GABA neurons in the cerebral cortex can be categorized into different neuronal subtypes defined by the presence of specific molecular, electrophysiologic, or anatomic properties. Cell type/input- and lamina-specific alterations of presynaptic and postsynaptic markers of specific circuits formed by certain of these cell types have been found in the DLPFC of subjects with schizophrenia. Early postmortem studies in patients with schizophrenia revealed an apparent reduction in inhibitory GABA neurons. These findings were largely in the cortex with the most robust changes seen in the calcium-binding protein parvalbumin (PV) containing neurons. However, it was never certain whether such reductions indicated a loss of cells or a down-regulation of the PV marker protein.[90] In particular, widely replicated findings of a reduced expression of GAD67, an enzyme required for the synthesis of GABA at inhibitory synapses, and GAT-1, the protein responsible for the reuptake of GABA at the presynaptic site, suggest alterations in the synthesis and reuptake of GABA in a subset of DLPFC inhibitory interneurons in schizophrenia.[91–93] The affected GABA neurons include those that contain PV, and the postsynaptic GABA$_A$ receptors that receive inputs from PV neurons are also altered in schizophrenia.[69] PV neurons and their postsynaptic GABA$_A$ receptors have a protracted period of development,[94] providing a broad window during which environmental events could disrupt their developmental trajectories.

It is the complex nature of interneuron development, migration, maturation, and synapse formation that makes these interneurons of specific interest to schizophrenia research. This research is now focusing on understanding how changes to the trajectory of interneuron specification, migration, or maturation might contribute to the etiopathogenesis of schizophrenia (**Box 3**).

INTEGRATING EPIDEMIOLOGY AND NEUROPATHOLOGY: WHAT CAN BE LEARNED FROM ANIMAL MODELS?

Several of the animal models related to schizophrenia have shown abnormalities in GABAergic interneurons. Postnatal exposure to various psychopharmacologic probes

---

Box 3
Cortical GABA neurons in schizophrenia

- Multiple markers of GABA inhibitory neurons are altered but the number of neurons in the cerebral cortex does not seem to be reduced.

- A subset of GABA neurons exhibit decreased GABA synthesis and uptake; these changes are best characterized in the PV-containing subset.

- Postsynaptic GABA receptors are also altered; these changes seem to be specific for different subunits and types of GABA$_A$ receptors.

- Lower expression levels of the gene for GAD67, which is responsible for most GABA synthesis, are found in multiple cortical regions.

has been associated with altered GAD67 or PV expression in regions of interest. Agents used include MK-801[95]; amphetamine[96]; phencyclidine[95]; and picrotoxin (a noncompetitive antagonist of the $GABA_A$ receptor).[97]

Altered GAD67 or PV expression has also been noted in transgenic animals of interest to schizophrenia research, including the heterozygous Reeler mouse[98] and DISC1 mutant mice.[99] An interesting recent approach has been to selectively target the function of these GABAergic interneurons directly. In one study when the expression of the NR1 subunit of the N-methyl-D-aspartate receptor was reduced selectively within inhibitory GABA neurons in mice, this seemed to confer a schizophrenia-like phenotype.[100] Impaired GABAergic function in schizophrenia could also be secondary to alterations in the striatal dopaminergic system. For example, Li and colleagues[101] developed a model in which increased striatal dopamine signaling has been linked with diminished prefrontal cortical inhibition, presumably caused by diminished GABA function.

Meyer and Feldon[102] have recently published a comprehensive assessment of epidemiologically informed animal models related to schizophrenia. To date, animal models have tried to emulate a range of exposures related to the neurodevelopmental hypothesis. These included obstetric complications,[103,104] immune activation,[105–107] low maternal vitamin D,[23,108] advanced paternal age,[51,109,110] and early life stress.[111,112] These models express surprisingly high face and predictive validity for schizophrenia. For example, maternal immune activation with the viral mimic Poly-IC leads to a reduction in reelin- and PV-positive interneurons and GABA content in the prefrontal cortex of adult offspring.[113,114] Similarly, when pregnant rats were exposed to the bacterial membrane component lipopolysaccharide a reduction in reelin and GAD67 interneurons in the hippocampus of their offspring was revealed.[115] Finally in models of postadolescent stress, such as social isolation, similar reductions in hippocampal or prefrontal cortical GABAergic neuron structure or content have been found.[116,117] In summary, there is evidence from animal models to suggest that disruption to GABA interneurons is a shared phenotype associated with diverse genetic and environmental stressors. As such, the orderly development of these cells may be a marker of early brain disruption.

SUMMARY

It has been previously argued that it is critical that schizophrenia epidemiology is firmly anchored to a neurobiologically informed framework.[118] Although clinical research is clearly important, animal models can play a key role in unraveling the biologic mechanisms linking early life disruptions to later neuropsychiatric disorders. Moreover, animal models provide an experimental platform that allows researchers to focus on more substrate-pure neurobiologic correlates of clinical syndromes.[119]

Research inspired by epidemiologic clues, such as prenatal nutrition and prenatal infection, is likely to lead to the identification of informative pathways. However, on its own, epidemiology will never be able to address the biocomplexity underpinning a poorly understood group of disorders like schizophrenia. The best returns will come from linking schizophrenia epidemiology with molecular, cellular, and behavioral neuroscience. Cross-disciplinary projects related to candidate genetic or nongenetic risk factors can address the biologic plausibility of these factors, and can also provide a road to new discoveries in neuroscience. There is a need for shared discovery platforms that encourage greater cross-fertilization between schizophrenia epidemiology and basic neuroscience research. We are confident that the neurodevelopmental hypothesis will continue to inspire research in epidemiology and neuroscience, and that this journey will continue to provide clues to the neurobiologic correlates of schizophrenia.

REFERENCES

1. Weinberger DR. Implications of normal brain development for the pathogenesis of schizophrenia. Arch Gen Psychiatry 1987;44(7):660–9.
2. Murray RM, Lewis SW. Is schizophrenia a neurodevelopmental disorder? Br Med J (Clin Res Ed) 1987;295(6600):681–2.
3. Thompson BL, Levitt P. Now you see it, now you don't–closing in on allostasis and developmental basis of psychiatric disorders. Neuron 2010;65(4):437–9.
4. McGrath JJ, van Os J, Hoyos C, et al. Minor physical anomalies in psychoses: associations with clinical and putative aetiological variables. Schizophr Res 1995;18(1):9–20.
5. Buckley PF, Dean D, Bookstein FL, et al. A three-dimensional morphometric study of craniofacial shape in schizophrenia. Am J Psychiatry 2005;162(3):606–8.
6. Compton MT, Chan RC, Walker EF, et al. Minor physical anomalies: potentially informative vestiges of fetal developmental disruptions in schizophrenia. Int J Dev Neurosci 2011;29(3):245–50.
7. Welham J, Isohanni M, Jones P, et al. The antecedents of schizophrenia: a review of birth cohort studies. Schizophr Bull 2009;35(3):603–23.
8. McGrath J, Feron F, Burne THJ, et al. The neurodevelopmental hypothesis of schizophrenia; a review of recent developments. Ann Med 2003;35(2):86–93.
9. Velakoulis D, Wood SJ, McGorry PD, et al. Evidence for progression of brain structural abnormalities in schizophrenia: beyond the neurodevelopmental model. Aust N Z J Psychiatry 2000;34(Suppl):S113–26.
10. Pantelis C, Yucel M, Wood SJ, et al. Structural brain imaging evidence for multiple pathological processes at different stages of brain development in schizophrenia. Schizophr Bull 2005;31(3):672–96.
11. Pantelis C, Velakoulis D, McGorry PD, et al. Neuroanatomical abnormalities before and after onset of psychosis: a cross-sectional and longitudinal MRI comparison. Lancet 2003;361(9354):281–8.
12. Jones P, Murray RM. The genetics of schizophrenia is the genetics of neurodevelopment. Br J Psychiatry 1991;158:615–23.
13. Owen MJ, O'Donovan MC, Thapar A, et al. Neurodevelopmental hypothesis of schizophrenia. Br J Psychiatry 2011;198(3):173–5.
14. Ripke S, Sanders AR, Kendler KS, et al. Genome-wide association study identifies five new schizophrenia loci. Nat Genet 2011;43(10):969–76.
15. Susser ES, Lin SP. Schizophrenia after prenatal exposure to the Dutch hunger winter of 1944-1945. Arch Gen Psychiatry 1992;49:938–88.
16. St Clair D, Xu M, Wang P, et al. Rates of adult schizophrenia following prenatal exposure to the Chinese famine of 1959-1961. JAMA 2005;294(5):557–62.
17. Xu MQ, Sun WS, Liu BX, et al. Prenatal malnutrition and adult schizophrenia: further evidence from the 1959-1961 Chinese famine. Schizophr Bull 2009; 35(3):568–76.
18. Brown AS, Susser ES. Prenatal nutritional deficiency and risk of adult schizophrenia. Schizophr Bull 2008;34(6):1054–63.
19. Brown AS, Bottiglieri T, Schaefer CA, et al. Elevated prenatal homocysteine levels as a risk factor for schizophrenia. Arch Gen Psychiatry 2007;64(1):31–9.
20. McGrath J. Hypothesis: is low prenatal vitamin D a risk-modifying factor for schizophrenia? Schizophr Res 1999;40(3):173–7.

21. McGrath JJ, Eyles DW, Pedersen CB, et al. Neonatal vitamin D status and risk of schizophrenia: a population-based case-control study. Arch Gen Psychiatry 2010;67(9):889–94.
22. Kesby JP, Eyles DW, Burne TH, et al. The effects of vitamin D on brain development and adult brain function. Mol Cell Endocrinol 2011;347(1–2):121–7.
23. Kesby JP, Cui X, O'Loan J, et al. Developmental vitamin D deficiency alters dopamine-mediated behaviors and dopamine transporter function in adult female rats. Psychopharmacology (Berl) 2010;208(1):159–68.
24. McGrath J, Iwazaki T, Eyles D, et al. Protein expression in the nucleus accumbens of rats exposed to developmental vitamin D deficiency. PLoS One 2008; 3(6):e2383.
25. Kesby JP, Burne TH, McGrath JJ, et al. Developmental vitamin D deficiency alters MK 801-induced hyperlocomotion in the adult rat: an animal model of schizophrenia. Biol Psychiatry 2006;60(6):591–6.
26. Feron F, Burne TH, Brown J, et al. Developmental vitamin D3 deficiency alters the adult rat brain. Brain Res Bull 2005;65(2):141–8.
27. Eyles D, Brown J, Mackay-Sim A, et al. Vitamin D3 and brain development. Neuroscience 2003;118(3):641–53.
28. Insel BJ, Schaefer CA, McKeague IW, et al. Maternal iron deficiency and the risk of schizophrenia in offspring. Arch Gen Psychiatry 2008;65(10):1136–44.
29. McGrath J, Brown A, St Clair D. Prevention and schizophrenia–the role of dietary factors. Schizophr Bull 2011;37(2):272–83.
30. Brown AS, Derkits EJ. Prenatal infection and schizophrenia: a review of epidemiologic and translational studies. Am J Psychiatry 2010;167(3):261–80.
31. McGrath J, Castle D. Does influenza cause schizophrenia? A five year review. Aust N Z J Psychiatry 1995;29(1):23–31.
32. Brown AS, Begg MD, Gravenstein S, et al. Serologic evidence of prenatal influenza in the etiology of schizophrenia. Arch Gen Psychiatry 2004;61(8):774–80.
33. Brown AS, Cohen P, Greenwald S, et al. Nonaffective psychosis after prenatal exposure to rubella. Am J Psychiatry 2000;157(3):438–43.
34. Brown AS, Schaefer CA, Quesenberry CP Jr, et al. Maternal exposure to toxoplasmosis and risk of schizophrenia in adult offspring. Am J Psychiatry 2005; 162(4):767–73.
35. Mortensen PB, Norgaard-Pedersen B, Waltoft BL, et al. Early infections of *Toxoplasma gondii* and the later development of schizophrenia. Schizophr Bull 2007; 33(3):741–4.
36. Buka SL, Tsuang MT, Torrey EF, et al. Maternal infections and subsequent psychosis among offspring. Arch Gen Psychiatry 2001;58:1032–7.
37. Brown AS, Schaefer CA, Quesenberry CP Jr, et al. No evidence of relation between maternal exposure to herpes simplex virus type 2 and risk of schizophrenia? Am J Psychiatry 2006;163(12):2178–80.
38. Patterson PH. Immune involvement in schizophrenia and autism: etiology, pathology and animal models. Behav Brain Res 2009;204(2):313–21.
39. Geddes JR, Verdoux H, Takei N, et al. Schizophrenia and complications of pregnancy and labor: an individual patient data meta-analysis. Schizophr Bull 1999; 25(3):413–23.
40. Cannon M, Jones PB, Murray RM. Obstetric complications and schizophrenia: historical and meta-analytic review. Am J Psychiatry 2002;159(7):1080–92.
41. Rehn AE, Van Den Buuse M, Copolov D, et al. An animal model of chronic placental insufficiency: relevance to neurodevelopmental disorders including schizophrenia. Neuroscience 2004;129(2):381–91.

42. Boksa P. Animal models of obstetric complications in relation to schizophrenia. Brain Res Brain Res Rev 2004;45(1):1–17.
43. Malaspina D, Harlap S, Fennig S, et al. Advancing paternal age and the risk of schizophrenia. Arch Gen Psychiatry 2001;58(4):361–7.
44. El-Saadi O, Pedersen CB, McNeil TF, et al. Paternal and maternal age as risk factors for psychosis: findings from Denmark, Sweden and Australia. Schizophr Res 2004;67(2–3):227–36.
45. Sipos A, Rasmussen F, Harrison G, et al. Paternal age and schizophrenia: a population based cohort study. BMJ 2004;329(7474):1070.
46. Hultman CM, Sandin S, Levine SZ, et al. Advancing paternal age and risk of autism: new evidence from a population-based study and a meta-analysis of epidemiological studies. Mol Psychiatry 2011;16(12):1203–12.
47. Vestergaard M, Mork A, Madsen KM, et al. Paternal age and epilepsy in the offspring. Eur J Epidemiol 2005;20(12):1003–5.
48. Saha S, Barnett AG, Buka SL, et al. Maternal age and paternal age are associated with distinct childhood behavioural outcomes in a general population birth cohort. Schizophr Res 2009;115(2–3):130–5.
49. Saha S, Barnett AG, Foldi C, et al. Advanced paternal age is associated with impaired neurocognitive outcomes during infancy and childhood. PLoS Med 2009;6(3):e40.
50. Miller B, Messias E, Miettunen J, et al. Meta-analysis of paternal age and schizophrenia risk in male versus female offspring. Schizophr Bull 2011;37(5): 1039–47.
51. Flatscher-Bader T, Foldi CJ, Chong S, et al. Increased de novo copy number variants in the offspring of older males. Translational Psychiatry 2011;1(e34).
52. McGrath J, Saha S, Welham J, et al. A systematic review of the incidence of schizophrenia: the distribution of rates and the influence of sex, urbanicity, migrant status and methodology. BMC Med 2004;2(1):13.
53. Cantor-Graae E, Selten JP. Schizophrenia and migration: a meta-analysis and review. Am J Psychiatry 2005;162(1):12–24.
54. Veling W, Hoek HW, Selten J, et al. Age at migration and future risk of psychotic disorders among immigrants in The Netherlands: a 7-year incidence study. Am J Psychiatry 2011;168:1278–85.
55. Marcelis M, Navarro-Mateu F, Murray R, et al. Urbanization and psychosis: a study of 1942-1978 birth cohorts in The Netherlands. Psychol Med 1998;28: 871–9.
56. Mortensen PB, Pedersen CB, Westergaard T, et al. Effects of family history and place and season of birth on the risk of schizophrenia. N Engl J Med 1999;340: 603–8.
57. McGrath J, Scott J. Urban birth and risk of schizophrenia: a worrying example of epidemiology where the data are stronger than the hypotheses. Epidemiol Psychiatr Soc 2006;15(4):243–6.
58. van Os J, Kenis G, Rutten BP. The environment and schizophrenia. Nature 2010; 468(7321):203–12.
59. Scott J, Varghese D, McGrath J. As the twig is bent, the tree inclines: adult mental health consequences of childhood adversity. Arch Gen Psychiatry 2010;67(2):111–2.
60. Moore TH, Zammit S, Lingford-Hughes A, et al. Cannabis use and risk of psychotic or affective mental health outcomes: a systematic review. Lancet 2007;370(9584):319–28.

61. McGrath J, Welham J, Scott J, et al. Association between cannabis use and psychosis-related outcomes using sibling pair analysis in a cohort of young adults. Arch Gen Psychiatry 2010;67(5):440–7.
62. Saha S, Varghese D, Slade T, et al. The association between trauma and delusional-like experiences. Psychiatry Res 2011;189(2):259–64.
63. Scott J, Chant D, Andrews G, et al. Association between trauma exposure and delusional experiences in a large community-based sample. Br J Psychiatry 2007;190:339–43.
64. Read J, van Os J, Morrison AP, et al. Childhood trauma, psychosis and schizophrenia: a literature review with theoretical and clinical implications. Acta Psychiatr Scand 2005;112(5):330–50.
65. Guerguerian R, Lewine RR. Brain torque and sex differences in schizophrenia. Schizophr Res 1998;30(2):175–81.
66. Harrison PJ. Schizophrenia: a disorder of neurodevelopment? Curr Opin Neurobiol 1997;7(2):285–9.
67. Harrison PJ. The neuropathology of schizophrenia. A critical review of the data and their interpretation. Brain 1999;122(Pt 4):593–624.
68. Harrison PJ, Lewis DA, Kleinman JE. Neuropathology of schizophrenia. In: Weinberger DR, Harrison PJ, editors. Schizophrenia. 3rd edition. Oxford (United Kingdom): Blackwell; 2001. p. 372–92.
69. Lewis DA, Curley AA, Glausier JR, et al. Cortical parvalbumin interneurons and cognitive dysfunction in schizophrenia. Trends Neurosci 2012;35(1):57–67.
70. Goldman-Rakic PS. Working memory dysfunction in schizophrenia. J Neuropsychiatry Clin Neurosci 1994;6(4):348–57.
71. Weinberger DR, Berman KF, Zec RF. Physiologic dysfunction of dorsolateral prefrontal cortex in schizophrenia. I. Regional cerebral blood flow evidence. Arch Gen Psychiatry 1986;43(2):114–24.
72. Perlstein WM, Carter CS, Noll DC, et al. Relation of prefrontal cortex dysfunction to working memory and symptoms in schizophrenia. Am J Psychiatry 2001; 158(7):1105–13.
73. Callicott JH, Mattay VS, Verchinski BA, et al. Complexity of prefrontal cortical dysfunction in schizophrenia: more than up or down. Am J Psychiatry 2003; 160(12):2209–15.
74. Goldman-Rakic PS. Cellular basis of working memory. Neuron 1995;14(3): 477–85.
75. Sawaguchi T, Matsumura M, Kubota K. Depth distribution of neuronal activity related to a visual reaction time task in the monkey prefrontal cortex. J Neurophysiol 1989;61(2):435–46.
76. Rao SG, Williams GV, Goldman-Rakic PS. Destruction and creation of spatial tuning by disinhibition: GABA(A) blockade of prefrontal cortical neurons engaged by working memory. J Neurosci 2000;20(1):485–94.
77. Alexander GE, Goldman PS. Functional development of the dorsolateral prefrontal cortex: an analysis utlizing reversible cryogenic depression. Brain Res 1978;143(2):233–49.
78. Luna B, Garver KE, Urban TA, et al. Maturation of cognitive processes from late childhood to adulthood. Child Dev 2004;75(5):1357–72.
79. Crone EA, Wendelken C, Donohue S, et al. Neurocognitive development of the ability to manipulate information in working memory. Proc Natl Acad Sci U S A 2006;103(24):9315–20.
80. Lewis DA, Levitt P. Schizophrenia as a disorder of neurodevelopment. Annu Rev Neurosci 2002;25:409–32.

81. Marin O, Rubenstein JL. A long, remarkable journey: tangential migration in the telencephalon. Nat Rev Neurosci 2001;2(11):780–90.
82. Marin O, Yaron A, Bagri A, et al. Sorting of striatal and cortical interneurons regulated by semaphorin-neuropilin interactions. Science 2001;293(5531):872–5.
83. Pleasure SJ, Anderson S, Hevner R, et al. Cell migration from the ganglionic eminences is required for the development of hippocampal GABAergic interneurons. Neuron 2000;28(3):727–40.
84. McKenna IM, Ramakrishna G, Diwan BA, et al. K-ras mutations in mouse lung tumors of extreme age: independent of paternal preconceptional exposure to chromium(III) but significantly more frequent in carcinomas than adenomas. Mutat Res 2001;490(1):57–65.
85. Marin O, Anderson SA, Rubenstein JL. Origin and molecular specification of striatal interneurons. J Neurosci 2000;20(16):6063–76.
86. Tanaka DH, Yanagida M, Zhu Y, et al. Random walk behavior of migrating cortical interneurons in the marginal zone: time-lapse analysis in flat-mount cortex. J Neurosci 2009;29(5):1300–11.
87. Murakami F, Tanaka D, Yanagida M, et al. Intracortical multidirectional migration of cortical interneurons. Novartis Found Symp 2007;288:116–25 [discussion: 125–9, 276–81].
88. Faux C, Rakic S, Andrews W, et al. Differential gene expression in migrating cortical interneurons during mouse forebrain development. J Comp Neurol 2010;518(8):1232–48.
89. Chen PL, Avramopoulos D, Lasseter VK, et al. Fine mapping on chromosome 10q22-q23 implicates Neuregulin 3 in schizophrenia. Am J Hum Genet 2009; 84(1):21–34.
90. Eyles DW, McGrath JJ, Reynolds GP. Neuronal calcium-binding proteins and schizophrenia. Schizophr Res 2002;57(1):27–34.
91. Beneyto M, Morris HM, Rovensky KC, et al. Lamina- and cell-specific alterations in cortical somatostatin receptor 2 mRNA expression in schizophrenia. Neuropharmacology 2012;62(3):1598–605.
92. Beneyto M, Abbott A, Hashimoto T, et al. Lamina-specific alterations in cortical GABAA receptor subunit expression in schizophrenia. Cereb Cortex 2011;21(5): 999–1011.
93. Lewis DA, Hashimoto T, Volk DW. Cortical inhibitory neurons and schizophrenia. Nat Rev Neurosci 2005;6(4):312–24.
94. Beneyto M, Lewis DA. Insights into the neurodevelopmental origin of schizophrenia from postmortem studies of prefrontal cortical circuitry. Int J Dev Neurosci 2011;29(3):295–304.
95. Turner CP, DeBenedetto D, Ware E, et al. Postnatal exposure to MK801 induces selective changes in GAD67 or parvalbumin. Exp Brain Res 2010;201(3): 479–88.
96. Peleg-Raibstein D, Knuesel I, Feldon J. Amphetamine sensitization in rats as an animal model of schizophrenia. Behav Brain Res 2008;191(2):190–201.
97. Berretta S, Gisabella B, Benes FM. A rodent model of schizophrenia derived from postmortem studies. Behav Brain Res 2009;204(2):363–8.
98. Pillai A, Mahadik SP. Increased truncated TrkB receptor expression and decreased BDNF/TrkB signaling in the frontal cortex of reeler mouse model of schizophrenia. Schizophr Res 2008;100(1–3):325–33.
99. Shen S, Lang B, Nakamoto C, et al. Schizophrenia-related neural and behavioral phenotypes in transgenic mice expressing truncated Disc1. J Neurosci 2008; 28(43):10893–904.

100. Belforte JE, Zsiros V, Sklar ER, et al. Postnatal NMDA receptor ablation in corticolimbic interneurons confers schizophrenia-like phenotypes. Nat Neurosci
2010;13(1):76–83.
101. Li YC, Kellendonk C, Simpson EH, et al. D2 receptor overexpression in the striatum leads to a deficit in inhibitory transmission and dopamine sensitivity in
mouse prefrontal cortex. Proc Natl Acad Sci U S A 2011;108(29):12107–12.
102. Meyer U, Feldon J. Epidemiology-driven neurodevelopmental animal models of
schizophrenia. Prog Neurobiol 2010;90(3):285–326.
103. Mallard EC, Rehn A, Rees S, et al. Ventriculomegaly and reduced hippocampal
volume following intrauterine growth-restriction: implications for the aetiology of
schizophrenia. Schizophr Res 1999;40(1):11–21.
104. Boksa P, El-Khodor BF. Birth insult interacts with stress at adulthood to alter
dopaminergic function in animal models: possible implications for schizophrenia and other disorders. Neurosci Biobehav Rev 2003;27(1–2):91–101.
105. Meyer U, Yee BK, Feldon J. The neurodevelopmental impact of prenatal infections at different times of pregnancy: the earlier the worse? Neuroscientist
2007;13(3):241–56.
106. Patterson PH. Maternal infection: window on neuroimmune interactions in
fetal brain development and mental illness. Curr Opin Neurobiol 2002;12(1):
115–8.
107. Zuckerman L, Rehavi M, Nachman R, et al. Immune activation during pregnancy
in rats leads to a postpubertal emergence of disrupted latent inhibition, dopaminergic hyperfunction, and altered limbic morphology in the offspring: a novel
neurodevelopmental model of schizophrenia. Neuropsychopharmacology
2003;28(10):1778–89.
108. Eyles DW, Feron F, Cui X, et al. Developmental vitamin D deficiency causes
abnormal brain development. Psychoneuroendocrinology 2009;34(Suppl 1):
S247–57.
109. Foldi CJ, Eyles DW, McGrath JJ, et al. Advanced paternal age is associated with
alterations in discrete behavioural domains and cortical neuroanatomy of
C57BL/6J mice. Eur J Neurosci 2010;31(3):556–64.
110. Smith RG, Kember RL, Mill J, et al. Advancing paternal age is associated with
deficits in social and exploratory behaviors in the offspring: a mouse model.
PLoS One 2009;4(12):e8456.
111. Rilling JK, Winslow JT, O'Brien D, et al. Neural correlates of maternal separation
in rhesus monkeys. Biol Psychiatry 2001;49(2):146–57.
112. Ellenbroek BA, van den Kroonenberg PT, Cools AR. The effects of an early
stressful life event on sensorimotor gating in adult rats. Schizophr Res 1998;
30(3):251–60.
113. Meyer U, Nyffeler M, Yee BK, et al. Adult brain and behavioral pathological
markers of prenatal immune challenge during early/middle and late fetal development in mice. Brain Behav Immun 2008;22(4):469–86.
114. Bitanihirwe BK, Peleg-Raibstein D, Mouttet F, et al. Late prenatal immune activation in mice leads to behavioral and neurochemical abnormalities relevant to the
negative symptoms of schizophrenia. Neuropsychopharmacology 2010;35(12):
2462–78.
115. Nouel D, Burt M, Zhang Y, et al. Prenatal exposure to bacterial endotoxin
reduces the number of GAD67- and reelin-immunoreactive neurons in the
hippocampus of rat offspring. Eur Neuropsychopharmacol 2012;22(4):300–7.
116. Bloomfield C, French SJ, Jones DN, et al. Chandelier cartridges in the prefrontal
cortex are reduced in isolation reared rats. Synapse 2008;62(8):628–31.

117. Harte MK, Powell SB, Swerdlow NR, et al. Deficits in parvalbumin and calbindin immunoreactive cells in the hippocampus of isolation reared rats. J Neural Transm 2007;114(7):893–8.
118. McGrath JJ, Richards LJ. Why schizophrenia epidemiology needs neurobiology–and vice versa. Schizophr Bull 2009;35(3):577–81.
119. Arguello PA, Gogos JA. Modeling madness in mice: one piece at a time. Neuron 2006;52(1):179–96.

Predicting Risk and the Emergence of Schizophrenia

Mary C. Clarke, PhD[a,b,*], Ian Kelleher, PhD[a],
Maurice Clancy, MB, MRCPsych[a,c], Mary Cannon, PhD, MRCPsych[a,c]

KEYWORDS

- Schizophrenia • Psychiatric risk factors • Environmental risk factors
- Genetic risk factors • Prenatal stress • Obstetric complications • Cannabis

KEY POINTS

- The presence of certain molecular, biological, and psychosocial factors at certain points in the life span, has been linked to later development of schizophrenia.
- Environmental risk factors for schizophrenia include prenatal exposures, obstetric complications (OCs), childhood trauma, urban birth, migrant status, and adolescent cannabis use.
- Identified risk factors are neither necessary nor sufficient causal factors for schizophrenia. The vast majority of people who are exposed to them do not develop schizophrenia and a majority of individuals with schizophrenia may not have had the specific exposure in question.
- These risk factors cannot be ignored because of their small effect and need to be considered in the context of schizophrenia as a lifelong brain disorder.

INTRODUCTION

The presence of certain molecular, biologic, and psychosocial factors at certain points in the life span, has been linked to later development of schizophrenia. These include common and rare genetic variants; prenatal exposures, such as infection, stress, and nutrition; OCs; childhood trauma; urban birth; migrant status; and adolescent cannabis use. Some of these risk factors operate on an individual level and some on a societal level but all need to be considered in the context of schizophrenia as a lifelong brain disorder. Research interest in schizophrenia is shifting to ever-earlier stages of the disease process, so the journey to discover the causes of schizophrenia is leading back to late childhood/early adolescence as the important time period in the disease process on which to focus screening and preventative measures.

[a] Department of Psychiatry, Royal College of Surgeons in Ireland, Education and Research Centre, Beaumont Hospital, Dublin 9, Ireland; [b] Department of Psychology, Division of Population Health Sciences, Beaux Lane House, Dublin 2, Ireland; [c] Department of Psychiatry, Beaumont Hospital, Dublin 9, Ireland
* Corresponding author. Department of Psychiatry, Royal College of Surgeons in Ireland, Education and Research Centre, Beaumont Hospital, Dublin 9, Ireland.
E-mail address: maryclarke@rcsi.ie

Psychiatr Clin N Am 35 (2012) 585–612
http://dx.doi.org/10.1016/j.psc.2012.06.003
0193-953X/12/$ – see front matter © 2012 Elsevier Inc. All rights reserved.

psych.theclinics.com

OBSTETRIC COMPLICATIONS

Historical findings show that OCs as a broad category of risk factor for schizophrenia has a modest but consistently found association with schizophrenia. Odds ratios (ORs) of 1.5 to 2.0 have been replicated in several population-based cohort studies using prospective data.[1] Within this broad category of complications there is good evidence of an association between 10 specific complications and schizophrenia—these are complications of pregnancy, such as bleeding, preeclampsia, diabetes, and rhesus incompatibility; abnormal fetal growth and development measures, such as low birth weight, congenital malformations, and small head circumference; and complications of delivery, such as asphyxia, uterine atony, and emergency cesarean section. The evidence supporting an association between these individual complications and schizophrenia comes from the largest studies with the most reliable epidemiologic data that have explored the link between prenatal/neonatal life and the development of schizophrenia in adulthood.

The past decade has seen few comparable studies conducted that have used population-based, prospective data. The only study to do so and to also examine a broad range of OCs was by Byrne and colleagues.[2] This large, nested, case-control study using Danish register–based data found an almost 2-0 fold increase in the rate of schizophrenia among those who had experienced any one of the following complications: maternal nonattendance at antenatal appointments, gestational age of 37 weeks or less, preeclampsia, threatened premature delivery, hemorrhage during delivery, manual extraction of the baby, and maternal sepsis of childbirth and the puerperium. The data was adjusted for the confounding effects of family psychiatric history and socioeconomic and demographic factors. The evidence for the association between OCs and schizophrenia coming from this large, well-controlled study with good quality data is in keeping with previous findings—an association exists but it is modest.

Several other cohort studies using population-based data have recently been conducted but they have only addressed specific OCs,[3,4] such as the association between fetal growth measures and schizophrenia (in a cohort of Swedish male conscripts); instead of, the association between prenatal exposure to maternal hypertension/diuretic treatment and schizophrenia; and the association between prenatal exposure to analgesics and schizophrenia (both in a Danish cohort using national population-based register data).[5,6] Finally, one study[7] examined the association between maternal-fetal blood incompatibility and schizophrenia in a large California-based cohort. Evidence from these studies suggests the following:

1. Birth weight is not associated with schizophrenia when gestational age is taken into account.
2. Maternal hypertension and diuretic treatment during pregnancy are OCs of note—experience of either one in the third trimester independently increases the odds of the exposed offspring developing schizophrenia 2-fold and experience of both increases the odds 4-fold.
3. Prenatal exposure to analgesics is an OC equally worthy of note with exposure increasing the odds of schizophrenia 4-fold, after adjustment for the confounding effects of parental history of schizophrenia, prenatal infection exposure, exposure to other drugs in the prenatal period, other pregnancy complications, and parental social status and parental age.
4. Maternal-fetal blood incompatibility leads to a 2-fold increase in the rate of schizophrenia in adulthood among exposed offspring.

It is possible that OCs have a direct effect on fetal neurodevelopment[8]—for example, evidence suggests that perinatal hypoxia may have lasting effects on dopaminergic function. The same data also suggest, however, a further indirect effect of OCs such that birth insults alter the manner in which dopamine function is regulated by stress in adulthood.[9] Cannon and colleagues[10] have recently found that neurotrophic factors, perhaps stimulated in response to fetal distress, may be important in the origin of schizophrenia. In this nested case-control study, assays from cord and maternal blood samples taken at delivery showed that, among schizophrenia patients, birth hypoxia was associated with a 20% decrease in brain-derived neurotrophic factor (BDNF) whereas among the matched healthy controls birth hypoxia was associated with a 10% increase in BDNF. The deleterious effects of OCs, such as hypoxia and hyperbilirubinaemia, on N-methyl-D-aspartate (NMDA) receptors have also been proposed as a potential mechanism.[11]

Hypoxia itself has been proposed to mediate the effects of other OCs. Cannon and colleagues[12] found a linear relationship between the number of hypoxia causing OCs, such as abnormal fetal heart rate, third-trimester heart rate, placental hemorrhaging, and risk of schizophrenia, suggesting that any association between these specific OCs and schizophrenia is accounted for by the effect of hypoxia on risk for schizophrenia. These data also suggest that hypoxia interacts with genetic susceptibility to further increase risk. The risk of schizophrenia increased with the number of hypoxia-related OCs within families—given genetic vulnerability to schizophrenia, those who were exposed to hypoxia were more likely to develop schizophrenia than family members not exposed to hypoxia.

CANNABIS USE

Over the past 5 years, robust epidemiologic studies with prospective data on cannabis use have shown that cannabis confers an increase in risk for schizophrenia. Several reviews and meta-analyses examining this association have been published since 2004 and all have concluded that the evidence supports cannabis as a component cause of schizophrenia.[13] The results of the meta-analyses varied from an overall 2-fold to a 2.9-fold increase in later schizophrenia outcomes in cannabis users. Early-onset or adolescent-onset cannabis use confers an even higher risk of later schizophrenia—approximately 4-fold.

The majority (90%) of adolescents who abuse cannabis do not develop schizophrenia. The risk for psychotic illness attached to cannabis use seems influenced by the amount used and the duration of use as well as the type or strength of cannabis.[14] Individual genetic susceptibility may also be important. Caspi and colleagues,[15] using data from the Dunedin Multidisciplinary Health and Development Study, showed that individuals with the high-activity allele (val) of the COMT gene were more likely to develop schizophrenia or schizophreniform disorder in adulthood if they had used cannabis in adolescence, with the effect more marked in those who had used cannabis earlier in adolescence, whereas this effect was not seen among individuals who were homozygous for the low-activity (Met) allele. Individuals who were heterozygous (Val/Met) were also found at increased risk, but the effect was less marked. Both self-report and informant reports of psychotic symptoms yielded a similar pattern of results,[16] with findings that cannabis use is associated with a greater frequency of hallucinogenic experiences in Val allele carriers who had high psychosis liability at baseline. It is not yet known how cannabis exerts its effect on risk of psychosis, but it seems likely to involve changes in dopamine transmission.

On balance, the evidence suggests that cannabis may only exert a modest increase in relative risk on an individual level but has a much greater effect at a population level given its widespread use in the general population. It has been estimated that 8% to 15% of all schizophrenia can be attributed to cannabis use.[17,18]

PRENATAL INFECTION

Mednick and colleagues[19] first reported an increased risk of schizophrenia among individuals exposed prenatally to the 1957 influenza epidemic in Helsinki. Most subsequent studies examining this issue have found a positive association but there have also been some negative findings (Brown[20] provides an extensive review of this literature). One reason for the inconsistent results is likely to be the differing methodologies used across studies, with earlier studies using ecologic designs in which large populations were deemed exposed if they were in utero at the time of an influenza epidemic and later studies taking advantage of archived maternal serum to establish individual exposure to the infection. Earlier studies pointed to the importance of exposure to infection during the second trimester of fetal development, but the more robust recent work places the window of vulnerability in the first trimester.[21,22] A wide variety of infections, such as influenza, herpes, polio, rubella, toxoplasmosis, and respiratory infections, have been implicated. The effect sizes reported for the association between prenatal exposure to infection and later schizophrenia have generally been in the region of a 1.5-fold to 2-fold increase in risk.[23,24] Studies using prenatal serum samples, however, have found that those exposed prenatally to rubella had a 10-20-fold increase in risk of adult schizophrenia[25] and that those exposed during the first trimester of gestation to influenza had a 7-fold increase in risk.[22] There is some evidence that prenatal exposure to infection may be interacting with another risk factor for schizophrenia, such as genetic risk, to produce its effect.[26] We found an additive effect of having a positive family history such that, when coupled with prenatal exposure to infection, the risk is significantly increased relative to either risk factor on its own. There was an almost 5-fold increase in the odds of having schizophrenia for individuals with both psychosis liability and prenatal infection exposure compared with individuals without either risk factor.

Despite much speculation, the mechanism by which prenatal infection increases the risk of schizophrenia has not yet been elucidated. An indirect effect of infection on fetal brain development seems the most plausible pathogenic mechanism. The wide range of infections associated with schizophrenia during the prenatal period indicates that some pathogenic mechanism common to many infections, such as the maternal immune response to infection, may be in operation. Possible indirect mechanisms include maternal IgG antibodies elicited by the infection or an infection-induced excess of maternal cytokines, either of which may damage the developing fetus.[27] A positive association between elevated maternal levels of the cytokine interleukin-8 during pregnancy and an increased risk of schizophrenia spectrum disorders in the offspring has been found.[22]

The findings of immune dysregulation in schizophrenia[28] and evidence of abnormal expression of immune-related genes in postmortem schizophrenia studies[29] support the idea of the maternal immune response as the important mechanism. Animal models of infection have provided evidence that the maternal immune response affects fetal brain development in ways that are consistent with neuropathology seen in schizophrenia. Abnormalities in the hippocampus and cortex as well as in cerebellar white matter and evidence of altered behavior, such as deficits in social interaction and prepulse inhibition of the startle response, have been found in animal models of maternal infection.[30] In addition, there is evidence that some of the behavioral deficits are ameliorated by administration of antipsychotic medication[30] and that several other risk factors for schizophrenia, such as winter birth, urban birth, fetal hypoxia, maternal stress, and maternal nutrition, elevate cytokine levels.[30] This finding suggests that perhaps maternal immune response may mediate the effects of other environmental risk factors that have been assumed to have independent effects on risk of schizophrenia.

PRENATAL STRESS

There is a growing body of literature examining the causal relationship between prenatal exposure to stress and the development of schizophrenia and other psychotic disorders in adulthood. The prenatal stress/schizophrenia association has been examined in several different ways. Death of spouse[31,32] and experience of catastrophic events, such as war[33] and nuclear explosion,[34] have been found to increase the risk of schizophrenia among those exposed. van Os and Selten[33] found an increased relative risk (RR) of schizophrenia (RR 1.28) among those in the Netherlands who were in their first or second trimester during the Nazi invasion in May 1940, and Malaspina and colleagues[35] found that those in their second month of gestation during the 1967 Arab-Israel War (Six-Day War) also had an increased risk of schizophrenia. Imamura and colleagues[34] found that those exposed in their second or third trimester to the nuclear explosion in Nagasaki were at increased risk of schizophrenia. Myhrman and colleagues[36] showed that the risk of schizophrenia among unwanted children was raised compared with wanted or mistimed children, even after adjustment for confounding by sociodemographic, pregnancy, and perinatal variables (odds ratio [OR] 2.4). This study examined self-ratings of a woman's desire to be pregnant. The ratings were gathered prospectively beginning in the sixth or seventh month of gestation. The association was present after accounting for both maternal depression and measures of fetal well-being at the time of the birth. Khashan and colleagues[32] found that death or serious illness of a relative during the first trimester was associated with an increased risk of developing schizophrenia, even when several potential confounders were controlled for. This partially replicates the classic finding of Huttunen and Niskanen.[31] This study showed that those whose fathers had died during their fetal period were at an increased risk of schizophrenia compared with those whose fathers had died during early childhood. This epidemiological evidence has been supported by recent animal work linking prenatal stress and impaired behavioral adjustment/emotional reactivity in the offspring.

As in the infection studies, the diversity of stress exposures associated with schizophrenia raises the possibility of a single pathophysiologic mechanism underlying the association. The common denominator could be the stress response and the resulting glucocorticoid hormones known to be precipitated by psychological stressors.[37] Animal models of prenatal stress have informed our understanding of the mechanisms at play. For example, it has been shown in humans that the greatest sensitivity of the developing fetus to stress is likely to be during late first or second trimester of pregnancy,[19] when, based on animal evidence, glucocorticoid receptor expression is commencing in the developing fetal brain. The precise timing of glucocorticoid receptor expression in the developing human brain, however, is currently unknown. Collectively, the findings from animal studies suggest that exposure of the developing brain to stress-induced glucocorticoid hormones generates a syndrome that recreates some aspects of the schizophrenia phenotype.[38]

The majority of studies, however, that have examined the prenatal stress/schizophrenia association have not had information on maternal adverse responses to stress, such as substance abuse, which may mediate the association. And there is evidence that the schizophrenia–risk-increasing effect of maternal stress during pregnancy may overlap with the risk-inducing effects of other environmental factors, thus making it hard to delineate independent effects of some of the risk factors discussed in this article. For example, psychological stress and neuroendocrine markers of stress can affect immune function and, therefore, susceptibility to infection[39]; maternal stress during pregnancy has been shown to increase the risk of fetal hypoxia,[40] which, in turn, has been show to increase the risk of schizophrenia; and stress has been shown to alter people's eating behavior, steering them toward sweet and fatty foods[41] and possibly leading to maternal micronutritional deficiencies during pregnancy.

CHILDHOOD TRAUMA

Recent evidence has shown that childhood trauma is a risk factor for the development of schizophrenia[42–44] and psychotic symptoms.[45] Although several previous studies have suffered from methodological limitations, such as small, highly selected samples and nonstandardized measures of trauma, a recent study has sought to overcome these problems. Heins and colleagues[46] examined exposure to childhood trauma among nonaffective psychosis patients from geographically representative clinics in Holland and Belgium. Siblings of patients and healthy control were recruited as comparison groups. The use of a sibling comparison group helped to control for any unmeasured familial confounding in the associations examined. Heins and colleagues showed that those with childhood trauma had 4 times the odds of developing a psychotic disorder and that there was a dose-response effect present such that patients had more trauma exposure than their siblings, who, in turn, had more trauma exposure than the healthy comparison group. In addition, childhood abuse, but not neglect, was significantly associated with the positive symptoms of psychosis; there was no such association with negative symptoms. This finding indicates that there may be symptom-specific and exposure-specific mechanisms at play.

Our work has shown significant associations between psychotic symptoms in early adolescence and reports of child physical abuse, exposure to domestic violence, and involvement in bullying[45] and that cannabis use and childhood trauma both independently increased the risk for psychotic symptoms in adolescence.[44] Both cannabis use and childhood trauma, however, additively interacted to increase the likelihood of psychotic symptoms in adolescence to a much greater extent than either risk factor independently. This indication of environmental factors working together to produce a synergistic effect on risk has been found in other studies. Cougnard and colleagues[47] examined data from 2 large European population cohort studies (1 adult cohort and 1 cohort aged 14–24 years) and calculated the additive interaction between 3 environmental risk factors for psychosis (cannabis use, childhood trauma, and urbanicity) and baseline psychotic experiences in predicting persistence of psychotic experiences. The authors concluded that level of environmental risk combines synergistically with subclinical psychotic symptoms to cause abnormal persistence of these symptoms.

PRENATAL NUTRITION

Evidence for the involvement of prenatal nutrition in the pathway to schizophrenia in some individuals has come from several sources. First, ecological evidence comes from the study of populations exposed to famine. Individuals exposed to the Dutch

Hunger Winter (1944–1945) and individuals exposed to the Great Chinese Famine (1958–1961) had a greater risk of developing schizophrenia compared with those not exposed to these famines. Although data of this ecological nature are open to methodologic criticisms, data from studies on micronutritional deficiencies and risk of schizophrenia come from more robust studies. There is evidence that deficiencies of folate, vitamin D, iron, and protein during the prenatal period all independently increase the risk of schizophrenia. Homocysteine levels are linked to folate in the metabolic cycle[48]; and elevated maternal homocysteine levels in the third trimester have been shown to be associated with a 2-fold increase in risk of schizophrenia in the offspring. McGrath and colleagues[49–51] have shown that vitamin D supplementation in males in Finland reduced the incidence among these individuals and that both low and high concentrations of neonatal vitamin D are associated with an increase risk of schizophrenia; and a large Danish showed that those exposed to prenatal iron deficiency had a 4-fold increase in risk of schizophrenia. There has been some evidence to suggest that polyunsaturated fatty acids deficiency during gestation increases the risk of schizophrenia but this evidence has largely been indirect and from animal studies. McGrath and colleagues have also shown that vitamin D–deficient rats have features characteristic of schizophrenia, such as enlarged ventricles, a thinner neocortex, and altered behavior in adulthood, such as hyperlocomotion and impaired latent inhibition.[52] There is also animal evidence suggesting that exposure to suboptimal levels of protein in utero leads to abnormalities in brain development that are similar to those seen in schizophrenia patients, such as a reduced number of hippocampal cells, and affects behavior in ways consistent with the schizophrenia phenotype, such as reduced prepulse inhibition and adverse effects on learning and memory.[53]

Several biological pathways, both direct and indirect, possibly mediate the association between prenatal nutritional deficiency and later schizophrenia. Direct effects are possible because many micronutrients are important components of molecules in neurodevelopment and indirect effects are possible because it is plausible that nutritional deficiencies could result in de novo mutations in genes critical for brain development.[54] **Table 1** outlines some of the recent studies examining environmental risk factors for schizophrenia.

EPILEPSY AS A RISK FACTOR FOR SCHIZOPHRENIA

The nature of the relationship between psychosis and epilepsy has been of great interest to psychiatrists for more than a century.[62–65] The majority of studies[66–68] have found a higher prevalence of psychosis in patients with epilepsy compared with the general population, but this finding varies greatly, with reported rates varying from 0.48%[69] to 35.7%.[70] A seminal Icelandic population study surveyed a complete population of all individuals with epilepsy in Iceland and reported a rate of psychosis of 7.2%.[71]

In a systematic review and meta-analysis that we conducted, the pooled prevalence rate for schizophrenia in epilepsy patients was 1.3% (95% CI, 0.7–1.7) (**Fig. 1**). This percentage was found after pooling a total of 17 articles. A large Danish population–based study found that people with a history of epilepsy have nearly 2.5 times the risk of developing schizophrenia and nearly 3 times the risk of developing a schizophrenia-like psychosis compared with the general population.[72] It was also found that both a family history of psychosis and a family history of epilepsy increase the risk of schizophrenia.

In a population-based family study examining shared susceptibility to epilepsy and psychosis, we found that individuals with epilepsy had a 5.5-fold increase in the odds

Table 1
A selection of recent studies examining the association between environmental risk factors and schizophrenia

Risk Factor	Author	Description
1. Obstetric complications		
Fetal growth	Gunnell et al,[3] 2003; Gunnell et al,[4] 2005	Swedish cohort study: no association when gestational age is taken into account
Medication	Sørensen et al,[6] 2004; Sørensen et al,[5] 2003	Danish cohort study: OR 4.7 (95% CI, 1.9–12.0) for prenatal exposure to analgesics in the second trimester Danish cohort study: OR 4.0 (95% CI, 1.4–11.4) for prenatal exposure to both hypertension and diuretic treatment in the third trimester
Rhesus incompatibility	Hollister et al,[55] 1996; Insel et al,[7] 2005	Case-control study: rate of 2.1% vs 0.8% for Rh incompatible vs Rh compatible Californian cohort study: RR 2.2 (95% CI, 1.1–4.4) for male offspring where there was maternal-fetal blood incompatibility
2. Cannabis use	Henquet et al,[17] 2005; Moore et al,[18] 2007	Meta-analysis of epidemiological studies with prospective data: pooled OR 2.1 (95% CI, 1.7–2.5) Meta-analysis of epidemiological studies with prospective data: pooled OR 1.4 (95% CI, 1.2–1.6)
3. Prenatal infection		
Influenza	Brown et al,[22] 2004	Serologic nested case-control study: OR 3.0 (95% CI, 0.9–10.1) for the first half of pregnancy
Taxoplasmosis	Brown et al,[56] 2005	Serologic nested case-control study: OR 2.6 (95% CI, 1.0–6.8) for high IgG antibody titre
Herpes	Brown et al,[57] 2006	Serologic nested case-control study: no association found
Rubella	Brown et al,[21] 2000	Birth cohort study: RR 5.2 (95% CI, 1.9–14.3) for nonaffective psychosis
Respiratory infection	Brown et al,[58] 2000	Birth cohort study: RR 2.1 (95% CI, 1.0–4.3) for secondnd trimester
Genital-reproductive infection	Babulas et al,[59] 2006	Birth cohort study: RR 5.0 (95% CI, 2.0–12.6) for periconceptional period

4. Prenatal stress

Risk factor	Reference	Findings
Death/illness of relative	Huttunen and Niskanen,[31] 1978; Khashan et al,[32] 2008	Finnish cohort study: significant increase in risk for prenatal compared with postnatal death of spouse Danish birth cohort: RR 1.67 (95% CI, 1.0–2.7) for death of relative during first trimester
War	van Os and Selten, 1998[33]; Malaspina et al,[35] 2008	Dutch birth cohort: RR 1.1 (95% CI, 1.0–1.2) for exposure in second trimester Jerusalem birth cohort: hazard ratio 2.3 (95% CI, 1.1–4.7) for first-trimester exposure
Unwanted pregnancy	Myhrman et al,[36] 1996	Finnish birth cohort: OR 2.5 (95% CI, 1.5–4.2) for children of unwanted pregnancies
5. Childhood trauma	Kelleher et al,[45] 2008; Harley et al,[44] 2010; Heins et al,[46] 2011	Irish cohort study: OR 5.9 (95% CI, 1.2–27.9) for childhood physical abuse and risk of psychotic symptoms in adolescence Irish cohort study: OR 6.1 (95% CI, 1.6–23.1) for childhood trauma and psychotic symptoms Case-control study: OR 4.5 (95% CI, 2.7–7.3) for childhood trauma and nonaffective psychotic disorder

6. Prenatal nutrition

Risk factor	Reference	Findings
Iron deficiency	Insel et al,[51] 2008; Sorensen et al,[60] 2010	Californian cohort study: RR 3.7 (95% CI, 1.4–9.8) for maternal mean hemoglobin of 10 g/dL or less Danish cohort study: OR 1.6 (95% CI, 1.2–2.2) for maternal anemia during pregnancy
Homocysteine	Brown et al,[48] 2007	Nested case-control study: OR 2.3 (95% CI, 1.1–4.8) for elevated third-trimester homocysteine levels
Vitamin D	McGrath et al,[61] 2003	Nested case-control study: OR 0.7 (95% CI, 0.5–1.0) for African American subgroup

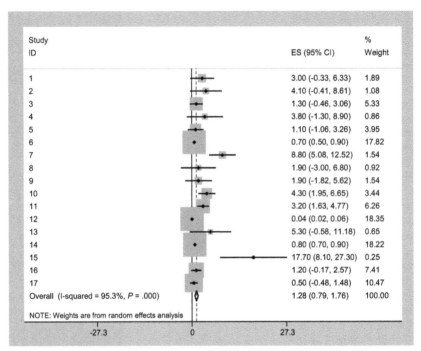

Fig. 1. Prevalence of schizophrenia in epilepsy (1.3%).

of having a broadly defined psychotic disorder and an almost 8.5-fold increase in the odds of having schizophrenia.[73] There was strong evidence of clustering of the association between epilepsy and psychosis within families. Individuals with a parental history of epilepsy had a 2-fold increase in the odds of developing a psychotic disorder compared with patients without a parental history of epilepsy. Reciprocally, individuals with a parental history of psychotic disorder had a 2.8-fold increase in the odds of having a diagnosis of generalized epilepsy compared with individuals without a parental history of psychosis.

This evidence suggests that epilepsy and psychotic illness may represent different outcomes of a common etiologic process. Neuropathologic, neuroimaging, and genetics findings show that similar structural brain abnormalities and genetic abnormalities are present in patients with schizophrenia and patients with epilepsy.[74–77] For instance, enlarged ventricles have been found common to first-episode psychosis and temporal lobe epilepsy patients without psychosis.[78] Neuronal migration defects have been proposed as a mechanism related to enlarged ventricles and this defect could be common to schizophrenia and epilepsy. From a neurobiological perspective, significant gray matter and white matter deficits occur in temporal lobe epilepsy with psychosis. Some of these deficits overlap with those found in schizophrenia. These include the medial temporal structures but also extend to lateral temporal and extratemporal regions.[79] Recent genetic work shows that a rare genetic mutation can lead to either epilepsy or schizophrenia. A microdeletion in the genomic area 15q13-14 containing the nicotine receptor was linked to development of either schizophrenia or juvenile epilepsy.[77]

In summary, a history of epilepsy in patients increases their risk of developing schizophrenia. An improved understanding of the mechanism underlying this association would be a fruitful line of inquiry and may yield useful information on the etiopathogenesis of both psychosis and epilepsy.

ACQUIRED BRAIN INJURY AS A RISK FACTOR FOR SCHIZOPHRENIA

Acquired brain injury (ABI) increases the risk of psychiatric illness[80–82] but the question of whether ABI is a risk factor for schizophrenia remains controversial. Earlier studies stated that there was a 2-fold to 3-fold increased risk of psychosis after an ABI.[83] More recent studies have contradicted this view and reported that there is limited evidence between an association between head injury and psychosis.[83–85] Consensus is divided and this can often lead to difficulties from a medicolegal viewpoint.

We conducted a recent systematic review and meta-analysis on population-based controlled studies and showed a significant association between traumatic brain injury and schizophrenia with an OR of 1.65 (95% CI, 1.17–2.32). It is difficult, however, to definitively establish causality. Patients who develop psychosis after head injury may already have been at risk of psychosis before the injury. Confounders include illicit substance use. In patients with a family history of psychosis, the contribution of head injury may be greater to susceptible patients. Two family studies yielded a pooled OR of 2.8 (95% CI, 1.17–2.32). The impact of head injuries seems to be greater among those with an inherited susceptibility to schizophrenia.[86,87] Studies have also found an increased rate of pre-existing psychosis among people with head injury and it is thought that psychosis increases the risk for ABI.[88] The apparent complexity of the causal pathway between ABI and schizophrenia adds to the difficulty of investigating this relationship. Influences of gene-environment interaction or an epigenenetic mechanism must be considered.

There does not seem to be a dose-response between the severity of the head injury and the subsequent risk of schizophrenia. When subdivided by severity of ABI, the pooled ORs were similar in studies providing rates for mild head injury specifically (1.17) to estimates for severe head injury (1.18). Achte and colleagues[89] followed-up 3552 Finnish soldiers who had received head injuries during World War II. During this period, 2.6% developed psychoses resembling schizophrenia, which is much higher than the incidence expected in the normal population. Soldiers with mild head injuries developed schizophrenia more frequently than those with severe head injuries. Factors independent of the injury may play a decisive role.

ANTI-NMDA RECEPTOR ENCEPHALITIS AS A RISK FACTOR FOR SCHIZOPHRENIA

Anti–NMDA receptor encephalitis is a severe form of encephalitis associated with antibodies against NR1 and NR2 subunits and occurs primarily in females. Prominent features on initial presentation include psychotic symptoms and may be misdiagnosed as first-onset schizophrenia.[90] There can be motor changes, such as catatonia, seizures, and dyskinesias. There are also behavioral changes, autonomic dysfunction, and impaired consciousness.[91] The combination of psychotic symptoms with catatonia and orofacial dyskinesias, which are indicators of dopaminergic involvement, are all consistent with the effects of the NMDA receptor antagonist, phencyclidine, which replicates many aspects of the presentation of schizophrenia.[92] It is also implicated in phencyclidine induced psychosis.

The psychiatric presentations of these cases of anti-NMDA receptor encephalitis thus provide important support for the NMDA receptor hypofunction hypothesis for psychosis and the possibility that autoantibodies to the NMDA receptor subunits may be implicated in the development of psychosis is novel.

GENETICS OF SCHIZOPHRENIA

Family Studies

Historically, the evidence from family studies of schizophrenia have shown that that a sibling or child of a person with schizophrenia has a 10-fold increased risk of developing schizophrenia compared with the risk in the general population.[93] The risk in a recent large register-based study has shown lower risks (ORs 2–4) and lack of specificity for schizophrenia among offspring of parents with nonaffective psychosis.[94] Adoption and cross-fostering studies show an increased risk of schizophrenia in the biological but not the adoptive families of schizophrenic adoptees.[95]

Twin Studies and the Heritability Index

Twin studies have shown that the concordance rates for schizophrenia in monozygotic (MZ) twins is approximately 40% to 50% whereas the concordance rate for dizygotic (DZ) twins is 6% to 10%.[96,97] Heritability estimates are approximately 80%, which make schizophrenia among the most heritable of psychiatric disorders. Heritability calculations assume, however, no interactions among genes or between gene and the environment—an assumption that may have significant implications for the validity of these estimations.[98] Another assumption is that MZ twins share their environment to an equal degree as DZ twins. This assumption may not be valid in particular when considering the prenatal environment because MZ pairs differ from DZ pairs in terms of sharing the placenta (ie, MZ twins are more likely to share a placenta). For this reason, MZ twins may share more of the prenatal environment than DZ twins and, as discussed in this article, prenatal life is a rich source of risk factors for later schizophrenia. The risk of schizophrenia and schizophrenia-related disorders is similar for the offspring of both affected and unaffected MZ twins,[99,100] providing support for the presence of unexpressed genotypes in schizophrenia and the importance of epigenetics.

Genome-Wide Association Studies

Over the past 2 decades there has been a concentration of effort and resources in investigating the molecular genetics of schizophrenia (for review, see the article by Gejman and colleagues[101]). The initial approach involved candidate gene studies and more than 1000 genes have been studied in schizophrenia (www.szgene.org) but with little replication of findings. The newer approach has been to use genome-wide association studies (GWAS), which interrogate the genome systematically and are independent of a prior hypothesis (**Table 2**). To date, 12 GWAS studies have been published, but, despite large sample sizes, the problem of nonreplication has not been eliminated. The largest study, a mega-analysis with a discovery sample of 21,856 and a replication of samples of 29,839 individuals, was published in October 2011 by the Schizophrenia Psychiatric Genome-Wide Association Study Consortium and found 5 new schizophrenia loci not previously identified in the other GWAS.[102] The best-replicated finding from GWAS is evidence for involvement of the major histocompatibility complex (MHC) locus. The MHC locus has a high gene density but genes with an immune function predominate—which links back to the epidemiologic data on infections and autoimmunity as risk factors for schizophrenia (discussed elsewhere). Another notable feature of these GWAS studies is the small effect sizes of the genes identified. ORs are usually approximately 1.10. An elegant analysis by the International Schizophrenia Consortium[103] estimated that hundreds (perhaps thousands) of genes may be involved in conferring risk for schizophrenia, each with small effect. The investigators showed that an aggregate score, derived from the

Table 2
Top genes or genomic regions identified in schizophrenia GWAS and ORs

Authors and Year	Sample (Case-Control)	Gene or Region	OR
Lencz et al,[159] 2007	178/144	CSF2RA, SHOX	3.23
Sullivan et al,[160] 2008	738/733	AGBL1	6.01
O'Donovan et al,[161] 2008	Discovery: 479/2937 Follow-up: 6829/9987	ZNF804A	1.12
Need et al,[162] 2009	Discovery: 871/863 Follow-up: 1460/12,995	ADAMTSL3	0.68
Purcell et al,[163] 2009 (ISC)	3322/3587	MHC	0.82
Stefansson et al,[164] 2009 (SGENE)	Discovery: 2663/13,498 Follow-up: 4999/15,555	MHC NRGN TCF4	1.16 1.15 1.23
Shi et al,[165] 2009 (MGS)	2681/2653 1286/973 (AA)	MHC CENTG2 ERBB4	0.88 1.23 0.73
Ikeda et al,[166] 2010	575/564	OAT	0.57
Yue et al,[167] 2011	Discovery: 746/1599 (AA) Follow-up: 4027/5603 (AA)	ZKSCAN4 NKAPL PGBD1 TSPAN18	0.79 0.78 0.79 1.29
Shi et al,[168] 2011	Discovery: 3750/6468 (AA) Follow-up: 4383/4539 (AA)	Rs10489202 Rs1060041 Rs11586522 Rs16887244 Rs1488935	1.12 1.11 1.04 0.83 0.871
Gejman et al,[101] 2011 (PGC)	Discovery: 9394/12,462 Follow-up: 8442/21,397	MIR137 PCGEM1 TRIM26 CSMD1 MMP16 CNNM2 NT5C2 STT3A CCDC68 TCF4	1.12 1.20 1.15 1.11 1.10 1.10 1.15 1.11 1.10 1.23

Abbreviations: AA, Asian ancestry; ISC, International schizophrenia consortium; MGS, molecular genetics of schizophrenia study; PGC, schizophrenia psychiatric genome-wide association study consortium; SGENE, A large scale genome-wide association study of schizophrenia addressing variation in expressivity and contribution from environmental factors.

top 10% to 50% of a set of 74,000 single-nucleotide polymorphisms (SNPs) from the association results in a discovery sample, can predict up to 3% of the variance in a target group. Using a different approach, Agerbo and colleagues[104] came to the same conclusion and reported that the percentage of excess risk associated with a family history of schizophrenia mediated through genome-wide SNP variation ranged up to a maximum of 4%. This raises the question, "Where is the missing heritability?"[105,106] It may be surmised that the "missing heritability" is likely to lie in the environment or gene-environment interaction, which is not captured by individual SNPs or their combination. The area of epigenetics is a promising area of investigation in the coming years.

Copy Number Variation Studies

In addition to the reports of common SNP variations, many rare structural genomic variants, such as copy number variants (CNVs), have been identified (for review, see the article by Gejman and colleagues[101]). These rare variants seem to have larger effect sizes than SNPs but many are private mutations confined to single families. These variants are not specific to schizophrenia and confer risk for a variety of conditions, such as epilepsy, autistic spectrum disorder, and attention-deficit/hyperactivity disorder. An interesting aspect of these structural variants is that so many affect genes are implicated in brain development, which links nicely with the neurodevelopmental hypothesis of schizophrenia described first in the late 1980s and discussed elsewhere in this article. Apart from their rarity, a problematic aspect of the large CNVs identified to date is that they span multiple genes and the contribution of each gene may be difficult to disentangle. Nevertheless, some commentators hold that these rare variants could hold the key to explaining the transmission of schizophrenia and argue that mutations with the largest effects in individuals, regardless of their frequency in the population, is the most informative as to the underlying pathogenesis of schizophrenia.

Several conclusions can be drawn from the GWAS and CNV studies so far:

- Common variants for schizophrenia identified to date are of small effect.
- There is substantial overlap between the genetic architecture of schizophrenia and bipolar disorder.
- There is a large unexplained gap between heritability estimates from family studies and the amount of genetic variation that can be attributed to genome-wide SNP variation.

GENE-ENVIRONMENT INTRERACTION

There are strong indications, from several sources, that gene/environment interactions are important in the cause of schizophrenia. There is evidence from animal work that neuregulin-1 and DISC1 may modify the consequences of prenatal immune activation[107,108] and that neuregulin 1 may modify the effect of exposure to social defeat.[107] There is also evidence from human studies that COMT may modify the effects of adolescent exposure to cannabis,[15] that individuals at high genetic risk for schizophrenia are particularly sensitive to the adverse effects of a negative family rearing environment,[109] and the effect of urbanicity is mediated by genetic liability to psychosis.[110] The urbanicity studies found that 60% to 70% of those in the sample who developed schizophrenia did so as a result of the synergistic action between urban dwelling and familial liability to psychosis.

Our study of prenatal infection and family history of psychosis found that up to half of the cases of schizophrenia in the sample could be attributed to the synergistic action of prenatal infection exposure and familial liability to psychotic disorder. The possibility of OCs interacting with underlying genetic vulnerability has been raised by several other lines of evidence.[111–114] In particular, recent findings show that many of the susceptibility genes identified for schizophrenia are affected by hypoxia.[115–117] Nicodemus and colleagues[116] performed a gene-environment interaction analysis in a family study of schizophrenia probands, siblings, and controls. The authors examined whether a set of schizophrenia candidate genes affected by hypoxia or involved in vascular function in the brain interacted with serious OCs to influence risk for schizophrenia. They found that 4 of the 13 genes examined showed evidence for significant serious OC-by-gene interaction. All of the OCs rated as serious had the potential to cause hypoxia—the most common were bleeding during pregnancy, extended labor, delivery problems, and respiratory distress at birth. The 4 genes found to interact with these OCs, AKT_1, BDNF, GRM3, and $DTNBP_1$, showed previous evidence of an association with schizophrenia and were affected by hypoxia. In keeping with the epidemiological findings discussed previously, the OCs identified in this study were diverse and occurred during both prenatal and perinatal periods. The overall evidence suggests that these exogenous environmental factors are working on a developmentally vulnerable brain in which endogenous factors have gone awry to produce synergistic increases in risk of schizophrenia in adulthood.

PREVENTION

If gene-environment interaction is important in the etiology of schizophrenia, then preventing the environmental exposures will reduce some of the risk associated with susceptibility genes as well as reducing the risk associated with the independent effects of the environmental exposures. It has been calculated that there is an infection population-attributable proportion of 30% in the samples used to analyze the associations between schizophrenia and influenza, toxoplasmosis, and genital-reproductive infections. If these 3 infections had been prevented, then there would have been 30% fewer cases of schizophrenia in the patient groups examined in these studies. It has also been suggested that the start of influenza immunization may have been responsible for a reduction in the rate of schizophrenia beginning in the 1950s.[118] Evidence like this has been used in support of suggestions that greater coverage of the pregnant population with wide-ranging immunization would decrease the incidence of schizophrenia in the general population. McGrath and colleagues[50] have calculated that almost 44% of the schizophrenia cases in a Danish cohort may have been due to nonoptimal neonatal vitamin D levels. McGrath and colleagues[49] had previously presented evidence that vitamin D supplementation in males in Finland was associated with a reduction in the incidence of schizophrenia in that population, indicating the potential usefulness of supplementation at a population level for micronutritional deficiencies. As noted by McGrath and Lawlor,[119] however, although infection and nutrition may be the exposures most amenable to public health intervention, the evidence is not yet robust enough to justify such action.

Fig. 2 shows the multifactorial, highly complex potential causal pathways to schizophrenia. It seems likely that some seemingly independent risk factors are actually taking place at different times along the same causal pathway. If the antecedent factors can be identified, perhaps through large cohorts with multiples exposures measured, then where best to aim preventative strategies can be investigated. For example, as discussed previously, there is evidence that maternal stress during pregnancy increases the risk of fetal hypoxia. If maternal stress during pregnancy can be prevented or reduced, then some of the risk associated with hypoxia may be able to be reduced.

CLINICAL PREDICTION OF PSYCHOSIS RISK: THE ULTRA–HIGH-RISK APPROACH

Psychosis is usually preceded by a prodromal period before full-blown illness. This period is characterized by the presence of psychotic symptoms at a subthreshold level of intensity and/or duration or frequency compared with established psychotic disorder. Although the psychosis prodrome is, by definition, a retrospective diagnosis, several research groups have developed criteria aimed at prospectively identifying young people during the prodrome, before onset of first-episode psychosis. These criteria have been formalized in several instruments, including the Comprehensive

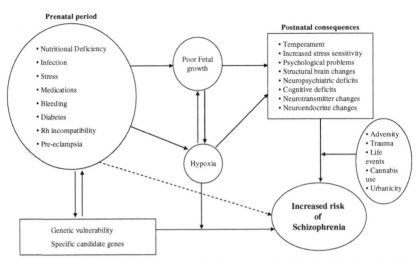

Fig. 2. Proposed pathways and mechanisms linking OCs and risk of schizophrenia. (*Reproduced from* Clarke MC, Roddy S, Cannon M. Obstetric complications and schizophrenia: historical overview and new directions. In: Brown AS, Patterson PH, editors. The origins of schizophrenia. New York: Columbia University Press; 2011. p. 96–119; with permission.)

Assessment of At-Risk Mental States[120] and the Structured Interview for Prodromal Syndromes.[121] Three prodromal risk syndromes have been described in these instruments, characterized by

1. Attenuated positive symptoms
2. Frank psychotic symptoms that are brief in duration or
3. Genetic risk combined with functional deterioration

Prospective studies have demonstrated that approximately 15% to 40% of young people who present to the clinic with these putative prodromal risk syndromes go on to develop a psychotic disorder within the proceeding 2 years.[122–126] As a result, these individuals are considered an ultra–high-risk (UHR) group for psychosis.[127]

Neurocognitive Manifestations of Psychosis Risk

A great deal of research has been conducted addressing neurocognitive risk factors associated with prodromal risk syndromes, which helps inform about the underlying pathophysiology associated with psychosis risk. This has included research on working memory, attention/vigilance, executive functioning, verbal learning/memory, and speed of processing. Research has shown impairments across most of these cognitive domains in UHR samples.

Working memory

Verbal and spatial working memory have both been shown to be impaired in UHR samples, using assessments, such as letter-number span tasks, delayed match-to-sample tasks, spatial board tasks, and hidden tokens tasks. Several different groups have demonstrated verbal and spatial working memory deficits in UHR samples.[128–133] Wood and colleagues,[134] for example, demonstrated spatial working memory deficits in an Australian sample of 38 UHR patients using a block-tapping test. Smith and colleagues[135] have also shown spatial working memory deficits in an American sample of 8 UHR patients. Hawkins and colleagues[136] demonstrated verbal working memory deficits on a letter-number sequencing task in a sample of 36 Canadian and American UHR patients, a finding recently replicated by Carrion and colleagues[137] in a larger sample of UHR patients (n = 127) also using the letter-number sequencing task.

Attention and vigilance

The Continuous Performance Test is the classic task used in neurocognitive assessments of attention and vigilance. Hambrecht and colleagues[138] conducted one of the earliest such tests in a sample of 51 putatively prodromal patients and found that the UHR sample demonstrated significantly poorer scores compared with healthy controls. Attention deficits have now been demonstrated many times across different studies.[131–134]

Executive function

Tasks, such as the Wisconsin Card Sorting Test (WCST) and the Tower of Hanoi, are among the most commonly used measures of executive functioning in UHR samples. Several groups have demonstrated executive function deficits in UHR patients.[130–132] Pukrop and colleagues[139] showed deficits on the WCST in a German sample of 90 UHR patients. Pflueger and colleagues,[129] using both the WCST and Tower of Hanoi tasks, also found executive functioning deficits in a sample of 60 UHR patients in Basel, Switzerland. Most recently, in one of the largest studies to date, Carrion and colleagues[137] showed deficits on the WCST in a sample of 127 UHR patients.

Verbal learning/memory

Several different tasks are used to assess verbal learning and memory, which include assessing the participants' ability to immediately recall words as well as their ability to recall the words after a delay. The California Verbal Learning Test, Hopkins Verbal Learning Test, and the Rey Auditory Verbal Learning Test are frequently used, with immediate and delayed testing trials, as well as the Wechsler Memory Scale. Verbal learning tasks regularly show some of the greatest levels of impairment relative to other neurocognitive domains.[137–142] Niendam and colleagues,[142] for example, showed pronounced verbal learning deficits in a sample of 45 12-year-old to 29-year-old UHR patients attending a prodromal clinic in California. Similarly, Jhashan and colleagues[143,144] demonstrated marked deficits in verbal learning in a sample of 48 12-year-old to 30-year-old patients with prodromal syndromes.

Processing speed

Tests of processing speed have been used less frequently than tests of other neurocognitive domains but have consistently demonstrated, in studies incorporating them, some of the most marked neurocognitive impairments. Processing speed tasks used have included the Trail Making Test, digit symbol-coding test, the Stroop Color and Word Test, and verbal fluency tests.[130] Hawkins and colleagues[136] found deficits in a sample of 36 American and Canadian UHR patients using a digit symbol-coding task and the Stroop Color and Word Test. Eastvold and colleagues[130] reported that a sample of 40 UHR patients performed significantly more poorly on the Stroop Color and Word Test compared with healthy controls. Simon and colleagues[140] reported poorer scores in a sample of 69 UHR patients on both the Trail Making Test and verbal fluency tests. Frommann and colleagues[132] found, in a sample of German patients who were in the early versus late stages of the prodrome, that although patients in the later stage of the prodrome demonstrated a range of neurocognitive deficits, early-stage prodromal patients uniquely showed processing speed deficits. The authors have recently conducted one of the first studies of prodromal syndromes outside the clinic setting.[145] Among a population sample of 11-year-old to 13-year-old patients, up to 8% fulfilled criteria for a prodromal risk syndrome. Using the Measurement and Treatment Research to Improve Cognition in Schizophrenia (MATRICS) consensus neurocognitive battery, young people who met criteria for prodromal risk syndromes demonstrated deficits in processing speed, including on the Trail Making Test, Part A, and the symbol-coding task from the Brief Assessment of Cognition in Schizophrenia, as well as deficits in nonverbal working memory, using the Wechsler Memory Scale spatial span task.[146] Deficits were most pronounced on the symbol-coding task from the Brief Assessment of Cognition in Schizophrenia (z score difference between UHR group and controls = 1), in line with the findings of Frommann and colleagues[132] that processing speed deficits are the main finding in the early UHR stages.

In the largest study to date of neurocognitive functioning in patients with prodromal syndromes, Seidman and colleagues[133] found that processing speed, measured with a symbol-coding task, was the most pronounced of all neurocognitive deficits. Most recently, Carrion and colleagues[137] have also shown in a large sample of American UHR patients that not only were processing speed deficits especially pronounced relative to most other neurocognitive deficits but also processing speed deficits were uniquely predictive of social and role functioning, independent of positive psychotic symptoms. This is interesting given that some researchers have suggested that symbol-coding deficits reflect the core of schizophrenia neurocognitive impairment.[147,148] In a meta-analysis of 40 studies, Dickinson[148] reported that the effect size of the impairment on a symbol-coding task significantly exceeded the effect sizes of tasks commonly used to measure more specific cognitive domains, including episodic memory, executive function, and working memory. This, they have argued, represents a systems-based dysfunction, which may be at the heart of psychosis risk, reflecting a process of disturbed integration and coordination between distributed brain networks.

The Community Approach

Although UHR research has been in progress in the clinic, a parallel stream of research has been ongoing in the general population, studying psychosis from a broader perspective, that is, individuals in the community who experience isolated psychotic symptoms. These symptoms are especially prevalent in young people, with meta-analyses demonstrating a median population prevalence of 17% among children ages 9 years to 12 years and 7.5% among adolescents ages 13 years to 18 years.[149] By comparison, a meta-analysis of (mainly) adult studies demonstrated a population prevalence of 5% for psychotic symptoms.[150] The presence of these symptoms at a subclinical level in the community is of clinical interest because, as in UHR studies, longitudinal research has demonstrated that these symptoms are associated with increased risk for psychotic disorder in adulthood, albeit not to the same degree as in UHR patients. In an influential article, Poulton and colleagues[151] demonstrated that community-based children who reported psychotic symptoms at age 11 were, at age 26, at a 5-fold to 16-fold increased risk of schizophreniform disorder. This finding was replicated by researchers in an Australian sample, who showed that self-reported auditory hallucinations at age 14 years were associated with increased risk for psychotic disorder at age 21.[152] Young people in the general population who report psychotic symptoms have been shown to share a wide range of risk factors with schizophrenia patients, including social, environmental, substance use, obstetric, developmental, anatomic, and intellectual risk factors.[153] For these reasons, this population has been considered to form part of an extended psychosis phenotype, comprised of ostensibly healthy community-based individuals with occasional psychotic symptoms on one end and schizophrenia patients on the other end. Researchers have argued that work on this extended psychosis phenotype may provide valuable insights into the etiology of clinical psychotic disorder.[154,155] Neurocognitive research has only recently begun on this population but some of the cognitive differences that are characteristic of the prodrome and first-episode psychosis have already been shown to also occur in this population. In particular, deficits in processing speed have been found pronounced in this group. Blanchard and colleagues,[156] for example, showed that, in addition to poorer scores in tests of receptive language and motor skills, young people with psychotic symptoms performed more poorly on the Trail Making Test, Part B. This is in line with a previous cohort study, which demonstrated that childhood performance on this task predicted schizophrenia in adulthood.[157] Using the MATRICS battery in a sample of more than 200 community-based adolescents, we have recently shown that psychotic symptoms are associated with significantly poorer scores in tests of processing speed and working memory, with performance on digit symbol-coding particularly pronounced.[158] This mirrors findings in UHR sample as well as in first-episode psychosis.

SUMMARY

There is strong evidence for involvement of a range of environmental risk factors in the pathway to schizophrenia. These include OCs, prenatal infection, prenatal stress, prenatal nutrition, and adolescent cannabis use. These risk factors, however, are neither necessary nor sufficient causal factors for schizophrenia. The majority of people who are exposed to them do not develop schizophrenia and a majority of individuals with schizophrenia may not have had the specific exposure in question. These risk factors are component causes embedded in highly complex pathways to schizophrenia in which some of these risk factors may add to, mediate, or moderate each other's effects. Just as with genetic risk factors, however, a risk factor should not be ignored because it is of small effect. It is likely that these environmental risk factors also affect the outcome of genetic risk factors for schizophrenia through gene/environment interaction and/or through epigenetic effects. In addition, work studying the etiologic overlap between neurodevelopmental disorders, such as epilepsy and schizophrenia, and work on the extended psychosis phenotype are starting to provide potentially valuable insights into the etiology of clinical psychotic disorder.

REFERENCES

1. Cannon M, Jones PB, Murray RM. Obstetric complications and schizophrenia: historical and meta-analytic review. Am J Psychiatry 2002;159:1080–92.
2. Byrne M, Agerbo E, Bennedsen B, et al. Obstetric conditions and risk of first admission with schizophrenia: a Danish national register based study. Schizophr Res 2007;97:51–9.
3. Gunnell D, Rasmussen F, Fouskakis D, et al. Patterns of fetal and childhood growth and the development of psychosis in young males: a cohort study. Am J Epidemiol 2003;158:291–300.
4. Gunnell D, Harrison G, Whitley E, et al. The association of fetal and childhood growth with risk of schizophrenia. Cohort study of 720,000 Swedish men and women. Schizophr Res 2005;79:315–22.
5. Sørensen HJ, Mortensen EL, Reinisch JM, et al. Do hypertension and diuretic treatment in pregnancy increase the risk of schizophrenia in offspring? Am J Psychiatry 2003;160:464–8.

6. Sørensen HJ, Mortensen EL, Reinisch JM, et al. Association between prenatal exposure to analgesics and risk of schizophrenia. Br J Psychiatry 2004;160: 366–71.

7. Insel BJ, Brown AS, Bresnahan MA, et al. Maternal-fetal blood incompatibility and the risk of schizophrenia in offspring. Schizophr Res 2005;80:331–42.

8. Boog G. Obstetrical complications and further schizophrenia of the infant: a new methodological threat to the obstetrician? J Gynecol Obstet Biol Reprod 2003; 32:720–7.

9. Boksa P, El-Khodor BF. Birth insult interacts with stress at adulthood to alter dopaminergic function in animal models: possible implications for schizophrenia and other disorders. Neurosci Biobehav Rev 2003;27:91–101.

10. Cannon TD, Yolken R, Buka S, et al. Collaborative study group on the perinatal origins of severe psychiatric D. Decreased neurotrophic response to birth hypoxia in the etiology of schizophrenia. Biol Psychiatry 2008;64:797–802.

11. Dalman C. Obstetric complications and risk of schizophrenia: an association appears undisputed, yet mechanisms are still unknown. Lakartidningen 2003; 100:1974–9.

12. Cannon TD, Rosso IM, Hollister JM, et al. A prospective cohort study of Genetic and perinatal influences in the etiology of schizophrenia. Schizophr Bull 2000; 26:249–56.

13. Casadio P, Di Forti M, Murray RM. Cannabis use as a component cause of schizophrenia. In: Brown AS, Patterson PH, editors. The origins of schizophrenia. Columbia University Press; 2011. p. 157–75.

14. Di Forti M, Morgan C, Dazzan P, et al. High-potency cannabis and the risk of psychosis. Br J Psychiatry 2009;195(6):488–91.

15. Caspi A, Moffitt TE, Cannon M, et al. Moderation of the effect of adolescent-onset cannabis use on adult psychosis by a functional polymorphism in the catechol-O-methyltransferase gene: longitudinal evidence of a gene X environment interaction. Biol Psychiatry 2005;57(10):1117–27.

16. Henquet C, Rosa A, Delespaul P, et al. COMT ValMet moderation of cannabis-induced psychosis: a momentary assessment study of 'switching on' hallucinations in the flow of daily life. New York: Columbia University Press; Acta Psychiatr Scand 2009;119(2):156–60.

17. Henquet C, Murray R, Linszen D, et al. The environment and schizophrenia: the role of cannabis use. Schizophr Bull 2005;31(3):608–12.

18. Moore TH, Zammit S, Lingford-Hughes A, et al. Cannabis use and risk of psychotic or affective mental health outcomes: a systematic review. Lancet 2007;370(9584):319–28.

19. Mednick SA, Machon RA, Huttunen MO, et al. Adult schizophrenia following prenatal exposure to an influenza epidemic. Arch Gen Psychiatry 1988;45: 189–92.

20. Brown AS. Maternal infection and schizophrenia. In: Brown AS, Patterson PH, editors. The origins of schizophrenia. New York: Columbia University Press; 2011. p. 25–57.

21. Brown AS, Cohen P, Greenwald S, et al. Nonaffective psychosis after prenatal exposure to rubella. Am J Psychiatry 2000;157:438–43.

22. Brown AS, Begg MD, Gravenstein S, et al. Serologic evidence of prenatal influenza in the etiology of schizophrenia. Arch Gen Psychiatry 2004;61: 774–80.

23. Cannon M, Kendell R, Susser E, et al. Prenatal and perinatal risk factors for schizophrenia. In: Murray RM, Jones PB, Susser E, et al, editors. The

epidemiology of schizophrenia. Cambridge (UK): Cambridge University Press Cambridge University Press; 2002. p. 74–99.

24. Clarke MC, Harley M, Cannon M. The role of obstetric events in schizophrenia. Schizophr Bull 2006;32:3–8.

25. Brown AS, Cohen P, Harkavy-Friedman J, et al. Prenatal rubella, premorbid abnormalities, and adult schizophrenia. Biol Psychiatry 2001;49(6):473–86.

26. Clarke MC, Tanskanen A, Huttunen M, et al. Evidence for an Interaction between familial liability and prenatal exposure to infection in the causation of schizophrenia. Am J Psychiatry 2009;166(9):1025–30.

27. Gilmore JH, Jarskog LF. Exposure to infection and brain development: cytokines in the pathogenesis of schizophrenia. Schizophr Res 1997;24(3): 365–7.

28. Sperner-Unterweger B. Immunological aetiology of major psychiatric disorders: evidence and therapeutic implications. Drugs 2005;65(11):1493–520.

29. Arion D, Unger T, Lewis DA, et al. Molecular evidence for increased expression of genes related to immune and chaperone function in the prefrontal cortex in schizophrenia. Biol Psychiatry 2007;62(7):711–21.

30. Patterson PH. Anmial models of the maternal infection risk factor. In: Brown AS, Patterson PH, editors. The origins of schizophrenia. Columbia University Press; 2011. p. 255–81.

31. Huttunen MO, Niskanen P. Prenatal loss of father and psychiatric disorders. Arch Gen Psychiatry 1978;35(4):429–31.

32. Khashan AS, Abel KM, McNamee R, et al. Higher risk of offspring schizophrenia following antenatal maternal exposure to severe adverse life events. Arch Gen Psychiatry 2008;65(2):146–52.

33. van Os J, Selten JP. Prenatal exposure to maternal stress and subsequent schizophrenia. The May 1940 invasion of The Netherlands. Br J Psychiatry 1998;172:324–6.

34. Imamura Y, Nakane Y, Ohta Y, et al. Lifetime prevalence of schizophrenia among individuals prenatally exposed to atomic bomb radiation in Nagasaki City. Acta Psychiatr Scand 1999;100(5):344–9.

35. Malaspina D, Corcoran C, Kleinhaus KR, et al. Acute maternal stress in pregnancy and schizophrenia in offspring: a cohort prospective study. BMC Psychiatry 2008;8:71.

36. Myhrman A, Rantakallio P, Isohanni M, et al. Unwantedness of a pregnancy and schizophrenia in the child. Br J Psychiatry 1996;169(5):637–71.

37. Koenig JI, Kirkpatrick B, Lee P. Glucocorticoid hormones and early brain development in schizophrenia. Neuropsychopharmacology 2002;27(2): 309–18.

38. Patterson PH. Anmial models of the maternal stress risk factor. In: Brown AS, Patterson PH, editors. The origins of schizophrenia. New York: Columbia University Press; 2011. p. 335–64.

39. Iampietro MC, Ellman LM. Maternal stress during pregnancy and schizophrenia. In: Brown AS, Patterson PH, editors. The origins of schizophrenia. Columbia University Press; 2011. p. 120–39.

40. Sharma S, Norris WE, Kalkunte S. Beyond the threshold: an etiological bridge between hypoxia and immunity in preeclampsia. J Reprod Immunol 2010; 85(1):112–6.

41. Epel E, Lapidus R, McEwen B, et al. Stress may add bite to appetite in women: a laboratory study of stress-induced cortisol and eating behavior. Psychoneuroendocrinology 2001;26(1):37–49.

42. Read J, van Os J, Morrison AP, et al. Childhood trauma, psychosis and schizophrenia: a literature review with theoretical and clinical implications. Acta Psychiatr Scand 2005;112:330–50.

43. Morgan C, Fisher H. Environmental factors in schizophrenia: childhood trauma—a critical review. Schizophr Bull 2007;33:3–10.

44. Harley M, Kelleher I, Clarke M, et al. Cannabis use and childhood trauma interact additively to increase the risk of psychotic symptoms in adolescence. Psychol Med 2010;40(10):1627–34.

45. Kelleher I, Harley M, Lynch F, et al. Associations between childhood trauma, bullying and psychotic symptoms among a school-based adolescent sample. Br J Psychiatry 2008;193:378–82.

46. Heins M, Simons C, Lataster T, et al. Childhood trauma and psychosis: a case-control and case-sibling comparison across different levels of genetic liability, psychopathology, and type of trauma. Am J Psychiatry 2011;168(12):1286–94.

47. Cougnard A, Marcelis M, Myin-Germeys I, et al. Does normal developmental expression of psychosis combine with environmental risk to cause persistence of psychosis? A psychosis proneness-persistence model. Psychol Med 2007; 37:513–27.

48. Brown AS, Bottiglieri T, Schaefer CA, et al. Elevated prenatal homocysteine levels as a risk factor for schizophrenia. Arch Gen Psychiatry 2007;64(1):31–9.

49. McGrath J, Saari K, Hakko H, et al. Vitamin D supplementation during the first year of life and risk of schizophrenia: a Finnish birth cohort study. Schizophr Res 2004;67(2–3):237–45.

50. McGrath JJ, Eyles DW, Pedersen CB, et al. Neonatal vitamin D status and risk of schizophrenia: a population-based case-control study. Arch Gen Psychiatry 2010;67(9):889–94.

51. Insel BJ, Schaefer CA, McKeague IW, et al. Maternal iron deficiency and the risk of schizophrenia in offspring. Arch Gen Psychiatry 2008;65(10):1136–44.

52. Cui X, Eyles DW, Burne TH, et al. Developmental Vitamin D deficiency as a risk factor for schizophrenia. In: Brown AS, Patterson PH, editors. The origins of schizophrenia. New York: Columbia University Press; 2011. p. 282–99.

53. Tarantino LM, Reyes TM, Palmer AA. Animal models of prenatal protein malnutrition relevant for schizophrenia. In: Brown AS, Patterson PH, editors. The origins of schizophrenia. Columbia University Press; 2011. p. 300–34.

54. Harper KN, Brown AS. Prenatal nutrition and the etiology of schizophrenia. In: Brown AS, Patterson PH, editors. The origins of schizophrenia. New York: Columbia University Press; 2011. p. 58–95.

55. Hollister JM, Laing P, Mednick SA. Rhesus incompatibility as a risk factor for schizophrenia in male adults. Arch Gen Psychiatry 1996;53:19–24.

56. Brown AS, Schaefer CA, Quesenberry CP Jr, et al. Maternal exposure to toxoplasmosis and risk of schizophrenia in adult offspring. Am J Psychiatry 2005; 162(4):767–73.

57. Brown AS, Schaefer CA, Quesenberry CP Jr, et al. No evidence of relation between maternal exposure to herpes simplex virus type 2 and risk of schizophrenia? Am J Psychiatry 2006;163(12):2178–80.

58. Brown AS, Schaefer CA, Wyatt RJ, et al. Maternal exposure to respiratory infections and adult schizophrenia spectrum disorders: a prospective birth cohort study. Schizophr Bull 2000;26(2):287–95.

59. Babulas V, Factor-Litvak P, Goetz R, et al. Prenatal exposure to maternal genital and reproductive infections and adult schizophrenia. Am J Psychiatry 2006; 163(5):927–9.

60. Sørensen HJ, Nielsen PR, Pedersen CB, et al. Association between prepartum maternal iron deficiency and offspring risk of schizophrenia: population-based cohort study with linkage of Danish national registers. Schizophr Bull 2011; 37(5):982–7.

61. McGrath J, Eyles D, Mowry B, et al. Low maternal vitamin D as a risk factor for schizophrenia: a pilot study using banked sera. Schizophr Res 2003;63(1–2):73–8.

62. Esquirol E. Des maladies mentales considerees sous les rapports medical. JB Balliere; 1838.

63. Kraeplin E. Psychiatrie: Ein Lehrbuch fur Studierende und Artze. Leipzig (Germany): Barth; 1913.

64. Flor-Henry P. Psychosis and temporal lobe epilepsy. A controlled investigation. Epilepsia 1969;10(3):363–95.

65. Trimble MR. The psychoses of epilepsy. New York: Raven Press; 1991.

66. Gibbs EL, Gibbs FA, Fuster B. Psychomotor epilepsy. Arch Neurol Psychiatry 1948;60(4):331–9.

67. Slater E, Beard AW, Glithero E. The schizophrenialike psychoses of epilepsy. Br J Psychiatry 1963;109:95–150.

68. Schmitz B. Psychosis in epilepsy: frequency and risk factors. J Epilepsy 1995;8: 295–305.

69. Swinkels WA, Kuyk J, van Dyck R, et al. Psychiatric comorbidity in epilepsy. Epilepsy Behav 2005;7(1):37–50.

70. Jensen I, Larsen JK. Mental aspects of temporal lobe epilepsy. Follow-up of 74 patients after resection of a temporal lobe. J Neurol Neurosurg Psychiatry 1979; 42(3):256–65.

71. Gudmundsson G. Epilepsy in Iceland. A clinical and epidemiological investigation. Acta Neurol Scand 1966;43(Suppl 25):1–124.

72. Qin P, Xu H, Laursen TM, et al. Risk for schizophrenia and schizophrenia-like psychosis among patients with epilepsy: population based cohort study. BMJ 2005;331(7507):23.

73. Clarke M, Tanskanen A, Huttunen MO, et al. Evidence for shared genetic susceptibility to epilepsy and psychosis: a population based family study. Biol Psychiatry 2012;71(9):836–9.

74. Bruton CJ, Stevens JR, Frith CD. Epilepsy, psychosis, and schizophrenia: clinical and neuropathologic correlations. Neurology 1994;44(1):34–42.

75. Helbig I, Mefford HC, Sharp AJ, et al. 15q13.3 Microdeletions increase risk of idiopathic generalized epilepsy. Nat Genet 2009;41(2):160–2.

76. Masurel-Paulet A, Andrieux J, Callier P, et al. Delineation of 15q13.3 microdeletions. Clin Genet 2010;78(2):149–61.

77. Vassos E, Collier DA, Holden S, et al. Penetrance for copy number variants associated with schizophrenia. Hum Mol Genet 2010;19(17):3477–81.

78. Barr WB, Ashtari M, Bilder RM, et al. Brain morphometric comparison of first-episode schizophrenia and temporal lobe epilepsy. Br J Psychiatry 1997;170: 515–9.

79. Sundram F, Cannon M, Doherty CP, et al. Neuroanatomical correlates of psychosis in temporal lobe epilepsy: voxel-based morphometry study. Br J Psychiatry 2010;197(6):482–92.

80. Bryant RA, O'Donnell ML, Creamer M, et al. The psychiatric consequences of traumatic brain injury. Am J Psychiatry 2010;167:312–20.

81. Fleminger S. Head injury. In: David A, Fleminger S, Kopelman MD, et al, editors. Lishman's organic psychiatry: a textbook of neuropsychiatry. 4th edition. Blackwell Publishing; 2009. p. 167–279.

82. Davidson K, Bagley CR. Schizophrenia-like psychosis associated with organic disorders of the central nervous system: a review of the literature. Current problems of neuropsychiatry. Br J Psychiatry 1969;(Special publication 4):S113–84.

83. David A, Prince M. Psychosis following head injury: a critical review. J Neurol Neurosurg Psychiatry 2005;76(Suppl 1):i53–60.

84. Kim E. Does traumatic brain injury predispose individuals to develop schizophrenia? Curr Opin Psychiatry 2009;21:286–9.

85. Hesdorffer DC, Rauch SL, Tamminga CA. Long-term psychiatric outcomes following traumatic brain injury: a review of the literature. J Head Trauma Rehabil 2009;24:452–9.

86. Malaspina D, Goertz RR, Friedman JH, et al. Traumatic brain injury and schizophrenia in members of schizoiphrenia and bipolar pedigrees. Am J Psychiatry 2001;158:440–6.

87. Nielsen AS, Mortensen PB, O'Callaghan E, et al. Is head injury a risk factor for schizophrenia? Schizophr Res 2002;55:93–8.

88. Fann JR, Burington MS, Leonetti A, et al. Psychiatric illness following traumatic brain injury in an adult health maintenance organisation population. Arch Gen Psychiatry 2004;61:53–61.

89. Achte KA, Hillbom E, Aalberg V. Psychoses following war brain injuries. Acta Psychiatr Scand 1969;225:1–94.

90. Dalmau J, Gleichman AJ, Hughes EG, et al. Anti-NMDA receptor encephalitis: case series and analysis of the effects of antibodies. Lancet Neurol 2008;7:1091–8.

91. Barry H, Hardiman O, Healy DG, et al. Anti-NMDA receptor encephalitis: an important differential diagnosis in psychosis. Br J Psychiatry 2011;199:508–9.

92. Baldridge EB, Bessen HA. Phencyclidine. Emerg Med Clin Morth Am 1990;8: 541–50.

93. Gottesman II, Shields J. Schizophrenia: the epigenetic puzzle. Cambridge (United Kingdom): Cambridge University Press; 1982.

94. Dean K, Stevens H, Mortensen PR, et al. Full spectrum of psychiatric outcomes among offspring with parental history of mental disorder. Arch Gen Psychiatry 2010;67:822–9.

95. Ingraham LJ, Kety SS. Adoption studies of schizophrenia. Am J Hum Genet 2000;97:18–22.

96. Cardno AG, Gottesman I. Twin studies of schizophrenia: from bow-and-arrow concordances to Star Wars Mx and functional genomics. Am J Med Genet 2000;97:12–7.

97. Sullivan PF, Kendler KS, Neale MC. Schizophrenia as a complex trait: evidence from a meta-analysis of twin studies. Arch Gen Psychiatry 2003;60:1187–92.

98. Schwartz S, Susser E. Twin studies of heritability. In: Susser E, Schwzrtz S, Morabia A, et al, editors. Psychiatric epidemiology. New York: Oxford University Press; 2006.

99. Kringlen E, Cramer G. Offspring of monozygotic twins discordant for schizophrenia. Arch Gen Psychiatry 1989;46:873–7.

100. Gottesman II, Bertelsen A. Confirming unexpressed genotypes for schizophrenia: risks in the offspring of Fischer's Danish identical and fraternal discordant twins. Arch Gen Psychiatry 1989;46:867–72.

101. Gejman PV, Sanders AR, Kendler KS. Genetics of schizophrenia: new findings and challenges. Annu Rev Genomics Hum Genet 2011;12:121–44.

102. PGC (Schizophrenia Psychiatric Genome-Wide Association Study Consortium). Genome-wide association study identifies five new schizophrenia loci. Nat Genet 2011;43(10):969–76.

103. ISC (International Schizophrenia Consortium). Common polygenic variation contributes to risk of schizophrenia and bipolar disorder. Nature 2009;460: 748–52.

104. Agerbo E, Mortensen PB, Wiuf C, et al. Modelling the contribution of family history and variation in singly nucleotide polymorphisms to risk of schizophrenia: a Danish national birth cohort-based study. Schizophr Res 2012; 134:246–52.

105. Maher B. Personal genomes: the case of the missing heritability. Nature 2008; 456:18–21.

106. Mitchell KJ, Porteous DJ. Rethinking the genetic architecture of schizophrenia. Psychol Med 2011;41:19–32.

107. O'Tuathaigh CM, Harte M, O'Leary C, et al. Schizophrenia-related endophenotypes in heterozygous neuregulin-1 'knockout' mice. Eur J Neurosci 2010; 31(2):349–58.

108. Ibi D, Nagai T, Koike H, et al. Combined effect of neonatal immune activation and mutant DISC1 on phenotypic changes in adulthood. Behav Brain Res 2010;206(1):32–7.

109. Tienari P, Wynne LC, Sorri A, et al. Genotype-environment interaction in schizophrenia-spectrum disorder. Long-term follow-up study of Finnish adoptees. Br J Psychiatry 2004;184:216–22.

110. van Os J, Pedersen CB, Mortensen PB. Confirmation of synergy between urbanicity and familial liability in the causation of psychosis. Am J Psychiatry 2004; 161:2312–4.

111. Mueser KT, McGurk SR. Schizophrenia. Lancet 2004;19:2063–72.

112. Devlin B, Klei L, Myles-Worsely M, et al. Genetic liability to schizophrenia Oceanic Palau: a search in the affected and maternal generation. Hum Genet 2007;121:675–84.

113. Mittal VA, Ellman LM, Cannon TD. Gene-environment interaction and co variation in schizophrenia: the role of obstetric complications. Schizophr Bull 2008; 34:1083–94.

114. Fatemi SH, Folsom TD. The neurodevelopmental hypothesis of schizophrenia, revisited. Schizophr Bull 2009;35:528–48.

115. Schmidt-Kastner R, van Os J, Steinbusch H, et al. Gene regulation by hypoxia and the neurodevelopmental origin of schizophrenia. Schizophr Res 2006; 84(2–3):253–71.

116. Nicodemus KK, Marenci S, Batten AJ, et al. Serious obstetric complications interact with hypoxia-regulated vascular expression genes to influence schizophrenia risk. Mol Psychiatry 2008;18:180–4.

117. Clarke MC, Roddy S, Cannon M. Obstetric complications and schizophrenia: Historical overview and new directions. In: Brown AS, Patterson PH, editors. The origins of schizophrenia. New York: Columbia University Press; 2011. p. 96–119.

118. Suvisaari JM, Haukka JK, Tanskanen AJ, et al. Decline in the incidence of schizophrenia in Finnish cohorts born from 1954 to 1965. Arch Gen Psychiatry 1999;56(8):733–40.

119. McGrath JJ, Lawlor DA. The search for modifiable risk factors for schizophrenia. Am J Psychiatry 2011;168(12):1235–8.

120. Yung AR, McGorry PD, McFarlane CA, et al. Monitoring and care of young people at incipient risk of psychosis. Schizophr Bull 1996;22(2):283–303.

121. McGlashan TH, Miller TJ, Woods SW. Pre-onset detection and intervention research in schizophrenia psychoses: current estimates of benefit and risk. Schizophr Bull 2001;27(4):563–70.

122. Woods SW, Addington J, Cadenhead KS, et al. Validity of the prodromal risk syndrome for first psychosis: findings from the North American Prodrome Longitudinal Study. Schizophr Bull 2009;35(5):894–908.

123. Cannon TD, Cadenhead K, Cornblatt B, et al. Prediction of psychosis in youth at high clinical risk: a multisite longitudinal study in North America. Arch Gen Psychiatry 2008;65(1):28–37.

124. Nelson B, Yung AR. Can clinicians predict psychosis in an ultra high risk group? Aust N Z Psychiatry 2010;44(7):625–30.

125. Ziermans TB, Schothorst PF, Sprong M, et al. Transition and remission in adolescents at ultra-high risk for psychosis. Schizophr Res 2011;126(1–3):58–64.

126. Addington J, Cadenhead KS, Cannon TD, et al. North American Prodrome Longitudinal Study: a collaborative multisite approach to prodromal schizophrenia research. Schizophr Bull 2007;33(3):665–72.

127. Yung AR, Phillips LJ, Yuen HP, et al. Psychosis prediction: 12-month follow up of a high-risk ("prodromal") group. Schizophr Res 2003;60(1):21–32.

128. Gschwandtner U, Pfluger M, Aston J, et al. Fine motor function and neuropsychological deficits in individuals at risk for schizophrenia. Eur Arch Psychiatry Clin Neurosci 2006;256(4):201–6.

129. Pflueger MO, Gschwandtner U, Stieglitz RD, et al. Neuropsychological deficits in individuals with an at risk mental state for psychosis—working memory as a potential trait marker. Schizophr Res 2007;97(1–3):14–24.

130. Eastvold AD, Heaton RK, Cadenhead KS. Neurocognitive deficits in the (putative) prodrome and first episode of psychosis. Schizophr Res 2007;93(1–3):266–77.

131. Kim KR, Park JY, Song DH, et al. Neurocognitive performance in subjects at ultrahigh risk for schizophrenia: a comparison with first-episode schizophrenia. Compr Psychiatry 2011;52(1):33–40.

132. Frommann I, Pukrop R, Brinkmeyer J, et al. Neuropsychological profiles in different at-risk states of psychosis: executive control impairment in the early—and additional memory dysfunction in the late—prodromal state. Schizophr Bull 2011;37(4):861–73.

133. Seidman LJ, Giuliano AJ, Meyer EC, et al. Neuropsychology of the prodrome to psychosis in the NAPLS consortium: relationship to family history and conversion to psychosis. Arch Gen Psychiatry 2010;67(6):578–88.

134. Wood SJ, Pantelis C, Proffitt T, et al. Spatial working memory ability is a marker of risk-for-psychosis. Psychol Med 2003;33(7):1239–47.

135. Smith CW, Park S, Cornblatt B. Spatial working memory deficits in adolescents at clinical high risk for schizophrenia. Schizophr Res 2006;81(2–3):211–5.

136. Hawkins KA, Addington J, Keefe RS, et al. Neuropsychological status of subjects at high risk for a first episode of psychosis. Schizophr Res 2004; 67(2–3):115–22.

137. Carrion RE, Goldberg TE, McLaughlin D, et al. Impact of neurocognition on social and role functioning in individuals at clinical high risk for psychosis. Am J Psychiatry 2011;168(8):806–13.

138. Hambrecht M, Lammertink M, Klosterkotter J, et al. Subjective and objective neuropsychological abnormalities in a psychosis prodrome clinic. Br J Psychiatry Suppl 2002;43:s30–7.

139. Pukrop R, Schultze-Lutter F, Ruhrmann S, et al. Neurocognitive functioning in subjects at risk for a first episode of psychosis compared with first- and multiple-episode schizophrenia. J Clin Exp Neuropsychol 2006;28(8):1388–407.

140. Simon AE, Cattapan-Ludewig K, Zmilacher S, et al. Cognitive functioning in the schizophrenia prodrome. Schizophr Bull 2007;33(3):761–71.

141. Lencz T, Smith CW, McLaughlin D, et al. Generalized and specific neurocognitive deficits in prodromal schizophrenia. Biol Psychiatry 2006;59(9):863–71.

142. Niendam TA, Bearden CE, Johnson JK, et al. Neurocognitive performance and functional disability in the psychosis prodrome. Schizophr Res 2006;84(1):100–11.

143. Jahshan C, Heaton RK, Golshan S, et al. Course of neurocognitive deficits in the prodrome and first episode of schizophrenia. Neuropsychology 2010;24(1): 109–20.

144. Keefe RS, Perkins DO, Gu H, et al. A longitudinal study of neurocognitive function in individuals at-risk for psychosis. Schizophr Res 2006;88(1–3):26–35.

145. Kelleher I, Murtagh A, Molloy C, et al. Identification and characterization of prodromal risk syndromes in young adolescents in the community: a population-based clinical interview study. Schizophr Bull 2012;38(2):239–46.

146. Kelleher I, Murtagh A, Murphy J, et al. Neurocognition in a community sample of young people at putative ultra high risk for psychosis assessed using the MATRICS consensus neurocognitive battery: processing speed as the core deficit. Cogn Neuropsychiatry, in Press.

147. Dickinson D, Ramsey ME, Gold JM. Overlooking the obvious: a meta-analytic comparison of digit symbol coding tasks and other cognitive measures in schizophrenia. Arch Gen Psychiatry 2007;64(5):532–42.

148. Dickinson D. Digit symbol coding and general cognitive ability in schizophrenia: worth another look? Br J Psychiatry 2008;193(5):354–6.

149. Kelleher I, Connor D, Clarke MC, et al. Prevalence of psychotic symptoms in childhood and adolescence: a systematic review and meta-analysis of population-based studies. Psychol Med 2012. [Epub ahead of print].

150. van Os J, Linscott RJ, Myin-Germeys I, et al. A systematic review and meta-analysis of the psychosis continuum: evidence for a psychosis proneness-persistence-impairment model of psychotic disorder. Psychol Med 2009;39(2):179–95.

151. Poulton R, Caspi A, Moffitt TE, et al. Children's self-reported psychotic symptoms and adult schizophreniform disorder: a 15-year longitudinal study. Arch Gen Psychiatry 2000;57(11):1053–8.

152. Welham J, Scott J, Williams G, et al. Emotional and behavioural antecedents of young adults who screen positive for non-affective psychosis: a 21-year birth cohort study. Psychol Med 2009;39(4):625–34.

153. Kelleher I, Cannon M. Psychotic-like experiences in the general population: characterizing a high-risk group for psychosis. Psychol Med 2011;41(1):1–6.

154. Polanczyk G, Moffitt TE, Arseneault L, et al. Etiological and clinical features of childhood psychotic symptoms: results from a birth cohort. Arch Gen Psychiatry 2010;67(4):328–38.

155. Laurens KR, Hodgins S, Maughan B, et al. Community screening for psychotic-like experiences and other putative antecedents of schizophrenia in children aged 9-12 years. Schizophr Res 2007;90(1–3):130–46.

156. Blanchard MM, Jacobson S, Clarke MC, et al. Language, motor and speed of processing deficits in adolescents with subclinical psychotic symptoms. Schizophr Res 2010;123(1):71–6.

157. Cannon M, Moffitt TE, Caspi A, et al. Neuropsychological performance at the age of 13 years and adult schizophreniform disorder: prospective birth cohort study. Br J Psychiatry 2006;189:463–4.

158. Kelleher I, Clarke MC, Rawdon C, et al. Neurocognition in the extended psychosis phenotype: performance of a community sample of adolescents with psychotic symptoms on the MATRICS neurocognitive battery. Schizophr Bull, in press.

159. Lencz T, Lambert C, DeRosse P, et al. Runs of homozygosity reveal highly pene-trant recessive loci in schizophrenia. Proc Natl Acad Sci 2007;104(50):19942–7.
160. Sullivan PF, Lin D, Tzeng JY, et al. Genomewide association for schizophrenia in the CATIE study: results of stage 1. Mol Psychiatry 2008;13(6):570–84.
161. O'Donovan MC, Craddock N, Norton N, et al. Identification of loci associated with schizophrenia by genome-wide association and follow-up. Nat Genet 2008;40(9):1053–5.
162. Need AC, Goldstein DB. Whole genome association studies in complex diseases: where do we stand? Dialogues Clin Neurosci 2010;12(1):37–46.
163. Purcell SM, Wray NR, Stone JL, et al. Common polygenic variation contributes to risk of schizophrenia and bipolar disorder. Nature 2009;460(7256):748–52.
164. Stefansson H, Ophoff RA, Steinberg S, et al. Common variants conferring risk of schizophrenia. Nature 2009;460(7256):744–7.
165. Shi J, Levinson DF, Duan J. Common variants on chromosome 6p22.1 are asso-ciated with schizophrenia. Nature 2009;460(7256):753–7.
166. Ikeda M, Aleksic B, Kirov G, et al. Copy number variation in schizophrenia in the Japanese population. Biol Psychiatry 2010;67(3):283–6.
167. Yue WH, Wang HF, Sun LD, et al. Genome-wide association study identifies a susceptibility locus for schizophrenia in Han Chinese at 11p11.2. Nat Genet 2011;43(12):1228–31.
168. Shi Y, Li Z, Xu Q, et al. Common variants on 8p12 and 1q24.2 confer risk of schizophrenia. Nat Genet 2011;43(12):1224–7.

Is Early Intervention for Psychosis Feasible and Effective?

Vinod H. Srihari, MD[a,b,]*, Jai Shah, MD[c],
Matcheri S. Keshavan, MD[d]

KEYWORDS

- Psychosis • Schizophrenia • Early intervention • Critical period

KEY POINTS

- Services that provide comprehensive, early intervention (EI) have shown promise in improving long-term outcomes in schizophrenia.
- Randomized trials in Northern Europe and the UK have demonstrated the long term effectiveness and economic viability of EI.
- Emerging data from the US confirms the feasibility of this model of care in the context of public-academic partnership.
- The project of improving early care in schizophrenia will benefit from a framework that integrates initiatives across traditional divisions of discovery-based and implementation research.

INTERVENING EARLY FOR PSYCHOSIS: WHY BOTHER?

Psychotic disorders are common, disabling, and costly under usual care. The prototypic psychotic illness, schizophrenia, affects between 0.55% and 1%[1,2] of people during their lives; typically manifests in adolescence or early adulthood (an especially formative period for social and vocational trajectories); and is among the

This work was supported by NIH grant MH088971 and a grant from the Donaghue Foundation (Srihari, PI); NIMH grants MH 64023 and MH 78113 (Keshavan, PI); and aDupont-Warren Research Fellowship, Harvard Medical School (Shah).

Disclosures: Dr Keshavan has received grant support from GSK and Sunovion.

[a] Department of Psychiatry, Yale University, New Haven, CT, USA; [b] Clinic for Specialized Treatment Early in Psychosis (STEP), 34 Park Street, Connecticut Mental Health Center, Room 273A, New Haven, CT 06519, USA; [c] Harvard Longwood Psychiatry Residency Training Program, Department of Psychiatry, Harvard Medical School, 330 Brookline Avenue, Rabb-2, Boston, MA 02215, USA; [d] Department of Psychiatry, Beth Israel Deaconess Medical Center and Massachusetts Mental Health Center, Harvard Medical School, Room 610, MMHC 75 Fenwood Road, Boston, MA 02115, USA

* Corresponding author.

E-mail address: vinod.srihari@yale.edu

top 10 causes worldwide of years lived with disability.[3] With routine care, less than one-fifth of patients achieve full recovery after a first episode of psychosis[4] and less than one-third achieve minimal age-appropriate employment or education.[5] Schizophrenia leads annual US mental illness expenditure, with $22.7 billion in direct healthcare costs (2002) attributed mostly to acute hospitalizations. This, however, represents only about a third of the larger estimated total costs that include the burden of unemployment, reduced workplace productivity, premature mortality from suicide, and family caregiving.[6]

Early intervention (EI) services can improve the poor outcomes of usual care. There are intuitively compelling arguments for intervening early in the course of schizophrenia-spectrum disorders. This article reviews these arguments within Birchwood's framework of the "critical period" hypothesis, presents evidence from experimental tests of this hypothesis, and reviews the effectiveness and feasibility of EI services. It concludes with a discussion of how further efforts in this active area of investigation can better address the public health challenge of caring for those with chronic psychotic disorders.

THE COURSE OF PSYCHOTIC ILLNESSES AND THE CRITICAL PERIOD

Beginning with Bleuler's[7] classic follow-up study of schizophrenic illnesses, which proposed stable rather than progressive functional decline as the norm in psychotic illnesses, the pessimistic prognostications embedded in early Kraepelinian classifications (exemplified by the term "dementia praecox") have been strongly challenged. The weight of evidence accumulating against a uniformly deteriorating, degenerative course was summarized in a seminal paper in 1988, which also introduced the concept of a critical period for psychotic illnesses.[8] This includes the three propositions elaborated next, with updated evidence.

Mental and Social Deterioration in Schizophrenia-Spectrum Illnesses is Nonlinear

Prospective studies have shown that most of the clinical and psychosocial deterioration occurs within the first 2 to 5 years after psychosis onset.[9] This period is notable for high risk for relapse, rehospitalization, and suicide. A 15-year follow-up study of first-episode nonaffective psychosis (in which 63% were eventually diagnosed with *Diagnostic and Statistical Manual III-R* schizophrenia) reported relapse rates of 43% (1 year); 55% (2 years); and 70% (5 years).[10] Two-thirds of completed suicides in schizophrenia occur within 6 years of diagnosis[11] with risk particularly elevated 1 year after a first psychiatric hospitalization.[12]

This early, turbulent period is not usually followed by progressive decline but rather a plateau in symptoms and impairment, even under usual systems of care. Long-term follow-up studies in predominantly chronic populations have confirmed this medium-term stability followed by gradual improvement for a third of patients.[13,14] A landmark study of 90 early psychosis patients followed for 10 years confirmed a steep decline to a stable 20% to 25% prevalence of residual positive or negative symptoms within 2 years of onset.[15] A recent meta-analysis of longitudinal studies of first-episode psychosis confirmed that the proportion of patients with poor outcomes does not increase over time.[5]

Desynchrony Between Clinical and Functional Variables is Evident Early in the Course of Schizophrenia

Although studies in chronic illness samples have demonstrated that symptom remission is not necessary for functional recovery,[16,17] early psychosis populations also express this desynchrony, albeit in the opposite direction: here, early symptomatic remission is often the norm and out of proportion to the levels of functional recovery, at least under usual care. Seventy-five percent or more of individuals with first-episode psychosis show symptom remission within the first year,[18,19] but less than one-third achieve minimal age-appropriate employment or educational functioning in the first few years after frank psychosis has emerged.[5]

The First Few Years Around the Onset of Psychosis Witness the Emergence of Several Important Predictors of Outcome

Several factors have been associated with poor long-term outcomes in schizophrenia. Some of these present opportunities for delivering or developing interventions, including prolonged untreated psychosis, social isolation, drug use, insidious onset, living in industrialized countries, and immigration.[16] More recent additions to the list of potentially modifiable factors are affective symptoms, nonadherence to medications, the presence of early negative symptoms, and cognitive dysfunction.[20] Although this list likely represents a mixed bag of factors that are either causally implicated in outcomes, secondary effects of the illness, or confounding variables, many are sources of distress at clinical presentation and have provoked efforts to better understand and modify the disease course.

One factor known for some time to be a correlate of relapse risk in psychosis is the level of expressed emotion (conceptualized as including emotional overinvolvement, hostility, and critical comments) by caregivers of affected individuals.[21] Hospitalized patients returning to high expressed emotion home settings have a relapse risk more than double those returning to low expressed emotion homes.[22] The association between expressed emotion and psychosis relapse seems to be valid in early psychosis[23] with evidence that critical engagement by relatives can increase as the illness becomes more chronic,[24] pointing to the potential use of EI.

A more recent addition to this list is the emergence of cardiovascular risk factors in early psychosis samples. The markedly premature mortality of patients with chronic psychotic disorders is primarily of cardiovascular origin, results in an estimated shortening of lifespan of up to 20 years,[25] with emerging evidence of a worsening of this mortality gap.[26] This cardiometabolic risk emerges quite early in treatment.[27] Along with antipsychotic choice, the emergence of established risk factors, such as smoking and obesity among younger patients,[28] offers an important opportunity for primary prevention of cardiovascular morbidity and mortality.

Increasing evidence in recent years also points to progressive brain changes during the early phases of psychosis. Structural alterations in medial temporal, prefrontal, anterior cingulate, and insular cortex might occur during the acute process of transition to psychosis.[29,30] However, other brain structural changes (ie, superior temporal gyrus volume reductions) found in early psychosis may progress during the early phase of the illness[31] but show no further reductions during the chronic phase.[32] Progressive gray matter reductions have been reported during the first several years after the onset of frank psychosis.[33]

Recent data suggest that brain structure and function (cerebral reserve) before or at the onset of illness may predict better response to treatment, perhaps because of availability of larger neural resources in the service of such adaptive neuroplasticity.[34–36] Earlier stages of psychotic illness, when significant gray and white matter alterations have not yet set in, may therefore respond better to therapeutic interventions. For example, Eack and colleagues[37] have recently shown a lack of progressive gray matter reductions and increases in gray matter in some brain regions in early course schizophrenia patients treated for 2 years with cognitive remediation by contrast to supportive interventions. Taken together, these observations support a neurobiologic basis for the critical period concept.

THE CRITICAL PERIOD HYPOTHESIS AND EI

This hypothesis suggests that intensive efforts to intervene during the critical period (ie, within 2–5 years) after the onset of psychosis can disproportionately alter the trajectory of schizophrenia-spectrum illnesses compared with usual models of care. Usual care is often organized around the dual tasks of acute management of relapses coupled with rehabilitative interventions that typically begin in earnest long after a plateau of functional loss has been reached. This hypothesis makes explicit what has long served as the intuitive basis for improving on such models of care.

The trajectories under usual care are depicted in **Fig. 1**. The three course types (A, B, and C) are a simplification imposed over the considerable heterogeneity reported in outcomes studies. This likely reflects heterogeneity within any diagnostic class but also the variable impact of environmental factors on genetic risk. Nevertheless, the replicated finding of a subset of patients who recover after a single episode (A) and those who are refractory to present treatments (C) is illustrated in this figure to make the point that current EI services are best positioned to target the various courses collapsed into B, which includes patients who, under ordinary care, suffer multiple relapses with variable and potentially malleable levels of return to premorbid functional trajectories.

EI for first-episode psychosis can be conceptualized as including one or more of an interlocking set of strategies composed of two main elements: reducing delay to treatment or reducing the duration of untreated psychosis (DUP), and the provision of more intensive intervention during the 2 to 5 years after identification of a psychotic disorder.[38] The second task includes the provision of phase-specific interventions that are adapted for younger, early course patients and their families. EI, for the rest of this discussion, is used to refer to service approaches that focus on these two tasks, primarily the second.

Outside of the scope of this discussion, but addressed by Clarke and colleagues elsewhere in this issue of the *Clinics*, are the important efforts to predict and prevent conversion to psychosis in high-risk samples. Such efforts to intervene before what is

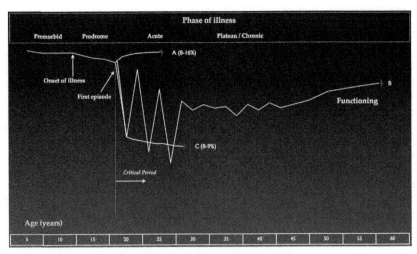

Fig. 1. The course of psychotic illnesses and the critical period.

an arbitrarily defined threshold of positive psychotic symptoms are consistent with a neurodevelopmental conception of schizophrenia-spectrum illnesses.[39–41] However, current limitations on accurate prediction and the lack of established preventive treatments make systematic implementation or assessment of feasibility outside research settings, premature.

Reducing the DUP

The largest experimental study of the impact of reducing DUP has been the impressive TIPS project.[42] A comprehensive education and detection system was delivered by randomized allocation to a healthcare sector in Norway, whereas two control sectors in Norway and Denmark delivered comparable care but without the benefit of efforts to reduce DUP. Although prior systematic reviews of observational studies had documented a strong correlation of DUP with outcome,[43,44] the TIPS project succeeded in experimentally manipulating DUP to address the question of whether this measure is a mere confound associated with poor prognosis cases or a causal mediator of outcomes. TIPS demonstrated that reducing DUP (from a median of 1.5 to 0.5 years) led to markedly improved clinical presentations and improved medium- and longer-term (5-year) outcomes.[45,46] Notably, when the intervention was interrupted, this resulted in measurable increases in DUP followed by attendant worsening in outcomes, further validating the causal inference.[47] Although one other study in Singapore used a broad, multifocal campaign that reduced DUP and improved pathways to care,[48] other less intensive attempts failed to reduce DUP, exemplifying the significant logistical challenge to replicating this finding.[49]

Providing Enriched (Multicomponent) Care During the Critical Period

Although TIPS demonstrated that intervening earlier improves outcomes, most studies have chosen to focus on the arguably more tractable goal of enriching care after presentation for treatment. Centers in Australia, Northern Europe, England, and Canada have pioneered the development and implementation of service models adapted for early psychosis samples.[50] Within this burgeoning area of research are multiple ongoing studies testing one or more of several pharmacologic and psychosocial approaches to improve outcomes in first-episode psychosis.[51] As is common in an area of intensive research, there are multiple definitions of first-episode[52] and multiple measures of outcome.[51] This diversity in samples, interventions, and definitions of outcome preclude any simple inferences about the overall success of the EI paradigm.[53]

The remainder of this article focuses on integrated EI services (ie, those that incorporate several component interventions designed to comprehensively serve the needs of individuals presenting early in the course of a chronic psychotic disorder). In contrast to trials testing the delivery of single treatments (pharmacologic or psychotherapeutic) or interventions focused on demonstrating changes in particular domains (eg, suicidality, comorbid substance use), we draw specifically on studies that evaluate overall, comprehensive services. These models of care are designed to address the wide range of needs presented by patients with early psychosis and their caregivers. Such work seeks to integrate care among the overlapping categories of medical and psychiatric treatment and referral, access to social service, case management, liaison with community supports, social and vocational rehabilitation and education, and support of caregivers. As such, these service models envision the multiple and variable needs of the heterogeneous samples identified as early or first-episode, and are thus the most relevant to a current evaluation of whether EI is effective and feasible.

DOES EI WORK?

We divide this question in four broad domains (**Box 1**) that require distinct responses. These are worth explicating in the context of EI before reviewing the salient evidence.

The first question raises the issue of efficacy or of whether and how much a treatment improves outcomes under relatively ideal conditions. In the context of a clinical trial, this implies recruiting a homogenous population, delivering well-defined treatments in as uniform a manner possible, and measuring outcomes that relate most closely to the putative mechanism of action of the treatment. Such explanatory trials, in essence, attempt to estimate the core therapeutic effects of a treatment.[54] This is in contrast to trials that seek to answer the second question about effectiveness or the impact of a treatment under conditions that are intended to more closely approximate real world clinical settings. With the example of a pharmacologic intervention in mind, it is easy to appreciate the argument that the core therapeutic effect needs to first be demonstrated in an efficacy trial, because a negative result might help avoid futile and expensive effectiveness trials in larger samples. Effects seen in more ideal efficacy conditions might become diluted in effectiveness studies that recruit patients who are more heterogeneous with respect to their response or collect outcomes that may be less closely related to the direct biologic effect of the drug. This linear progression from the establishment of efficacy to the study of effectiveness in more generalizable clinical samples is, however, often not appropriate for complex interventions, such as EI services.

Although initial efficacy or proof of concept trials by pioneer EI programs have sought to demonstrate the value of one or more interventions or models of care in selected early psychosis populations,[50] these have varied in terms of their definition of the sample, intervention, and outcome measures and their success at minimizing common sources of systematic bias and generating adequate power to precisely measure effects. A recent systematic review concluded that this presented the risk that the implementation of EI services will far outpace the strength of the supporting evidence.[51] One argument, based on the logic of knowledge development described previously, would seek to thus limit further implementation of services until the active ingredients or essence of these new approaches to care can be better understood and codified. An alternative appraisal is that legitimate differences in goals and attendant methodologic decisions in efficacy versus effectiveness trials should encourage appropriate deviations from this hierarchical convention.[55] Given the inevitable heterogeneity introduced by the current best diagnostic practice in early psychosis populations and the variety of their treatment needs, the more pragmatic position of determining whether a realistically defined service works for a recognizable target population is more relevant to evaluating the value of EI. This would allow empirically based improvements in service delivery to continue even as the effort to better define pathophysiologically meaningful subtypes continues.[56]

The pragmatic randomized trial[57] operationalizes an approach that combines elements of traditional explanatory trials with considerations of real-world effectiveness

---

Box 1
Evaluating healthcare interventions

1. Efficacy: Can it work?

2. Effectiveness: Does it work?

3. Costs: Is it worth it?

4. Translation: Can it be disseminated?

that is well suited to the current state of knowledge in schizophrenia. Subjects are randomly allocated to alternative service options, thus deviating from real-world clinical practice, but allowing minimization of selection bias. However, these studies embrace more biologically heterogenous samples that seek to mirror those that actually present to systems of care; use interventions that attempt to reflect what could be realistically delivered in such systems; and assess outcomes, often long term, that are most salient to stakeholders in such systems, including patients, families, and policy-makers.

There are four such second-generation trials in the EI literature that are focused on determining the effects of integrated EI service models. Consistent with the pragmatic focus, these trials from four different countries reflect local system resources and constraints in their design and fall on different positions along the efficacy–effectiveness continuum in the domains of sample, intervention, and outcome measurement (**Table 1**).

The UK-based Lambeth Early Onset (LEO) study randomized individuals with early psychosis to an intensive and case-managed treatment regimen of assertive community-based interventions comprising cognitive behavioral therapy, family counseling, vocational services, and low-dose antipsychotic medication. Subjects receiving specialized services had lower rates of relapse and dropout, improved measures of social and vocational functioning, satisfaction, quality of life, and medication adherence at 18-month follow-up.[58,59] The Danish OPUS study offered a similar set of specialized interventions, using a model of home-based assertive case management integrated with pharmacotherapy that favored lower-dose antipsychotics, and included family and individual psychoeducation with social skills training and vocational assistance as needed. This enriched intervention was applied for 2 years and, compared with involvement with a standard community mental health team,[60] delivered benefits in positive and negative symptom control, secondary substance abuse, treatment adherence, and higher satisfaction with care.[61] A Norwegian study of a similar home-based integrated approach compared with standard office-based care reported 2-year improvements in the number and duration of hospitalizations and the frequency of excellent outcomes (a composite that included relapse in symptoms and adherence to treatment) in the group receiving the enriched intervention. Finally, the ongoing STEP trial, directed by one of the authors, delivers an office-based integrated package that includes structured family psychoeducation, cognitive behavioral individual and group therapy, antipsychotic medications, and vocational and educational supports as needed. The treatment is delivered in a US community mental health center and compared with usual care will soon report similar trends in reduction of hospital use and improvement in vocational and social outcomes.[62]

All four studies used a rigorous, albeit pragmatic, randomized design and demonstrated measurable and nontrivial improvements in outcomes across four distinct healthcare systems. Although the first three trials used a particularly resource-intensive model of home-based outreach with enriched clinician/patient ratios ($\sim$1:01) that could be sustained only for a limited period of 2 years, the last trial has used a more pragmatic intervention that is office-based, with a clinician/patient ratio that mirrors the usual care arm ($\sim$1:30). This has allowed the integrated intervention to be sustained without a time limit but instead with gradual transfer to usual services in a stepped, individualized manner.

In OPUS and LEO, much of the demonstrated benefit was not durable at 5-year follow-up (ie, approximately 3 years after specialized care was discontinued).[62,63] This has raised questions of how long intensive care should be sustained and how to mitigate the presumed adverse effects of transferring care from specialized services. Some have raised ethical concerns about offering such enriched

Table 1
Pragmatic randomized controlled trials of integrated early intervention services: design characteristics

Study	Sample	Interventions	Outcomes Measured
LEO: Lambeth (United Kingdom)	Setting: Mental Health Service in Lambeth, London, UK. Recruitment January 2000 to October 2001. Broad inclusion criteria: 16–40 year olds with first or second presentation for nonaffective psychosis and no previous routine community mental health treatment.	1. Specialized multidisciplinary team: assertive outreach team with patient/clinician ratio of ~10:1/LD-SGAs/family counseling/CBT. 2. Standard care from community mental health teams with LD-SGA.	Broad, including clinical (eg, relapse, readmission); functional (eg, vocational functioning); and economic (eg, service use).
OPUS: Copenhagen (Denmark)	Setting: community-based mental health services in Copenhagen and Aarhus Counties. Recruitment from January 1998 to December 2000. Inclusion criteria: 18–45 years, schizophrenia-spectrum diagnosis by ICD-10/F2 category, no more than 12 weeks of continuous antipsychotic drug treatment.	1. Specialized multidisciplinary team assertive outreach team with patient/clinician ratio of ~10:1/LD-SGA/MFG, SST group/vocational strategies. 2. Standard care in a community mental health center, patient/clinician ratio ~30:1.	As above
Grawe–Sør–Trøndelag County (Norway)	Setting: community-based county mental health services. Recruitment initiated in 2001. Inclusion criteria: consecutive referrals ages 18–30 years, DSM-IV schizophrenia-spectrum disorders, within 2 years of psychosis onset.	1. Integrated treatment: home-based outreach with patient/clinician ratio of 10:1, multidisciplinary team; family psychoeducation, CBT- based communication strategies for families and individual therapy for patients and LD-A. 2. Standard care: office-based, focused on pharmacotherapy and problem-based case management.	Clinical (relapse, readmission); functional (GAF); and economic.
STEP-New Haven (United States)	Setting: community mental health center in New Haven county. Broad inclusion criteria: psychosis onset within past 5 years, no more than 12 weeks lifetime exposure to antipsychotic treatment.	1. Integrated care: specialized multidisciplinary team, office-based, patient/clinician ratio ~30:1; structured family psychoeducation; CBT-based group and individual problem solving, vocational and educational assistance as needed and pharmacotherapy. 2. Standard care: office-based, focused on pharmacotherapy and rehabilitative case management.	Broad, including clinical (eg, relapse, readmission); functional (eg, vocational functioning); and economic (eg, service use).

Abbreviations: CBT, cognitive-behavioral therapy; DSM, Diagnostic and Statistical Manual; GAF, Global Assessment of Functioning scale; ICD, International Classification of Diseases; LD-A, low-dose antipsychotics; LD-SGA, low-dose second-generation antipsychotics; MFG, Multi-Family Group psycho-education; SST, social skills training.

interventions for less than 5 years, given that this can be a particularly vulnerable period in development.[64] The STEP approach of offering a less resource-intensive approach that can be sustained longer with an individualized and gradual transition out of specialized care was designed to test an alternative approach. Similar approaches of using stepped reductions in intensity to prolong care through 5 years after entry have demonstrated durable effects in a Canadian public-sector program.[65]

ARE EI SERVICES WORTH THE COST?

The emergence of psychotic disorders in adolescence and young adulthood, their chronicity, and their widespread effects on cognitive functioning make them immensely disabling over the lifespan, placing them in the top 10 causes of disability in developed countries worldwide.[3] The direct healthcare ($22.7 billion) and total ($62.7 billion) costs in the United States[6] are comparable with estimates for far more common depressive disorders.[66] Similar cost estimates undertaken in the United Kingdom have shown a comparable economic burden.[67] Although there is a clear need to improve outcomes to reduce these costs, the fact of limited healthcare resources implies that investments in one area of public health need to be diverted from another. Economic analyses are emerging as the dominant way to quantify such "opportunity costs" and to inform the relative value placed on healthcare services, such as EI.

Several methodologic choices determine whether an economic analysis can provide valid justification for resource allocation.[68]

Measure Costs

First, is the measurement of costs. Focusing solely on direct expenditures or the costs of providing treatment (including inpatient, outpatient, and community health and social services) may seriously underestimate the overall costs of a serious mental illness. In a study of schizophrenia in England, such expenses accounted for less than a fifth of the total cost estimate.[69] The latter ideally includes comprehensive measures of indirect costs, such as lost opportunities for work and leisure and the cost of informal care provided by caregivers.

Measure Benefits

Second, choices made in the measurement of benefits can prejudice the scope of cost analyses. For instance, the surrogate outcomes of symptom control in psychosis may or may not adequately predict vocational functioning or overall quality of life, although these are far more challenging to measure.

Define Comparator

Third, it is important to define an adequate comparator to EI services against which economic gains or losses can be measured. The best available local alternative would provide the most stringent test of an EI service, whereas a poor-quality comparator might inflate estimates of the effectiveness of an integrated approach.

Integrate Life Expectancy Gains with Quality-of-Life Gains

Fourth, economic analyses attempt to integrate life expectancy gains with quality of life gains experienced during a particular time window. In the most common type of evaluation, or cost utility analyses,[70] interventions are assigned a weighted score representing quality of life over a time period, measured in terms of quality-adjusted life-years (QALYs). Comparing interventions in a ratio of currency (eg, dollars) per QALY allows for assessment of the relative benefits conferred by treatments across diseases. During the last decade QALYs have been frequently used in the evaluation of health benefits.[71] The UK-based National Institute for Health and Clinical Excellence, which provides service planners in England with QALY-based guidance, has endorsed EI services and recommends that they include "a full range of relevant pharmacologic, psychological, social, occupational and educational interventions for people with psychosis."[72] The use of QALYs has, however, met with criticism, especially in their lack of responsivity to real improvements in mental distress and disability.[73]

Take a Broad Societal Perspective

Finally, it is generally recommended that economic evaluations take a broad societal perspective. This is in contrast to measuring costs solely from the perspective of an insurer, provider, caregiver, or consumer of mental health care, which each bear only a fraction of the costs exacted by psychotic illnesses. With respect to EI, even small reductions in unemployment and family burden with long-term implications (indirect costs) might offset more immediate but larger per-patient costs of intensive, integrated care (direct costs). Aside from quantifying these costs, a societal rather than a provider perspective would be required to favor resource allocation to such an EI service whose greatest gains might manifest many years after initiation of the intervention.[68]

With these considerations in mind, available evidence on the potential for EI to deliver cost-effective care is not definitive.[74] An initial analysis from PEPP-Montreal investigated differences in expenditures before and after initiation of EI services, showing cost reductions but with uncertainty about whether this could be attributed to the EI service.[75] A similar pre and post study design for new EI services in Hong Kong and Italy found intervention to be good value for money as measured by limited outcomes and costs for the short-term (24 months, Hong Kong)[76] and medium-term (5 years, Italy).[77] In Sweden and Australia, specialized EI services were found to have lower costs (mostly because of decreased inpatient hospitalizations) and improved symptomatic and functional outcomes, although the durability of these differences remained questionable.[78,79] Extending their analysis to 8 years in a smaller sample, the Australian group subsequently found lower levels of positive symptomatology, improved remission rates and illness course, trends toward increased employment, and significantly lower direct service costs among the EI group.[80] This study is important in that it suggests that EI confers long-term advantages if more comprehensive indirect costs are taken into account.

Additional data from the LEO study evaluated a range of costs in detail.[81] Baseline and 18-month mental health service contacts and service use costs were overall higher for individuals receiving EI, with a small but insignificant total cost savings (primarily caused by reduced hospitalization). EI subjects trended toward greater vocational recovery and significantly elevated quality of life, effects that if sustained in longer-term follow-up deliver significant indirect costs reductions.

The notion of whether a broad societal perspective is possible for a system to adopt and to thereby promote the goals of public health for the generally shorter-term and narrower incentives faced by specific agents in the healthcare arena, highlights the importance of appreciating the cultural and policy context in which inferences about cost-effectiveness are made.[80] Health systems ensuring universal coverage (through either social insurance or single-payer schemes) might be more enabled to adopt such a perspective compared with systems in which healthcare coverage is less consistent. In latter systems, such as in the United States, strong incentives exist to shift costs between different payers with measurably adverse outcomes for patients and their families early in the course of psychotic illnesses.[82] Also, service use patterns and the costs associated with them can vary between sites and across countries.[83] This severely limits extrapolation of economic analyses across systems of care.

IS EI FEASIBLE?

It is worth noting that the development of multiple EI services across the globe has occurred in response to a pervasive dissatisfaction with standard services that were well known to be inadequately addressing the needs of these patients and their families.[84] After weighing the emerging evidence for these new approaches, the United Kingdom's National Health Service announced in 2000 the implementation of 50 EI teams across the country.[85] This signaled a commitment toward resourcing EI, which although meeting stakeholder demand has made possible further study and refinement of models of care.

The large number and range of innovative EI services in several countries has in effect demonstrated the acceptability of this approach to a wide range of stakeholders.[86] A more stringent requirement for feasibility, however, might also reference the last question (see **Box 1**) (ie, whether EI services can be disseminated across usual systems of care). Services that are demonstrated to work but cannot be implemented on a wide scale have marginal public health impact. This implementation gap has been documented in the United States for several mental illnesses[87,88] and for schizophrenia in particular.[89,90] This experience has suggested the impact of a complex set of barriers and the tasks of dissemination and implementation of effective interventions has itself become an active focus of study.[91]

Healthcare systems in the United Kingdom, Northern Europe, and Australia have already made substantial commitments to specialized EI services, whereas in the United States a comparable national strategy for improving systems of care is conspicuously absent. Although a detailed consideration of the barriers specific to the different regions in the United States is beyond the scope of this article, certain factors known to many clinicians are illustrative.

1. First is the public-private sector divide. Privately insured patients struggling with the emergence of a serious mental illness can rapidly lose health insurance[82] and typically arrive at the public state mental health system long after the critical period for EI has elapsed.
2. Second, several states care for adolescents and young adults by separate agencies, thus fragmenting care during the peak ages of risk for psychosis onset. Working across organizational cultures with their different emphases on protection of vulnerable children versus the treatment of serious mental illness proves challenging.
3. Third, the division of public mental health care by geographic catchments in the public sector can limit the collection of a critical mass of patients with early psychosis around which to organize care.

Reassuring cost data from other countries, reviewed previously, have had limited impact so far on EI service development in the United States. An important factor, as explicated in the previous section, is that there are powerful nonsocietal perspectives on economic burden at play in US healthcare delivery. Added to this is a paucity of US data on reduction of direct costs that would respond to the perspectives of private and public insurance providers in this country. The feasibility of EI, as for any complex intervention, thus depends as much on the particular perspective adopted within a particular system of care as the data on locally relevant costs. Such data, from the most salient pragmatic trials reviewed previously, suggest consistently positive effects on a variety of domains of outcome but only one such trial will deliver US-based data. Given this, there is reason to remain uncertain about the feasibility of disseminating EI in the United States, beyond research-funded settings.

WHAT NEXT: DOING WHAT IS KNOWN WHILE KNOWING BETTER WHAT TO DO

There are important gaps in knowledge of psychotic disorders that span the range from basic knowledge of cause, pathogenesis, and clinical classification to the more complex domains of dissemination and implementation. A few examples of basic uncertainties in the first domain are instructive.

1. First is the knowledge that early exposures to biologic or psychosocial stressors in utero, during the perinatal period, or around childhood could be causal and may be difficult to address or modify by the time of a first episode of psychosis in early adolescence or adulthood. Truly EI for these neurodevelopmental processes may thus have to await knowledge that allows action in the perinatal period or long before the currently discernible critical period.
2. Second, cognitive impairments can be broad and established by the time of a first episode[92]; the opportunity to prevent or ameliorate these deficits awaits more reliable identification of patients before their first break.[93]
3. Third, ongoing structural brain alterations have been reported up to 20 or more years after the onset of symptoms and are associated with poor outcomes.[94,95] This suggests that whatever the claims made for early course corrections, active attention needs to be paid over the longer term to ensure optimal outcomes.

In the second domain is the recognition, across disorders, that the success of disseminating a model of care (what is referred to as "feasibility" in this article) depends on a host of factors that range from the more generic challenges of changing clinician behavior to the more specific, parochial concerns of individual healthcare systems. Furthermore, there are distinct methodologic challenges in evaluating complex interventions, such as EI services, which deploy multiple interventions that are variably used by different participants. This makes it difficult and sometimes impossible for even large trials to confirm the active ingredients of the integrated service.[96]

It is important to recognize that gaps in the areas of knowledge (knowing what to do) and implementation (doing what is known) impair the ability to most effectively intervene in the early phases of illness. Distinct attention to both these areas is necessary. However, this distinction between knowledge and its translation can itself present a barrier to progress. Especially in the field of EIs for schizophrenia-spectrum disorders, reified divisions between discovery and translate- or implementation-oriented activities present another potential barrier.

Current consensual standards of evidence among US experts that result, for instance, in recommendations for broader implementation of models, such as Assertive Community Treatment or Supported Employment,[89] do not endorse EI. Commentators have reasonably questioned what the essential ingredients of EI might be and whether existing models of EI are merely providing what should be normal best practice. Such knowledge, which would permit more personalized and illness phase-specific treatment, requires access to populations who are early in the course of psychotic illness. Such populations are well known to be extremely difficult to recruit and retain in studies, a project that would be greatly aided by the kinds of EI services that have demonstrably improved pathways into and through care.

The current dichotomy between implementation and research can thus lead to an impasse. There are several lines of work that suggest a way forward. First, managers of healthcare resources, especially in the United States, should pay attention to how nationalized health systems elsewhere have responded to the suggestive, even if not definitive, evidence on secondary prevention in psychosis. Programs in the United Kingdom and Australia have demonstrated that vital information (across the domains of disease physiology to cost-effectiveness of models of care) can emerge from implementations of EI services. The ongoing STEP trial (see **Table 1**) and the large ongoing RAISE initiative[97] will deliver more US-relevant economic data. In an important respect, at least limited implementation may be necessary to generate locally actionable evidence on the range of questions relevant to early intervention.

The Knowledge Translation framework[98] used by the Canadian Institutes of Health Research suggests a more reciprocal organization of knowledge creation and implementation in an "action cycle." In the context of meeting the dual challenge of delivering better early care and improving the ability to study the early course of schizophrenia, we propose a further weakening of this division with three elements that could help advance the field. Given the context specificity of feasibility discussed previously, this proposal is specific to the United States, but likely of relevance to other countries that are less able to rely on a societal perspective for resource allocation:

- The implementation of EI services within public-academic collaborations. Ideally the intensity and range of clinical services would be supported but also limited by the available resources of the public community center. Such an ecologically real-world model would also be protected from changes in grant funding and could revive and draw on a traditional hub of community psychiatry in the United States.[99]
- The use of a pragmatic randomized controlled trial design to select locally relevant samples, deliver manageable interventions, and measure locally salient outcomes with a minimum of extra resourcing.[100]
- A commitment to measure outcomes, including costs, and to use this information to alter local processes of care. Ineffective or overly expensive services, from the perspective of the local healthcare agency, could then be discontinued or refined as necessary.

An important aspect of this proposal is the attempt to decentralize the development and implementation of EI services and to embrace the reality of the differing perspectives of actors in the current healthcare system. The perspective of the public-academic collaboration is suggested as the most likely to advance public health goals. This is suggested in contrast to the traditional approach of developing, testing, refining, and then manualizing services in mostly research settings before devising strategies to have these adopted more widely. This "develop then disseminate" approach is slow, cumbersome, inflexible to emerging knowledge, and does not adequately address the different incentives that agencies may have toward particular problems or populations. Also, as evidenced in successive national reports for schizophrenia, this approach has not been successful in increasing the uptake of empirically based interventions.[89,90]

The enthusiasm generated by work in EIs for psychotic disorders is evidenced by the wide implementation of services and the wealth of data accumulating from studies across the translational continuum. Beyond having an impact on schizophrenia-spectrum disorders, this work can suggest frameworks for other serious mental illnesses. Most are chronic diseases of adolescence[101] and as such offer similar opportunities for societal investment in health.[102]

REFERENCES

1. Goldner EM, Hsu L, Waraich P, et al. Prevalence and incidence studies of schizophrenic disorders: a systematic review of the literature. Can J Psychiatry 2002;47(9):833–43.
2. Perala J, Suvisaari J, Saarni SI, et al. Lifetime prevalence of psychotic and bipolar I disorders in a general population. Arch Gen Psychiatry 2007;64(1):19–28.
3. Lopez AD. A comprehensive assessment of mortality and disability from diseases, injuries, and risk factors in 1990 and projected to 2020. In: Murray CJ, Lopez AD, editors. Global burden of disease and risk factors. Boston: Harvard University Press; 1996.
4. Geddes J. Prevention of relapse in schizophrenia. N Engl J Med 2002;346(1):56–8.
5. Menezes NM, Arenovich T, Zipursky RB. A systematic review of longitudinal outcome studies of first-episode psychosis [review]. Psychol Med 2006; 36(10):1349–62.
6. Wu EQ, Birnbaum HG, Shi L, et al. The economic burden of schizophrenia in the United States in 2002. J Clin Psychiatry 2005;66(9):1122–9.
7. Bleuler M. The schizophrenic disorders: long term patient and family studies. New Haven (CT): Yale University Press; 1978 [Clements S, Trans.].
8. Birchwood M, Todd P, Jackson C. Early intervention in psychosis. The critical period hypothesis. Br J Psychiatry Suppl 1998;172(33):53–9.
9. Lieberman JA, Perkins D, Belger A, et al. The early stages of schizophrenia: speculations on pathogenesis, pathophysiology, and therapeutic approaches. Biol Psychiatry 2001;50(11):884–97.
10. Harrison G, Hopper K, Craig T, et al. Recovery from psychotic illness: a 15- and 25-year international follow-up study. Br J Psychiatry 2001;178(6):506–17.
11. Westermeyer JF, Harrow M, Marengo JT. Risk for suicide in schizophrenia and other psychotic and nonpsychotic disorders. J Nerv Ment Dis 1991;179(5):259–66.
12. Mortensen PB, Juel K. Mortality and causes of death in first admitted schizophrenic patients. Br J Psychiatry 1993;163:183–9.
13. Carpenter WT Jr, Strauss JS. The prediction of outcome in schizophrenia. IV: eleven-year follow-up of the Washington IPSS cohort. J Nerv Ment Dis 1991; 179(9):517–25.
14. McGlashan TH. A selective review of recent North American long-term followup studies of schizophrenia. Schizophr Bull 1988;14(4):515–42.
15. Eaton WW, Thara R, Federman B, et al. Structure and course of positive and negative symptoms in schizophrenia. Arch Gen Psychiatry 1995;52(2):127–34.
16. Strauss JS, Carpenter WT Jr. Prediction of outcome in schizophrenia. III. Five-year outcome and its predictors. Arch Gen Psychiatry 1977;34(2):159–63.
17. Shepherd M, Watt D, Falloon I, et al. The natural history of schizophrenia: a five-year follow-up study of outcome and prediction in a representative sample of schizophrenics. Psychol Med Monogr Suppl 1989;15:1–46.
18. Tohen M, Strakowski SM, Zarate C, et al. The McLean–Harvard first-episode project: 6-month symptomatic and functional outcome in affective and nonaffective psychosis. Biol Psychiatry 2000;48(6):467–76.
19. Lieberman J, Jody D, Geisler S, et al. Time course and biologic correlates of treatment response in first-episode schizophrenia. Arch Gen Psychiatry 1993; 50(5):369–76.
20. Green MF, Kern RS, Heaton RK. Longitudinal studies of cognition and functional outcome in schizophrenia: implications for MATRICS. Schizophr Res 2004;72(1): 41–51.

21. Brown GW, Birley JL, Wing JK. Influence of family life on the course of schizophrenic disorders: a replication. Br J Psychiatry 1972;121(562):241–58.
22. Hooley JM. Expressed emotion and relapse of psychopathology. Annu Rev Clin Psychol 2007;3:329–52.
23. Butzlaff RL, Hooley JM. Expressed emotion and psychiatric relapse: a meta-analysis. Arch Gen Psychiatry 1998;55(6):547–52.
24. Hooley JM, Richters JE. Expressed emotion: a developmental perspective. In: Cichetti D, Toth SL, editors. Emotion, cognition, and representation. Rochester (NY): University of Rochester Press; 1995. p. 133.
25. Brown S, Kim M, Mitchell C, et al. Twenty-five year mortality of a community cohort with schizophrenia. Br J Psychiatry 2010;196(2):116–21.
26. Saha S, Chant D, McGrath J. A systematic review of mortality in schizophrenia: is the differential mortality gap worsening over time? Arch Gen Psychiatry 2007; 64(10):1123–31.
27. Foley DL, Morley KI. Systematic review of early cardiometabolic outcomes of the first treated episode of psychosis. Arch Gen Psychiatry 2011;68(6):609–16 [Epub 2011 Feb 7].
28. Phutane VH, Tek C, Chwastiak L, et al. Cardiovascular risk in a first-episode psychosis sample: a 'critical period' for prevention? Schizophr Res 2011; 127(1–3):257–61.
29. Pantelis C, Velakoulis D, McGorry PD, et al. Neuroanatomical abnormalities before and after onset of psychosis: a cross-sectional and longitudinal MRI comparison. Lancet 2003;361(9354):281–8.
30. Smieskova R, Fusar-Poli P, Allen P, et al. Neuroimaging predictors of transition to psychosis: a systematic review and meta-analysis. Neurosci Biobehav Rev 2010;34(8):1207–22.
31. Kasai K, Shenton ME, Salisbury DF, et al. Differences and similarities in insular and temporal pole MRI gray matter volume abnormalities in first-episode schizophrenia and affective psychosis. Arch Gen Psychiatry 2003;60(11): 1069–77.
32. Yoshida T, McCarley RW, Nakamura M, et al. A prospective longitudinal volumetric MRI study of superior temporal gyrus gray matter and amygdala–hippocampal complex in chronic schizophrenia. Schizophr Res 2009; 113(1):84–94.
33. Thompson PM, Vidal C, Giedd JN, et al. Mapping adolescent brain change reveals dynamic wave of accelerated gray matter loss in very early-onset schizophrenia. Proc Natl Acad Sci U S A 2001;98(20):11650–5.
34. Koenen KC, Moffitt TE, Roberts AL, et al. Childhood IQ and adult mental disorders: a test of the cognitive reserve hypothesis. Am J Psychiatry 2009;166(1):50–7.
35. Barnett JH, Salmond CH, Jones PB, et al. Cognitive reserve in neuropsychiatry. Psychol Med 2006;36(8):1053–64.
36. Keshavan MS, Eack SM, Wojtalik JA, et al. A broad cortical reserve accelerates response to cognitive enhancement therapy in early course schizophrenia. Schizophr Res 2011;130(1–3):123–9.
37. Eack SM, Hogarty GE, Cho RY, et al. Neuroprotective effects of cognitive enhancement therapy against gray matter loss in early schizophrenia: results from a 2-year randomized controlled trial. Arch Gen Psychiatry 2010;67(7): 674–82.
38. Joseph R, Birchwood M. The national policy reforms for mental health services and the story of early intervention services in the United Kingdom. J Psychiatry Neurosci 2005;30(5):362–5.

39. Weinberger DR. Implications of normal brain development for the pathogenesis of schizophrenia. Arch Gen Psychiatry 1987;44(7):660–9.

40. Murray RM, Lewis SW. Is schizophrenia a neurodevelopmental disorder? Br Med J (Clin Res Ed) 1987;295(6600):681–2.

41. Keshavan MS, Anderson S, Pettegrew JW. Is schizophrenia due to excessive synaptic pruning in the prefrontal cortex? the Feinberg hypothesis revisited. J Psychiatr Res 1994;28(3):239–65.

42. Johannessen JO, McGlashan TH, Larsen TK, et al. Early detection strategies for untreated first-episode psychosis. Schizophr Res 2001;51(1):39–46.

43. Marshall M, Lewis S, Lockwood A, et al. Association between duration of untreated psychosis and outcome in cohorts of first-episode patients: a systematic review. Arch Gen Psychiatry 2005;62(9):975–83.

44. Perkins DO, Gu H, Boteva K, et al. Relationship between duration of untreated psychosis and outcome in first-episode schizophrenia: a critical review and meta-analysis. Am J Psychiatry 2005;162(10):1785–804.

45. Melle I, Larsen TK, Haahr U, et al. Prevention of negative symptom psychopathologies in first-episode schizophrenia: two-year effects of reducing the duration of untreated psychosis. Arch Gen Psychiatry 2008;65(6):634–40.

46. Larsen TK, Melle I, Auestad B, et al. Early detection of psychosis: positive effects on 5-year outcome. Psychol Med 2011;41(07):1461.

47. Joa I, Johannessen JO, Auestad B, et al. The key to reducing duration of untreated first psychosis: information campaigns. Schizophr Bull 2008;34(3): 466–72.

48. Chong S, Mythily S, Verma S. Reducing the duration of untreated psychosis and changing help-seeking behaviour in Singapore. Soc Psychiatry Psychiatr Epidemiol 2005;40(8):619–21.

49. Lloyd-Evans B, Crosby M, Stockton S, et al. Initiatives to shorten duration of untreated psychosis: systematic review. Br J Psychiatry 2011;198(4):256–63.

50. Edwards J, McGorry PD. Multi-component early intervention: models of good practice. In: Edwards J, McGorry PD, editors. Implementing early intervention in psychosis. London: Martin Dunitz; 2002. p. 63.

51. Marshall M, Rathbone J. Early intervention for psychosis. Cochrane Database Syst Rev 2011;(6):CD004718.

52. Breitborde NJ, Srihari VH, Woods SW. A review of the operational definition for first-episode psychosis. Early Interv Psychiatry 2009;3(4):259–65.

53. Review: more research needed on early intervention for psychosis. Evid Based Ment Health 2012;15(1):23.

54. Everitt B, Wessely S. Clinical trials in psychiatry. Chichester (England): John Wiley & Sons; 2008.

55. Wells KB. Treatment research at the crossroads: the scientific interface of clinical trials and effectiveness research. Am J Psychiatry 1999;156(1):5–10.

56. Insel T, Cuthbert B, Garvey M, et al. Research domain criteria (RDoC): toward a new classification framework for research on mental disorders. Am J Psychiatry 2010;167(7):748–51.

57. Hotopf M, Churchill R, Lewis G. Pragmatic randomised controlled trials in psychiatry. Br J Psychiatry 1999;175(3):217–23.

58. Craig TK, Garety P, Power P, et al. The Lambeth Early Onset (LEO) Team: randomised controlled trial of the effectiveness of specialised care for early psychosis. BMJ 2004;329(7474):1067.

59. Garety PA, Craig TK, Dunn G, et al. Specialised care for early psychosis: symptoms, social functioning and patient satisfaction. Br J Psychiatry 2006;188(1):37–45.

60. Jorgensen P, Nordentoft M, Abel MB, et al. Early detection and assertive community treatment of young psychotics: the Opus Study rationale and design of the trial. Soc Psychiatry Psychiatr Epidemiol 2000;35(7):283–7.
61. Petersen L, Jeppesen P, Thorup A, et al. A randomised multicentre trial of integrated versus standard treatment for patients with a first episode of psychotic illness. BMJ 2005;331(7517):602.
62. Bertelsen M, Jeppesen P, Petersen L, et al. Five-year follow-up of a randomized multicenter trial of intensive early intervention vs standard treatment for patients with a first episode of psychotic illness: the OPUS trial. Arch Gen Psychiatry 2008;65(7):762–71.
63. Gafoor R, Nitsch D, McCrone P, et al. Effect of early intervention on 5-year outcome in non-affective psychosis. Br J Psychiatry 2010;196(5):372–6.
64. Linszen D, Dingemans P, Lenior M. Early intervention and a five year follow up in young adults with a short duration of untreated psychosis: ethical implications. Schizophr Res 2001;51(1):55–61.
65. Norman RM, Manchanda R, Malla AK, et al. Symptom and functional outcomes for a 5 year early intervention program for psychoses. Schizophr Res 2011; 129(2–3):111–5.
66. Greenberg PE, Kessler RC, Birnbaum HG, et al. The economic burden of depression in the United States: how did it change between 1990 and 2000? J Clin Psychiatry 2003;64(12):1465–75.
67. Mangalore R, Knapp M. Cost of schizophrenia in England. J Ment Health Policy Econ 2007;10(1):23–41.
68. Meltzer D. Perspective and the measurement of costs and benefits for cost-effectiveness analysis in schizophrenia. J Clin Psychiatry 1999;60(Suppl 3): 32–5 [discussion: 36–7].
69. Davies LM, Drummond MF. Economics and schizophrenia: the real cost. Br J Psychiatry Suppl 1994;(25):18–21.
70. Barrett B, Byford S. Economic evaluations in evidence based healthcare. Evid Based Ment Health 2009;12(2):36–9.
71. Kind P, Lafata JE, Matuszewski K, et al. The use of QALYs in clinical and patient decision-making: issues and prospects. Value Health 2009;12:S27–30.
72. National Institute for health and clinical excellence. Available at: http://www.nice.org.uk/nicemedia/pdf/CG82NICEGuideline.pdf. 2009;2012(1/7). Accessed July 14, 2012.
73. Knapp M, Mangalore R. The trouble with QALYs. Epidemiol Psichiatr Soc 2007; 16(4):289–93.
74. Malla A, Pelosi AJ. Is treating patients with first-episode psychosis cost-effective? Can J Psychiatry 2010;55(1):3–7 [discussion: 7–8].
75. Goldberg K, Norman R, Hoch J, et al. Impact of a specialized early intervention service for psychotic disorders on patient characteristics, service use, and hospital costs in a defined catchment area. Can J Psychiatry 2006;51(14):895–903.
76. Wong KK, Chan SK, Lam MM, et al. Cost-effectiveness of an early assessment service for young people with early psychosis in Hong Kong. Aust N Z J Psychiatry 2011;45(8):673–80.
77. Angelo C, Vittorio M, Anna M, et al. Cost-effectiveness of treating first-episode psychosis: five-year follow-up results from an Italian early intervention programme. Early Interv Psychiatry 2011;5(3):203–11.
78. Cullberg J, Mattsson M, Levander S, et al. Treatment costs and clinical outcome for first episode schizophrenia patients: a 3-year follow-up of the Swedish "parachute project" and two comparison Groups. Acta Psychiatr Scand 2006;114(4):274–81.

79. Mihalopoulos C, McGorry PD, Carter RC. Is phase-specific, community-oriented treatment of early psychosis an economically viable method of improving outcome? Acta Psychiatr Scand 1999;100(1):47–55.

80. Mihalopoulos C, Harris M, Henry L, et al. Is early intervention in psychosis cost-effective over the long term? Schizophr Bull 2009;35(5):909–18.

81. McCrone P, Craig TKJ, Power P, et al. Cost-effectiveness of an early intervention service for people with psychosis. Br J Psychiatry 2010;196(5):377–82.

82. Dodds TJ, Phutane VH, Stevens BJ, et al. Who is paying the price? Loss of health insurance coverage early in psychosis. Psychiatr Serv 2011;62(8):878–81.

83. Knapp M, Chisholm D, Leese M, et al. Comparing patterns and costs of schizophrenia care in five European countries: the EPSILON study. European psychiatric services: inputs linked to outcome domains and needs. Acta Psychiatr Scand 2002;105(1):42–54.

84. Norman RM, Malla AK, Verdi MB, et al. Understanding delay in treatment for first-episode psychosis. Psychol Med 2004;34(2):255–66.

85. Department of Health. The NHS plan: a summary. London: Department of Health; 2000.

86. Edwards J, McGorry PD. Implementing early intervention in psychosis: a guide to establishing early psychosis services. London: Martin Dunitz; 2002.

87. Drake RE, Goldman HH, Leff HS, et al. Implementing evidence-based practices in routine mental health service settings. Psychiatr Serv 2001;52(2):179–82.

88. Torrey WC, Drake RE, Dixon L, et al. Implementing evidence-based practices for persons with severe mental illnesses. Psychiatr Serv 2001;52(1):45–50.

89. Dixon LB, Dickerson F, Bellack AS, et al. The 2009 schizophrenia PORT psychosocial treatment recommendations and summary statements. Schizophr Bull 2010;36(1):48–70.

90. Lehman AF, Kreyenbuhl J, Buchanan RW, et al. The schizophrenia Patient Outcomes Research Team (PORT): updated treatment recommendations 2003. Schizophr Bull 2004;30(2):193–217.

91. Bero LA, Grilli R, Grimshaw JM, et al. Getting research findings into practice. Closing the gap between research and practice: an overview of systematic reviews of interventions to promote the implementation of research findings. Br Med J 1998;317(7156):465–8.

92. Mesholam-Gately RI, Giuliano AJ, Goff KP, et al. Neurocognition in first-episode schizophrenia: a meta-analytic review. Neuropsychology 2009; 23(3):315–36.

93. Rund BR. A review of longitudinal studies of cognitive functions in schizophrenia patients. Schizophr Bull 1998;24(3):425–35.

94. Hulshoff Pol HE, Kahn RS. What happens after the first episode? A review of progressive brain changes in chronically ill patients with schizophrenia. Schizophr Bull 2008;34(2):354–66.

95. Mitelman SA, Brickman AM, Shihabuddin L, et al. A comprehensive assessment of gray and white matter volumes and their relationship to outcome and severity in schizophrenia. Neuroimage 2007;37(2):449–62.

96. Campbell NC, Murray E, Darbyshire J, et al. Designing and evaluating complex interventions to improve health care. BMJ 2007;334(7591):455–9.

97. National Institute of Mental Health. Recovery after an initial schizophrenic episode RAISE 2009. Available at: http://www.nimh.nih.gov/health/topics/schizophrenia/raise/index.shtml. Accessed July 14, 2012.

98. Straus SE, Tetroe J, Graham I. Defining knowledge translation. Can Med Assoc J 2009;181(3–4):165–8.

99. Talbott JA. The evolution and current status of public-academic partnerships in psychiatry. Psychiatr Serv 2008;59(1):15–6.
100. Hotopf M. The pragmatic randomised controlled trial. Adv Psychiatr Treat 2002; 8(5):326–33.
101. Insel TR. Translating scientific opportunity into public health impact: a strategic plan for research on mental illness. Arch Gen Psychiatry 2009;66(2):128–33.
102. Fielding JE, Teutsch SM. An opportunity map for societal investment in health. JAMA 2011;305(20):2110–1.

Can Structural Neuroimaging be Used to Define Phenotypes and Course of Schizophrenia?

John G. Kerns, PhD[a], John Lauriello, MD[b],*

KEYWORDS

- Structural neuroimaging • Functional magnetic resonance imaging
- Single-photon emission computed tomography • Psychiatric diagnosis
- Psychiatric prognosis • Schizophrenia • Psychosis

KEY POINTS

- To date there is no compelling evidence that structural neuroimaging measures taken in first-episode patients predict the course and outcome of schizophrenia.
- There is evidence suggesting that neuorimaging phenotypes can be associated with outcome in schizophrenia based on progressive brain changes. The preponderance of evidence appears to support an association between progressive changes in specific brain regions and poor outcome.
- Much research to date has focused on structural magnetic resonance imaging; however, many other imaging measures could be used, such as event-related brain potentials.
- Nonstructural imaging studies have found evidence that dopamine levels measured with single-photon emission computed tomography at baseline in first-episode patients predicts poor outcome.

INTRODUCTION

There is a wide variety of neuroimaging techniques that hold great promise for understanding neuropsychiatric disorders. Theoretically it is possible that neuroimaging techniques could be used to aid psychiatric diagnosis. At the same time, it is also possible that neuroimaging techniques could be used for prognosis, to predict treatment response, and to better understand the heterogeneity of disorders. This review examines research that has attempted to use structural neuroimaging measures to understand the course and outcome of schizophrenia.

A review published 5 years ago[1] attempted to answer the question of whether any brain-imaging measure predicted outcome and course in schizophrenia. Based on

[a] Psychological Sciences Department, University of Missouri, 214 McAlester Hall, Columbia, MO 65211, USA; [b] Department of Psychiatry, University of Missouri, One Hospital Drive, DC067.00, Columbia, MO 65212, USA
* Corresponding author.
E-mail address: LaurielloJ@health.missouri.edu

Psychiatr Clin N Am 35 (2012) 633–644
http://dx.doi.org/10.1016/j.psc.2012.06.005
0193-953X/12/$ – see front matter © 2012 Elsevier Inc. All rights reserved.

research conducted up to that time, the answer to that question was a clear "no," because there were no neuroimaging phenotypes with enough research support to justify their use in making predictions for individual patients in clinical practice. Five years later, the answer to the question of whether neuroimaging measures can be used to predict outcome and course in schizophrenia remains negative. Overall, previous research has yet to find compelling evidence that an initial neuroimaging scan at any time in the illness predicts future outcome.

By contrast, there is fair evidence that the degree of brain changes, as measured in serial brain scans over time, correlates with poor outcome in schizophrenia. Although it is unclear whether this method could be used to predict clinical outcome, such evidence does suggest that neuroimaging phenotypes can be related to the course of the disorder. In particular, in schizophrenia there may be one or more phenotypes involving deleterious progressive brain changes over time that are related to poor outcome of the disorder.

This article reviews the status of research that has attempted to use structural neuroimaging measures as predictors or correlates of the course of schizophrenia. The authors first discuss some of the various ways that neuroimaging measures have been used to understand the course of schizophrenia. For instance, although there are many types of brain-imaging techniques, only a subset have been frequently used in researching the course of schizophrenia. Next, a focused review evaluates the evidence for whether particular brain measures can be used to understand the course of schizophrenia. Finally, recommendations are made regarding future research on using neuroimaging measures to predict the course of schizophrenia.

OVERVIEW OF PREVIOUS RESEARCH

It is possible that a neuroimaging measure related to outcome at one phase of the disorder may or may not be related to outcome at another phase of the disorder. Previous research has attempted to use neuroimaging to predict outcomes in several different phases of schizophrenia. For example, some studies have attempted to predict which individuals considered at ultra-high risk for psychosis develop a psychotic disorder or more specifically develop schizophrenia. Other studies have attempted to use neuroimaging to predict the long-term outcome in people experiencing their first episode of psychosis with schizophrenia. Others have used neuroimaging to predict outcome in chronic patients, or have examined whether changes in brain imaging over time are correlated cross-sectionally with outcome in the disorder.

In reviewing studies that have attempted to predict outcome of the disorder, the overwhelming majority have focused on structural neuroimaging involving magnetic resonance imaging (MRI) or computed tomography. It has been rare for studies to have used magnetic resonance spectroscopy (MRS), neurotransmitter receptor binding, functional MRI (fMRI), or other types of imaging techniques. More commonly, these other methods have examined cross-sectional relationships between neuroimaging and measures of symptoms or levels of functional impairment. Therefore, the main focus of this review involves structural imaging, although some evidence for other imaging modalities is also briefly reviewed.

Most studies also have tended to focus on a particular set of brain regions or neural measures (eg, total volume of gray matter). The most common has been lateral ventricle size, followed by total gray matter or whole brain size. Regarding particular brain regions, the most commonly reported have been the frontal and temporal cortices and the hippocampus. When structure has been examined it has usually included its entirety, as opposed to more specific subareas of the structure (or for that matter for measure of structural shape). It remains to be seen whether more detailed investigations of particular brain structures would provide stronger evidence for relationships between neuroimaging measures and course. This review focuses first on the most common regions that have been examined across studies, but any results for regions examined only in one study are also mentioned.

With regard to measuring the course of schizophrenia, studies have reported a wide variety of measures, including global symptoms, positive or negative symptoms, or various measures of real-world functioning such as impairments in daily functioning, length of time hospitalized, or global assessment of functioning (and some of these measures are combinations of both symptom and real-world functioning measures). This review groups these aspects into measures of symptoms and measures of real-world functioning outcomes.

PREDICTING DISORDER ONSET IN ULTRA–HIGH-RISK INDIVIDUALS

The question of whether structural neuroimaging studies can predict the development of psychosis in ultra–high-risk individuals has been examined in several studies. The development of psychosis does not completely overlap with an eventual diagnosis of schizophrenia. These psychoses can be time limited or a symptom of another mental illness, but they may be reflective of what might be anticipated for those who go on to develop schizophrenia. There have been several reviews of these types of studies (eg, Ref.[2]). Two of the most recent and novel studies that have examined disorder onset in ultra–high-risk individuals are reviewed here.

As has been noted in previous reviews, results from neuroimaging ultra–high-risk studies have not necessarily provided a consistent picture of which regions predict disorder onset, which might be due to at least 2 factors. One is that many of these studies have had small sample sizes; a second is that these studies have focused on predicting a heterogeneous set of disorders: all psychotic disorders (an even more heterogeneous category than schizophrenia). Two recent studies have attempted to address these 2 factors.

In the first study,[3] data from several sites were pooled, resulting in an initial ultra–high-risk group of 182 subjects, of whom 48 developed a psychotic disorder within 2 years. A smaller volume of the parahippocampal cortex at baseline was found to predict development of a psychotic disorder. By contrast, bilateral decreased volume of the frontal cortex was found to differentiate ultra–high-risk individuals from controls at baseline, but the frontal cortex did not predict disorder onset. In a second study,[4] the researchers specifically examined which neuroimaging measures at baseline would predict the development of schizophrenia rather than predicting all psychotic disorders. In this study, 17 ultra–high-risk individuals developed schizophrenia (a smaller group of 7 developed affective psychosis, with different results found for the two disorder groups). For those who developed schizophrenia, at baseline they exhibited decreased volume in frontal and parietal cortex, with a trend for decreased volume in temporal cortex (by contrast, affective psychosis was associated with decreased subgenual cingulate). Hence, there was some evidence from this study that a decrease in widespread cortical volume predicts onset of schizophrenia.

PREDICTION OF OUTCOME IN FIRST-EPISODE PATIENTS

Other studies have examined persons undergoing their first episode of diagnosed schizophrenia and have examined whether baseline brain-imaging measures predict outcome in the disorder. As shown in **Table 1**, the authors have identified 9 studies that have obtained structural neuroimaging measures at first episode and have

Table 1
Studies using structural neuroimaging to predict long-term outcome in patients with first-episode schizophrenia

Authors,[Ref.] Year	Sample Size	Average Follow-Up (Years)
Bodnar et al,[14] 2010	57	0.5
Boonstra et al,[9] 2011	48	5
Cahn et al,[10] 2006	31	5
Lieberman et al,[5] 2001	56	2.5
Milev et al,[6] 2003	123	5
Prasad et al,[11] 2005	27	2
van Haren et al,[7] 2003	109	2
Wobrock et al,[8] 2009	23	1
Wood et al,[12] 2006	46	1.5

attempted to predict subsequent outcome. There is a wide variation in the sample sizes of these studies. In addition, the average length of follow-up is typically not very long, with 3 studies having an average length of greater than 3 years. The results for the brain regions most commonly reported in studies examining the relationship between neuroimaging and course (eg, lateral ventricles, frontal cortex) are reviewed here, with a mention of any other isolated significant results.

Lateral Ventricles

Five studies have reported results for whether size of the lateral ventricle predicts the course of the disorder. Four of these 5 studies reported no significant results.[5–8] These 4 studies include that with the longest duration and the 2 with the largest sample sizes. A fifth study did find an association with increased positive symptoms at 5-year follow-up.[9] However, in this study positive symptoms were actually associated with smaller lateral ventricles (and with a larger cerebellum). There is also the possibility of chance results in this study, as only 3 of 36 correlations between brain measures and outcome variables were significant.

One other study[10] did report a significant relationship between increased size of lateral ventricle and poorer functional outcome. However, this study did not use baseline brain measures and instead focused on the extent of changes in brain measures after 1 year as their predictor of outcome 5 years later. The extent of increase in the lateral ventricle at 1 year predicted subsequent poor functional outcome. Therefore, this study arguably cannot be taken as evidence of baseline structural measures predicting outcome, but instead found that structural changes over time predict poor outcome.

Total Gray Matter

Another commonly examined brain measure in studies attempting to link neuroimaging with course is total gray matter. Four studies have examined whether total gray matter in first-episode patients predicts outcome. Three studies using baseline total volume of gray matter[5,7,9] did not find any significant relationships with outcome. The fourth study did find that change in total gray matter in 1 year predicted poorer functioning and more total symptoms 5 years later.[10] As with the lateral ventricle, on the whole there is no evidence that total gray matter in first-episode patients predicts outcome, but the change in volume of total gray matter in 1 year was related to outcome.

Frontal Cortex

Four studies examined whether structural measures of the frontal cortex are associated with outcome. Two studies did not find any relationship between baseline frontal cortex measures and outcome.[6,10] One study found that volume of the left dorsolateral prefrontal cortex predicted poor outcome at 1 year, but this was not significant at year 2.[11] One study did find that an MRS measure of poor neural integrity in the left frontal cortex (lower N-acetylaspartate/creatine ratio) was associated with poorer outcome.[12] Hence, on the whole there is as yet limited evidence that frontal cortex structural measures at baseline are associated with outcome.

Finally, in one study of childhood-onset schizophrenia, decreased volume of left orbitofrontal cortex (and decreased temporal lobe volume) predicted worse symptoms at the time of hospital discharge.[13] Specifically, at the time of hospital discharge those children who had remitted (n = 16) differed from children who had not remitted (n = 40). Of note, this was clearly not a first-episode group (although presumably the first hospitalization, the average duration of illness at time of scan being 3.8 years). This finding is preliminary evidence that one region of the frontal lobe, as well as the temporal lobe, might predict short-term outcome in childhood-onset schizophrenia.

Temporal Lobe

Of the 2 studies that examined temporal cortex measures in first-episode patients, one study found that it predicted hallucinations 5 years later.[6] However, this study and another[12] found no evidence that it was related to any other measure of outcome.

Hippocampus

Four studies have examined the hippocampus in first-episode patients, with 2 reporting no significant association with outcome.[5,8] A third study did find that decreased volume, specifically in the hippocampal tail, predicted who would remit.[14] However, other parts of the hippocampus (and the amygdala) were unrelated to outcome. This result suggests that although the hippocampus as a whole may be unrelated to outcome, potentially a subregion of the hippocampus may well be. In a fourth study with a psychotic disorder group, smaller right hippocampal volume was associated with increased symptoms and a poorer clinical outcome.[15] However, in this study the majority of the participants had affective psychosis (18 of 28).

White Matter

Four studies have examined whether measures of white matter are associated with outcome. Two found no relationship between white matter and outcome.[7,9] A third found that an increase in white matter at 1 year predicted poor functioning 5 years later.[10] The fourth measured the volume of a specific white matter structure, the anterior limb of the internal capsule (ALIC), which is thought to be important for connectivity between the frontal cortex and the thalamus. Reduced area of the left ALIC was associated with absence of a clinically relevant change in symptoms over 1 year.[8] Hence, there is as yet no evidence that a global measure of white matter at baseline predicts outcome in first-episode patients, but some evidence does exist that changes in white matter over time might predict outcome and that a specific white matter region might predict poor outcome.

In summary, there is weak evidence at best that structural neuroimaging measures in first-episode patients correlate with the course of the disorder or predict outcome. There is as yet no consistently replicated evidence that associates neuroimaging measures with outcome. On the other hand, there is some preliminary evidence that some neuroimaging measures (eg, deterioration in 1 year, hippocampal tail, ALIC) might be related to some aspects of outcome.

PROGRESSIVE BRAIN CHANGES AND ASSOCIATION WITH OUTCOME

One other set of studies potentially touches on the issue of whether neuroimaging measures may be associated with course and outcome. Several studies have measured progressive changes in brain structure over time and have then examined whether those changes are correlated with outcome. These studies differ from the ones reviewed thus far because they are not attempting to predict a patient's outcome in the future. Instead, these studies examine whether cross-sectionally there is evidence that brain changes over time are related to present symptoms or to the current level of daily functioning (or to a measure of functioning encompassing the follow-up period, such as amount of time hospitalized). As shown in **Table 2**, these studies have been involved both first-episode and chronic patients. To aid in reaching conclusions about the associations between changes in particular brain regions and outcome, studies on both first-episode and chronic patients are reviewed here.

Lateral Ventricles

A common finding across many of these studies is an apparent increase in the size of the lateral ventricles over time, with this being by far the most well established brain-imaging measure change found in an earlier review.[16] Several of the studies in **Table 2** also examined whether changes in lateral ventricle size were associated with symptoms and with real-world functioning. In first-episode samples, 4 studies reported that increases in lateral ventricle size over time were associated with increased symptoms, with evidence of a relation to increased positive symptoms,[17] increased negative symptoms,[18,19] or both.[5] A fifth study found no association between changes in lateral ventricle size and outcome.[9] By contrast, an additional study found that

Table 2 Studies examining relationship between changes in structural neuroimaging measures over time and correlation with outcome		
Authors,[Ref.] Year	Sample Size	Average Follow-Up (Years)
First-Episode Patient Samples		
Boonstra et al,[9] 2011	41	5
DeLisi et al,[20] 1998	50	5
DeLisi et al,[21] 2004	26	10
Ebdrup et al,[18] 2011	22	0.5
Gur et al,[26] 1998	20	2
Lieberman et al,[5] 2001	56	2.5
Nakamura et al,[19] 2007	17	1.5
Chronic Patient Samples		
Davis et al,[24] 1998	53	5
Gur et al,[26] 1998	20	2
Mathalon et al,[27] 2001	24	3.6
Mitelman et al,[25] 2011	49	4
Saijo et al,[22] 2001	15	15.1
van Haren et al,[23,28,42] 2007, 2008, 2011	96	2

increased lateral ventricle size over time was associated with decreased symptoms at 5 years,[20] with this result being replicated in a subset of the original sample at 10 years.[21] However, in this study, increased lateral ventricle size was also associated with more time in hospital, consistent with it being associated with some aspect of clinical functioning (although it was not associated with any other measure of real-world functioning). Overall, there is some evidence that increases in lateral ventricle size over time in first-episode patients is associated with increasing symptoms, although there is one strong piece of negative evidence, and the studies are not necessarily consistent as far as relationship to positive or negative symptoms is concerned.

In one study of chronic patients, there was no significant association between increases in lateral ventricle size and symptoms.[22] However, this study had a small sample size and there was a nonsignificant trend for an association with negative symptoms. In addition, 3 studies that reported associations did find that increases in lateral ventricle size were associated with impairments in real-world functioning. In one study, increases in lateral ventricle size were associated with increased hospitalizations, with lower Global Assessment of Functioning (GAF) scores and poorer daily living skills.[23] In the 2 other studies, having Kraepelinian (ie, very poor outcome) schizophrenia with marked self-care deficits was associated with increases in lateral ventricle size.[24,25] Hence, it appears that increases in lateral ventricle size might be associated with symptoms in first-episode patients and with real-world functioning in chronic patients.

Frontal Cortex

One study of first-episode patients found that decreases in frontal areas was associated with poorer performance of executive functioning tasks.[17] A second study reported that decreases in frontal areas were associated with poorer cognition across a range of cognitive measures.[26] Hence, there is some evidence that decreases in frontal areas are associated with poorer cognitive performance in first-episode patients. Regarding symptoms, Gur and colleagues[26] reported mixed results. Decreases in frontal lobe areas were associated with decreases in some symptoms (delusions and thought disorder) but increases in other symptoms (affective flattening, alogia, and hallucinations).

In chronic patients, one study found inconsistent evidence that frontal decreases were associated with poor cognition. This study also found that frontal decreases tended to be associated with decreased symptoms.[26] By contrast, another study found evidence that frontal decreases were associated with increasing positive and negative symptoms and with increased time in hospital.[27] In another study, volume loss specifically in the left superior frontal gyrus was associated with increased number of hospitalizations.[23] Overall, there is some evidence for frontal decreases to be associated with poor cognition in first-episode patients and for frontal decreases to be associated with increased hospitalization in chronic patients, although one study found an association between frontal decreases and decreased symptoms.

Temporal Lobe

There is some evidence that decreases in the temporal lobe are associated with more symptoms and poorer functioning. A study of first-episode patients found mixed evidence, with temporal volume decreases associated with decreases in some symptoms (delusions and thought disorder), but increases in a range of negative symptoms (affective flattening, alogia, avolition, and attention) and also an association with poorer cognition.[26] However, in the same study, in a chronic sample temporal region decreases were, if anything, only associated with fewer symptoms. By contrast, one study reported that volume loss in the superior temporal gyrus was associated with increased negative symptoms.[27] Moreover, in a large sample of chronic patients, increased cortical thinning in the superior temporal gyrus was associated with both increased symptoms and poorer real-world functioning.[28] Hence, there appears to be fair evidence that volume losses in the superior temporal gyrus may be associated with increased symptoms, especially negative symptoms, and with poor real-world functioning, although again there is inconsistent evidence from one study with chronic patients.

Other Brain-Change Measures

There have been at least 3 other brain regions that have been examined in studies measuring changes in brain volume over time: gray matter, white matter, and the hippocampus. For gray matter changes, one small-sample first-episode study found that decreased gray matter was associated with increased British Psychiatric Rating Scale symptoms, especially the thought disturbance factor.[19] By contrast, a second first-episode study did not report any significant associations between gray matter changes and outcome measures.[9] In 2 studies, white matter changes have been associated with outcome variables. In a first-episode sample, white matter change in frontal areas was associated with increased negative symptoms.[17] In a chronic sample, increased total white matter volume was associated with more hospitalizations.[23] By contrast, another first-episode study did not find an association between white matter changes and outcome variables.[9] In a first-episode sample, hippocampal volume decreases were associated with decreases in overall symptom levels.[5]

In summary, although the results are not completely consistent, there is evidence that lateral ventricle enlargement is associated with symptom increases and with poor real-world functioning. There is some evidence that frontal lobe decreases are associated with poorer cognition in schizophrenia. There is fair evidence that volume losses in the superior temporal gyrus are associated with increased symptoms, especially negative symptoms, and with poor real-world functioning. Finally, changes in white matter have also been associated with poor outcome in 2 of 3 studies.

FUTURE RESEARCH

To date there is no compelling evidence that structural neuroimaging measures taken in first-episode patients predict the course and outcome of schizophrenia. For most specific measures that have been examined (ie, lateral ventricle size or frontal cortex volume), there is more negative evidence than positive evidence. By contrast, there is evidence suggesting that progressive brain changes are correlated with poor outcomes in schizophrenia. For most of the most frequently studied brain regions, specifically lateral ventricle size, frontal volume loss, superior temporal gyrus volume loss, and white matter changes, the preponderance of evidence seems to support an association between these progressive changes and poor outcome. Hence, there is some evidence that neuroimaging phenotypes may be associated with outcome of the disorder.

The limitation with using these measures is that they necessitate a longitudinal investigation of brain changes, making them less useful as predictors in the short term and less practical for making long-term predictions in clinical practice. Perhaps research that focused on predicting risk for progressive brain changes might uncover other neuroimaging measures that would also predict future outcome. For example, some brain measures taken at baseline might predict the likelihood of both progressive brain changes and poor outcome.

Another related issue for future research is to examine the nature of the phenotype involving progressive brain changes and poor outcome.[16,29] Does it reflect a single neurodegenerative process throughout the brain or more discrete changes to specific brain regions? Greater understanding of this process could further help our ability to predict outcomes.

Broadening the range of neuroimaging measures should also be considered. Much of the research to date has focused on structural MRI. However, there are many other imaging measures that could be used. For example, an event-related brain potential measure, mismatch negativity (MMN), recorded using scalp electrodes, has been associated in multiple studies with poor outcome cross-sectionally.[30] Multiple studies have also found that MMN is also correlated with progressive brain changes in the temporal lobe.[31,32] This finding suggests that event-related brain potentials could be used to help predict future outcome in schizophrenia. At the same time, there is a host of fMRI measures that cross-sectionally have been associated with poor outcomes and that could be used to help understand the course of the disorder (eg, see the recent series of articles by the CNTRICS working group[33]).

In addition, at least one study has examined whether fMRI predicted outcome.[34] In this study, 23 neuroleptic-naïve first-episode patients performed a working memory task with practice. After 10 weeks of treatment, 12 were considered treatment nonresponders. These nonresponders exhibited a lesser practice effect (ie, less of a decrease in fMRI activation) in the dorsolateral prefrontal cortex. This finding is preliminary evidence that a functional neuroimaging measure might be useful as a predictor of short-term outcome.

The authors have located 2 nonstructural imaging studies presenting evidence that dopamine levels measured with single-photon emission computed tomography at baseline in first-episode patients predicts poor outcome. One study examined dopamine D2 receptor (D2R) binding.[35] In this study, most of the patients at baseline were diagnosed with schizophreniform disorder and not with schizophrenia (n = 14 of 18). After 2 years, the majority had progressed to a diagnosis of schizophrenia (n = 11; the other 7 had other psychotic-disorder diagnoses). Increased D2R binding in medication-naïve patients at baseline was associated with meeting a schizophrenia diagnosis at 2 years. These results are generally similar to ultra–high-risk studies in that a neuroimaging measure predicted who would develop (or maintain) a diagnosis of schizophrenia over time (as opposed to predicting outcome just in those people with schizophrenia). It is also interesting this study replicated a previous result that D2R binding was associated with poor premorbid functioning, which also seems consistent with D2R binding being associated with a schizophrenia diagnosis among people with initial schizophrenia-spectrum diagnoses.

A second first-episode study examined striatal dopamine transporter (DAT) binding. Increased DAT binding was associated with both poorer functioning and increased negative symptoms at 4-year follow-up.[36] Hence, in 2 studies, albeit with small sample sizes and using different measures of dopamine, there is evidence that dopamine transmission in first-episode patients is associated with poorer outcome.

In addition to using multiple imaging modalities, another suggestion for future research is to use more specific brain measures. For example, there is evidence that hippocampal tail volume, but not the rest of the hippocampus, might predict poor outcome.[14] Therefore, more specific brain measures might be more predictive. It is also possible that more specific brain measures might be more predictive of only specific aspects of schizophrenia outcome. For example, previous research has consistently found that disorganization symptoms are correlated with cognitive and neuroimaging measures reflecting dorsolateral prefrontal cortex dysfunction (eg, Refs.[37,38]). This finding suggests that specific measures targeting functioning of the dorsolateral prefrontal cortex might specifically predict persistent disorganization symptoms. Another guideline for selecting brain measures is which measures have been associated with poor premorbid functioning. Given that poor premorbid functioning predicts poor outcome, potentially any brain measure that is also associated with poor premorbid functioning, such as D2R binding, might also then be expected to be associated with poor future outcome. This research would also help to expand our understanding of the relation between the neuroimaging phenotype across the course of the disorder from the premorbid phase to post onset.

One limitation of this review is the absence of quantitative meta-analytical assessments of which findings have replicated empiric support. Another possible limitation is the possibility of a "file drawer problem," as the authors do not know how many studies did not report the absence of an association between brain measures and outcome. In addition, the labels given herein for brain regions and measures lack some precision. For example, the frontal lobe is a very large region and different measures grouped as "frontal measures" may not indentify a consistent phenotype. In addition, a large set of studies has examined cross-sectional associations between neuroimaging measures and outcome that are the beyond the scope of this review (eg, Ref.[39]). This other cross-sectional analysis should help inform research on the course of schizophrenia. For example, research on cross-sectional relationships between superior temporal gyrus measures and outcome should help inform research on whether the superior temporal gyrus predicts the course of the disorder. Finally, the influence of medication might be a further important factor in understanding the relationship between neuroimaging and outcome, as some studies have found evidence of relationships between medication and neuroimaging measures (eg, Refs.[40,41]).

SUMMARY

Overall, baseline neuroimaging measures in first-episode patients have not been found to predict the course of the disorder. Instead, progressive brain changes over time have been associated with poor outcome. Hence, neuroimaging research has thus far found support for the course of schizophrenia to involve deleterious progressive brain changes associated with increased symptoms and poorer real-world functioning over time.

REFERENCES

1. Waddington JL. Neuroimaging and other neurobiological indices in schizophrenia: relationship to measurement of function outcome. Br J Psychiatry 2007;50:s50–7.
2. Wood SJ, Pantelis C, Velakoulis D, et al. Progressive changes in the development toward schizophrenia: studies in subjects at increased symptomatic risk. Schizophr Bull 2008;34:322–9.
3. Mechelli A, Riecher-Rossler A, Meisenzahl EM, et al. Neuroanatomical abnormalities that predate the onset of psychosis: a multicenter study. Arch Gen Psychiatry 2011;68:489–95.
4. Dazzan P, Soulsby B, Mechelli A, et al. Volumetric abnormalities predating the onset of schizophrenia and affective psychoses: an MRI study in subjects at ultra-high risk of psychosis. Schizophr Bull, in press.
5. Lieberman J, Chakos M, Wu H, et al. Longitudinal study of brain morphology in first episode schizophrenia. Biol Psychiatry 2001;49:487–99.
6. Milev P, Ho BC, Arndt S, et al. Initial magnetic resonance imaging volumetric brain measurements and outcome in schizophrenia: a prospective longitudinal study with 5-year follow-up. Biol Psychiatry 2003;54:608–15.

7. van Haren NE, Chan W, Pol HE, et al. Brain volumes as predictor of outcome in recent-onset schizophrenia: a multi-center MRI study. Schizophr Res 2003;64: 41–52.

8. Wobrock T, Gruber O, Schneider-Axmann T, et al. Internal capsule size associated with outcome in first-episode schizophrenia. Eur Arch Psychiatry Clin Neurosci 2009;259:278–83.

9. Boonstra G, Cahn W, Schnack HG, et al. Duration of untreated illness in schizophrenia is not associated with 5-year brain volume change. Schizophr Res 2011; 132:84–90.

10. Cahn W, van Haren NE, Hulshoff Pol HE, et al. Brain volume changes in the first year of illness and 5-year outcome of schizophrenia. Br J Psychiatry 2006;189: 381–2.

11. Prasad KM, Sahni SD, Rohm BR, et al. Dorsolateral prefrontal cortex morphology and short-term outcome in first-episode schizophrenia. Psychiatry Res 2005;140: 147–55.

12. Wood SJ, Berger GE, Lambert M, et al. Prediction of functional outcome 18 months after a first psychotic episode. Arch Gen Psychiatry 2006;63:969–76.

13. Greenstein DK, Wolfe S, Gochman P, et al. Remission status and cortical thickness in childhood-onset schizophrenia. J Am Acad Child Adolesc Psychiatry 2008;47:1133–40.

14. Bodnar M, Malla AK, Czechowska Y, et al. Neural markers of remission in first-episode schizophrenia: a volumetric neuroimaging study of the hippocampus and amygdala. Schizophr Res 2010;122:72–80.

15. de Castro-Manglano P, Mechelli A, Soutullo C, et al. Structural brain abnormalities in first-episode psychosis: differences between affective psychoses and schizophrenia and relationship to clinical outcome. Bipolar Disord 2011;13:545–55.

16. Hulshoff Pol HE, Kahn RS. What happens after the first episode? A review of progressive brain changes in chronically ill patients with schizophrenia. Schizophr Bull 2008;34:354–66.

17. Ho BC, Andreasen NC, Nopoulos P, et al. Progressive structural brain abnormalities and their relationship to clinical outcome. Arch Gen Psychiatry 2003;60:585–94.

18. Ebdrup BH, Skimminge A, Rasmussen H, et al. Progressive striatal and hippocampal volume loss in initially antipsychotic-naive, first-episode schizophrenia patients treated with quetiapine: relationship to dose and symptoms. Int J Neuropsychopharmacol 2011;14:69–82.

19. Nakamura M, Salisbury DF, Hirayasu Y, et al. Neocortical gray matter volume in first-episode schizophrenia and first-episode affective psychosis: a cross-sectional and longitudinal MRI study. Biol Psychiatry 2007;62:773–83.

20. DeLisi LE, Sakuma M, Ge S, et al. Association of brain structural change with the heterogeneous course of schizophrenia from early childhood through five years subsequent to a first hospitalization. Psychiatry Res 1998;84:75–88.

21. DeLisi LE, Sakuma M, Maurizio AM, et al. Cerebral ventricular change over the first 10 years after the onset of schizophrenia. Psychiatry Res 2004;130:57–70.

22. Saijo T, Abe T, Someya Y, et al. Ten year progressive ventricular enlargement in schizophrenia: an MRI morphometrical study. Psychiatry Clin Neurosci 2001;55: 41–7.

23. van Haren NE, Hulshoff Pol HE, Schnack HG, et al. Progressive brain volume loss in schizophrenia over the course of the illness: evidence of maturational abnormalities in early adulthood. Biol Psychiatry 2008;63:106–13.

24. Davis KL, Buchsbaum MS, Shihabuddin L, et al. Ventricular enlargement in poor-outcome schizophrenia. Biol Psychiatry 1998;43:783–93.

25. Mitelman SA, Canfield EL, Brickman AM, et al. Progressive ventricular expansion in chronic poor-outcome schizophrenia. Arch Gen Psychiatry 2011;68:1207–17.

26. Gur RE, Cowell P, Turetsky BI, et al. A follow-up magnetic resonance imaging study of schizophrenia. Relationship of neuroanatomical changes to clinical and neurobehavioral measures. Arch Gen Psychiatry 1998;55:145–52.

27. Mathalon DH, Sullivan EV, Lim KO, et al. Progressive brain volume changes and the clinical course of schizophrenia in men. Arch Gen Psychiatry 2001;58: 148–57.

28. van Haren NE, Schnack HG, Cahn W, et al. Changes in cortical thickness during the course of illness in schizophrenia. Arch Gen Psychiatry 2011;68:871–80.

29. Kempton MJ, Stahl D, Williams SC, et al. Progressive lateral ventricular enlargement in schizophrenia: a meta-analysis of longitudinal MRI studies. Schizophr Res 2010;120:54–62.

30. Wynn JK, Sugar C, Horan WP, et al. Mismatch negativity, social cognition, and functioning in schizophrenia patients. Biol Psychiatry 2010;67:940–7.

31. Rasser PE, Schall U, Todd J, et al. Gray matter deficits, mismatch negativity, and outcomes in schizophrenia. Schizophr Bull 2011;37:131–40.

32. Salisbury DF, Kuroki N, Kasai K, et al. Progressive and interrelated functional and structural evidence of post-onset brain reduction in schizophrenia. Arch Gen Psychiatry 2007;64:521–9.

33. Carter CS, Barch DM, Bullmore E, et al. Cognitive neuroscience treatment research to improve cognition in schizophrenia II: developing imaging biomarkers to enhance treatment development for schizophrenia and related disorders. Biol Psychiatry 2011;70:7–12.

34. van Veelen NM, Vink M, Ramsey NF, et al. Prefrontal lobe dysfunction predicts treatment response in medication-naive first-episode schizophrenia. Schizophr Res 2011;129:156–62.

35. Corripio I, Perez V, Catafau AM, et al. Striatal D2 receptor binding as a marker of prognosis and outcome in untreated first-episode psychosis. Neuroimage 2006; 29:662–6.

36. Mané A, Gallego J, Lomeña F, et al. A 4-year dopamine transporter (DAT) imaging study in neuroleptic-naive first episode schizophrenia patients. Psychiatry Res 2011;194:79–84.

37. Becker TM, Cicero DC, Cowan N, et al. Cognitive control components and speech symptoms in people with schizophrenia. Psychiatry Res 2012;196:20–6.

38. MacDonald AW III, Carter CS, Kerns JG, et al. Specificity of prefrontal dysfunction and context processing deficits to schizophrenia in never-medicated patients with first-episode psychosis. Am J Psychiatry 2005;162:475–84.

39. Goghari VM, Sponheim SR, MacDonald AW III. The functional neuroanatomy of symptom dimensions in schizophrenia: a qualitative and quantitative review of a persistent question. Neurosci Biobehav Rev 2010;34:468–86.

40. Leung M, Cheung C, Yu K, et al. Gray matter in first-episode schizophrenia before and after antipsychotic drug treatment. Anatomical likelihood estimation meta-analyses with sample size weighting. Schizophr Bull 2011;37:199–211.

41. Lieberman JA, Tollefson GD, Charles C, et al. Antipsychotic drug effects on brain morphology in first-episode psychosis. Arch Gen Psychiatry 2005;62:361–70.

42. van Haren NE, Hulshoff Pol HE, Schnack HG, et al. Focal gray matter changes in schizophrenia across the course of the illness: a 5-year follow-up study. Neuropsychopharmacology 2007;32:2057–66.

Reliable Biomarkers and Predictors of Schizophrenia and its Treatment

Anilkumar Pillai, PhD[a], Peter F. Buckley, MD[b],*

KEYWORDS

- Biomarker • Brain-derived neurotrophic factor • Schizophrenia • Treatment

KEY POINTS

- Identification of biomarkers in schizophrenia is still in the early stages of development compared with other areas in medicine.
- Several opportunities are available to develop and validate schizophrenia-specific biomarkers.
- Brain-derived neurotrophic factor is a candidate biomarker, although several questions need to be addressed concerning its validity.

INTRODUCTION

The term biomarker was defined by the National Institutes of Health as a "characteristic that is objectively measured and evaluated as an indicator of normal biologic processes, pathogenic processes, or pharmacologic responses to a therapeutic intervention." Thus, biomarkers include markers of risk, disease states, or surrogate end points for response to treatment. Moreover, biomarkers represent any information derived from characterizing an individual's gene, protein, metabolite, disease markers, and metabolic end products. Biomarkers can be broadly classified into 3 types:

1. Screening biomarkers to identify individuals at high risk for a disease
2. Diagnostic biomarkers to verify the presence of a disease
3. Prognostic biomarkers to monitor response to therapy

Recent advances in genetics, genomics, and proteomics offer a great opportunity for the identification of new biomarkers for schizophrenia. Accurate prediction and

Disclosures: None.
[a] Department of Psychiatry and Health Behavior, Medical College of Georgia, Georgia Health Sciences University, 997 Saint Sebastian Way, Augusta, GA 30912, USA; [b] School of Medicine, Department of Psychiatry and Health Behavior, Medical College of Georgia, Georgia Health Sciences University, 1120 15th Street, Augusta, GA 30912, USA
* Corresponding author.
E-mail address: pbuckley@georgiahealth.edu

identification of schizophrenia using biomarkers is a key factor for disease prevention, so that therapy can be provided to those individuals who are most likely to develop the disease or who are in early stages of the disease.

DISEASE BIOMARKERS

Compared with many other medical conditions, the diagnosis and treatment of schizophrenia is more haphazard, observational, and even trial-and-error. There is a lack of diagnostic or prognostic tests, and of any valid test that might indicate a different therapeutic strategy and/or a greater likelihood of success. This situation does not prevail at present in other areas of medicine. The understanding and treatment of breast cancer has been powerfully influenced.[1] Molecular typing has characterized broad types of breast cancers:

1. Tumors that express either estrogen or progesterone receptors
2. Tumors that express human epidermal receptor 2 in amplified form (HER2)
3. Tumors that lack expression of these receptors

Correspondingly, primary and especially adjuvant cancer chemotherapy have been informed by initial tumor characterization and matching of HER2 therapies thereupon. Anti-HER2 therapies (eg, the monoclonal antibody trastuzumab) are targeted for HER2-expressing tumors. The success of tamoxifen for estrogen-sensitive tumors has been well documented. Clinical trials on breast cancer have now progressed to a level of sophistication that is enviable in psychiatry: molecular characterization of tissue and detailed disease staging predefines treatment options. Treatment strategies are selected based on the molecular sensitivities of the tumor, and treatment progress is carefully evaluated using multimodality imaging as well as serial evaluation of tumor hormonal-monoclonal antibody biomarkers. In turn, this process is informing and influencing the current and future drug development for breast cancer.[2] There are many areas of similar successes, especially increasingly the incorporation of genetic testing into therapeutic dosing and treatment strategies.[3] Snyderman[4] has described the emergence of personalized medicine based on population-based preemptive care as well as individualized molecular and environmentally informed, risk-based targeted treatments. Even a cursory appraisal of schizophrenia therapeutics indicates that we have indeed a long way to go.

BIOMARKERS FOR SCHIZOPHRENIA

It is increasingly important, and difficult, to determine which biomarkers are promising for use in schizophrenia, owing to the complex nature of the pathophysiology of this disease. The selection of biomarkers can be hypothesis driven (ie, based on measurements of selected biomarkers from relevant pathophysiological pathways) or hypothesis free (ie, based on measurements of large numbers of biomarkers using novel technologies without a previously decided pathogenetic basis). Several recent studies of cognition in schizophrenia indicate well the potential for incorporating putative biomarkers into treatment studies.[5–7]

Opportunities

Given the complex pathophysiology of schizophrenia, biological markers representing neurochemical pathways, endophenotypes, or imaging markers have been investigated regarding their potential to aid in risk prediction.

Endophenotypes

Endophenotypes are trait markers that exist independently of the manifestation of the disease. The major endophenotypes well investigated in schizophrenia include cognitive measures,[8–12] neurophysiological measures,[13–18] and structural and functional brain abnormalities.[19–21] **Box 1** summarizes some important structural and functional endophenotypes in schizophrenia. In addition, combinations of different endophenotypes have been shown to provide better predictive outcomes than a single endophenotype.[22] Although endophenotypes are thought to reflect genetic vulnerability in schizophrenia, some endophenotypes are found on an intermediate level between genes and overt behavioral symptoms. It must be noted that the genetic component alone is insufficient to explain the pathophysiology of schizophrenia. A large body of evidence indicates that in addition to genetic abnormalities, a second level of environmental or other generalized/specific stressors probably must act as a second "hit" in the central nervous system. For example, a possible interaction between fetal hypoxia and predisposing genes has been suggested in the etiology of schizophrenia (see the article by Clarkes and colleagues elsewhere in this issue). Therefore, one cannot rule out the role of nongenetic factors as well as the interaction between environmental stressors and a genetic disposition in the onset and course of schizophrenia.

Biological markers

Several studies have examined the role of neurotransmitters and neuronal signaling molecules as useful biomarkers in schizophrenia.

Dopamine

The dopamine hypothesis of schizophrenia suggests an overactivity of dopamine signaling as the underlying mechanism of schizophrenia pathophysiology. Based on

---

Box 1
Selected candidate endophenotypes in schizophrenia

Cognition

Attention[8]

Spatial working memory[10]

Face memory and emotion processing[11]

Prefrontal executive/working memory phenotype[12]

Verbal memory deficit[9]

Neurophysiology

Sensorimotor gating (P50)[14]

Prepulse inhibition of startle reflex[16]

Saccadic dysfunction[13]

Mismatch negativity[17]

Eye-tracking dysfunction[15]

P300 amplitude reduction and latency delay[18]

Neuroimaging

Magnetic resonance imaging (MRI) whole-brain nonlinear pattern classification[20]

Frontal hypoactivation in response to cognitive tasks[19]

Functional MRI response to working memory tasks[21]

this robust relationship between the abnormal activity of dopaminergic systems and schizophrenia psychoses, treatment with dopamine D2 receptor (DRD2) antagonists has become the main therapeutic strategy in schizophrenia. Several studies reported increased accumulation of DOPA in the striatum of patients with schizophrenia and high dopamine accumulation in patients with paranoid psychosis. Although baseline levels of synaptic dopamine and the dopamine release in response to amphetamine are increased in schizophrenia,[23] the use of measures of dopamine and/or its metabolites directly have not served use particularly well thus far as potential biomarkers in the diagnosis or treatment of schizophrenia. This fact is as surprising as it is disappointing, given how robust is the link between dopamine and psychosis.

Glutamate

Seminal studies by Kim and colleagues[24] in 1980 suggested the glutamatergic hypothesis for schizophrenia, wherein they showed markedly reduced cerebrospinal fluid (CSF) glutamate levels in patients with schizophrenia. It has been shown that N-methyl-D-aspartate (NMDA) receptors stimulate dopamine release on presynaptic dopamine terminals, whereas they stimulate γ-aminobutyric acid (GABA) release on GABAergic neurons, which again inhibits dopamine release.[25] A significant increase in glutamine (a product derived from glutamate) was found in untreated schizophrenia patients, but not in patients treated with neuroleptics.[26] Studies have also explored the effect of glycine, which acts as a coagonist in NMDA-receptor activation, added to conventional antipsychotics, which has been shown to improve symptoms, but this has not been so in schizophrenia.[27] On the other hand, LY2140023, a selective agonist at metabotropic mGluR2 and mGluR3 glutamate receptors, is being considered as a potential treatment for schizophrenia, based on their ability to modulate NMDA-receptor–mediated neurotransmission.[28] Other similar agents are also under consideration.[29] Thus, receptor physiology has guided drug development. However, illness subtyping based on the expression of glutamine dysfunction has not been successful.

GABA

GABAergic interneurons play an important role in orchestrating the intermittent synchronous population-firing pattern of pyramidal neurons, which appears to be important for cortical somatosensory information processing. The synthesis of GABA from glutamate in GABAergic neurons depends on the expression of 2 molecular forms of glutamic acid decarboxylase (GAD67 and GAD65), and postmortem studies have reported decreases in GAD67 and parvalbumin.[30] It has also been suggested that the overexpression of DNA (cytosine-5-)-methyltransferase 1 (DNMT1) in cortical GABAergic interneurons of schizophrenia subjects may be presumably responsible for the transcriptional downregulation of specific gene promoters such as GAD67.[31] This work has yet to yield a valid biomarker of either disease or therapeutic potential.

Neuronal signaling molecules

Abnormalities in brain development and ongoing neuroplasticity play important roles in the pathogenesis of schizophrenia (see article by McGrath and colleagues elsewhere in this issue). In addition, molecules regulating neuroplasticity-related functions such as neuronal positioning, neurogenesis, and cognitive functions are directly or indirectly linked to glutamatergic, GABAergic, or dopaminergic neurotransmission or neuroprotection. The major neuroplasticity-associated molecules in schizophrenia are reelin, DISC1 (disrupted-in-schizophrenia 1), serine/threonine protein kinase AKT1 (V-akt murine thymoma viral oncogene homologue 1, oncogene AKT1), dysbindin, neuregulin/ErbB4, and brain-derived neurotrophic factor (BDNF). Postmortem and human genome-wide association (GWA) studies have shown abnormalities in these neurodevelopmental indices.

For example, reelin, a secreted extracellular matrix protein, regulates processes of neuronal migration and early development, and modulates the synaptic plasticity by enhancing the induction and maintenance of long-term potentiation. Reduced reelin expression levels and hypermethylation of the RELN promoter have been found in schizophrenia.[32] DISC1 has been shown to participate in several functions in neurodevelopment.[33] DISC1 haplotypes were reported to be associated with altered hippocampal function, including working memory and cognitive deficits in individuals with schizophrenia.[34] AKT, the most important downstream target of phosphatidylinositol-3-kinase (PI3K), plays an important role in various cellular functions, including metabolism, cell stress, and cell-cycle regulation. Akt1, one of the 3 isoforms of Akt, has been the primary focus of the studies examining the role of Akt in schizophrenia.[35] Akt is also involved in normal dopaminergic transmission and expression of dopamine-associated behavior.[36] Genetic studies have shown an association of *AKT1* gene polymorphisms with schizophrenia in diverse populations.[37,38] In addition, reductions in Akt levels were found in lymphocytes derived from people with schizophrenia as well as in the hippocampus and frontal cortex, using postmortem brain samples from those with schizophrenia.[35]

The dystrobrevin-binding protein 1 (DTNBP1)-encoded dysbindin-1 was first identified as a member of the dystrophin-associated protein complex[39] and later as a member of the biogenesis of lysosome-related organelles complex 1 (BLOC-1).[40] Despite some inconsistent observations, the association between variants in DTNBP1 and schizophrenia has been replicated by several independent studies.[41,42] In addition, postmortem findings have reported decreases in dysbindin expression in the prefrontal cortex and hippocampus of schizophrenia patients.[43,44] NRG1 plays an important role in neuronal functions such as myelination, development of GABAergic interneurons, formation of dendritic spines, migration of radial glial cells during cortical development, neuronal plasticity via NMDA receptor function, and expression of dopamine and serotonin receptors and monoamine transporters.[45] *NRG1* was identified as a potential risk gene for schizophrenia in an Icelandic genome-wide linkage analysis.[46] Despite some discrepancies, many studies have reported *NRG1* association with endophenotypes such as decreased PPI[47] and reduced integrity of the white matter.[48,49]

Another important molecule involved in neuroplasticity is BDNF. BDNF plays critical role in neuronal growth, differentiation, and survival, as well regulation of neuronal structure and function. The role of BDNF in schizophrenia is discussed in detail here.

BDNF AS AN EXAMPLE OF A PUTATIVE SCHIZOPHRENIA MARKER

BDNF protein is synthesized as a precursor, proBDNF, which is cleaved to the mature 14-kDa form (m-BDNF) by protease tissue plasminogen activator (tPA)-mediated activation of plasmin.[50] BDNF is expressed throughout the adult mammalian brain including the hippocampus, cerebral cortex, basal forebrain, striatum, hypothalamus, brainstem, and cerebellum.[51,52] BDNF has been shown to mediate hippocampal long-term potentiation (LTP), a process of synaptic strengthening associated with learning and memory.[53] In addition to its prominent role in synaptic plasticity and cognition, BDNF signaling has been implicated in the regulation of adult neurogenesis.[54] BDNF promotes the development of GABA neurons and induces the expression of GABA-related proteins such as GAD67 and GAT1.[55,56] BDNF is a key regulator in GABAergic signaling in cortex and other brain regions.[57-59] BDNF regulates the GABAergic system in the hippocampus,[60] and enhances the elongation and branching of axons of GABAergic neurons.[61]

Preclinical Studies

The role of BDNF in the pathophysiology and treatment of schizophrenia has been examined in rodent models. Deficits in spatial learning and memory have been found in BDNF knockout mice or in mice administered with function-blocking anti-BDNF antibodies.[62,63] Studies have also found deficits in LTP in BDNF gene–deleted mice.[64,65] BDNF levels have been extensively studied in various animal models of schizophrenia. It has been shown that animals with neonatal ibotenic acid lesions of the ventral hippocampus or amygdala have decreased BDNF mRNA levels in the prefrontal cortex and hippocampus.[66] Gestational methylazoxymethanol acetate (MAM) exposure induced deficits in both the acquisition and retention phases of the Morris maze, and these behavioral changes were associated with significant changes in BDNF.[67] In addition, chronic administration of D-amphetamine has been shown to reduce BDNF levels in the occipital cortex and hypothalamus in rats.[68] Moreover, administration of NMDA receptor antagonist MK-801 in rats decreased BDNF mRNA in the hippocampus and cerebral cortex.[69]

Several studies have examined the effect of antipsychotic drugs on BDNF levels in rodents. Data from rodent studies indicate that short-term treatment with antipsychotics differentially affects the expression of BDNF in rat brain.[70–72] Typical antipsychotics, such as haloperidol, have been shown to reduce BDNF levels in the rat brain,[73] whereas atypical antipsychotics, including clozapine and olanzapine, elevate BDNF levels in the rat brain.[74] Treatment with the atypical antipsychotic olanzapine markedly restored reductions in BDNF protein levels in the hippocampus associated with haloperidol treatment.[71,72] In addition, quetiapine treatment has been shown to prevent immobilization stress–induced decrease in levels of BDNF mRNA in rodents.[75] Because antipsychotics are likely to be used for the very long-term (over 10–50 years) management of schizophrenia, it is important to investigate the long-term treatment effects of these antipsychotics on BDNF levels. A significant reduction in BDNF protein levels was found in rat hippocampus with haloperidol, but not with olanzapine, after 90 days of treatment.[72] In addition, a corrective effect of atypical antipsychotics on BDNF expression following switching from typical antipsychotics (haloperidol and chlorpromazine) to atypical antipsychotics (olanzapine and risperidone) was also found in these studies. Such differences between typical and some atypical drugs regarding neurotrophic and neuroprotective mechanisms can have implications on the long-term treatment and management of schizophrenia.

Clinical Studies

BDNF is one of most studied neurotrophic factors for their role in the pathophysiology of schizophrenia, including studies on postmortem brain samples and peripheral tissues, and genetic association studies (**Table 1**). Postmortem studies have examined both mRNA and protein levels in different brain regions from schizophrenia and control subjects. Decreases in BDNF levels were found in the prefrontal cortex of subjects with schizophrenia.[77,78,80,81] Studies have shown mixed results on BDNF levels in hippocampus.[76,79,89,90] The discrepancies between these observations could be due to the methods, sample population, and the confounding variables such as pH and history of medication.

Studies on BDNF in first-episode psychosis

Several studies have examined peripheral BDNF levels in schizophrenia. Although many of the studies have investigated BDNF levels in chronic schizophrenia subjects, a few recent studies have examined BDNF profile in first-episode subjects. The authors found a significant decrease in plasma BDNF levels in drug-naïve first-episode

Table 1 Studies on BDNF levels in schizophrenia		
Authors,[Ref.] Year	Tissue/Region	Effect
Postmortem Brain Samples		
Thompson Ray et al,[76] 2011	Hippocampus	Decrease
Weickert et al,[77] 2003	Dorsolateral prefrontal cortex	Decrease in mRNA and protein
Hashimoto et al,[78] 2005	Prefrontal cortex	Decrease
Dunham et al,[79] 2009	Hippocampus	No change in proBDNF protein
Pillai,[80] 2008	Prefrontal cortex	Decrease
Issa et al,[81] 2010	Prefrontal cortex	Decrease
Serum/Plasma Samples		
Carlino et al,[82] 2011	Serum	Decrease
Buckley et al,[83] 2007	Plasma	Decrease
Pillai et al,[84] 2010	Plasma	Decrease
Jindal et al,[85] 2010	Serum	Decrease
Chen da et al,[86] 2009	Serum	Decrease
Xiu et al,[87] 2009	Serum	Decrease
Reis et al,[88] 2008	Serum	Increase
CSF Samples		
Issa et al,[81] 2010	CSF	Decrease
Pillai et al,[84] 2010	CSF	Decrease

subjects.[83] A significant association between plasma BDNF levels and Positive and Negative Syndrome Scales (PANSS) scores was also observed in these subjects. In addition, several recent studies have also examined BDNF levels in serum samples in first-episode subjects using different study populations. A significant decrease in serum BDNF levels was found in first-episode patients with schizophrenia.[76] This study also found a significant positive correlation between BDNF levels and PANSS-positive subscore in these subjects. Jindal and colleagues[85] found a significant decrease in serum BDNF levels in patients with schizophrenia, but not in patients with nonschizophrenia psychosis. However, no significant correlation between BDNF levels and the severity of positive and negative symptoms or overall functioning was found in this study. In addition to plasma and serum samples, the role of BDNF in schizophrenia has also been investigated in the CSF of schizophrenia subjects. A recent study of drug-naïve first-episode subjects found a significant decrease in CSF BDNF levels, and the CSF levels correlated well with changes in plasma BDNF levels.[84] In addition, a significant negative correlation of BDNF levels with the scores of baseline PANSS-positive symptom subscales was also found in the CSF and plasma samples.

Studies on BDNF in chronic schizophrenia

Studies on BDNF levels in subjects with chronic schizophrenia have reported mixed results. Moreover, changes in BDNF levels have also been found in studies of antipsychotic drug treatment. Serum BDNF levels were significantly low in chronic patients with schizophrenia than in healthy control subjects.[87] BDNF levels were found to be lower in patients treated with risperidone compared with those treated with clozapine and typical antipsychotics.[88] No significant change in plasma BDNF levels was found in schizophrenia subjects after treatment with olanzapine for 8 weeks.[91] Moreover, risperidone treatment for 4 weeks did not alter plasma BDNF levels in schizophrenia patients.[92] Recently, increased serum proBDNF and mBDNF levels, and reduced truncated-BDNF levels were found in schizophrenia subjects in comparison with controls.[82] Moreover, reduced truncated-BDNF correlated well with higher positive and lower negative PANSS scores and a worst performance in all cognitive assays, but not with antipsychotic type.

BDNF Val/Met polymorphism studies in schizophrenia

In humans, the *BDNF* gene is located on chromosome 11. Val66Met (rs6265) is a single-nucleotide polymorphism (SNP) in the gene where adenine and guanine alleles vary, resulting in valine (Val) to methionine (Met) substitution at codon 66. Val66-Met is probably the most investigated SNP of the *BDNF* gene, but besides this variant, other SNPs in the gene are C270T, rs7103411, rs2030324, rs2203877, rs2049045, and rs7124442. It is known that cleavage of proBDNF to mBDNF is essential for long-term hippocampal plasticity.[93] Studies have shown that the variant BDNFMet leads to altered BDNF trafficking and less efficient BDNF sorting in neurons.[94] Despite inconsistent observations on the association of the BDNF Val66Met variant with schizophrenia, several studies have linked this polymorphism to brain morphology in schizophrenia.[95–100] Although several previous studies have indicated an association between Val66Met and cognitive functions in healthy as well as schizophrenia subjects,[101–104] a recent meta-analysis failed to find any such relationship.[105]

Where We Stand Considering BDNF as a Putative Biomarker

Because of the complex nature of the central nervous system, it is often unclear whether a specific biomarker such as BDNF is directly correlated to the pathophysiology or simply associated with other factors related to schizophrenia. Despite some evidence supporting that BDNF can cross the blood-brain barrier, the transport of BDNF across the blood-brain barrier is still a topic of debate. As already discussed, clinical studies along with a large body of evidence from basic neuroscience studies indicate that BDNF may hold considerable promise for the development of novel therapeutic strategies for the treatment of schizophrenia. However, the role of peripheral BDNF as a biomarker needs further investigation. Several scientific questions should be considered in future studies.

Is the assay to measure peripheral BDNF levels a well-standardized method?
Do peripheral BDNF levels correlate well with the known psychiatric symptoms?
Do peripheral BDNF levels establish diagnosis for schizophrenia?
Do peripheral BDNF levels reliably predict response to treatment?
Is BDNF analysis shown to be cost-effective?

Furthermore, more studies need to be performed to understand the role of BDNF in structural and functional plasticity in schizophrenia. Such investigations should focus on studies to examine the role of BDNF in structural abnormalities of the brain such as alterations in regional brain area volume found in schizophrenia subjects, as well as cognitive measurements and their relation to psychopathology. As data from fields such as genetics, molecular and cellular biology, neuroimaging, and behavioral research converge from the bench and the bedside, it is expected that more systematic studies similar to those discussed herein will provide clinicians the proper tools to diagnose and manage schizophrenia.

CHALLENGES

To date, no validated biomarker exists as a measure and/or clinical marker for schizophrenia. As discussed herein, while several molecules and pathways can be considered as potential biomarkers for schizophrenia, aspects of clinical validation, such as the relationship of a biomarker to disease mechanism and its correlation with prognosis, disease severity, or treatment, remain obscure. Moreover, it is appreciated that discrepancies in results between published clinical studies often can be attributed to the differences in well-defined healthy controls, as well as how carefully these are matched. Other serious confounds to detecting a robust biomarker include the reliability of clinical diagnosis; comorbidity with other disorders; variations in age, pH, and postmortem interval; and, of course, the inherent variability in methodology and quality of samples across studies in schizophrenia. It remains speculative as to whether changes in molecular signaling pathways or in functional/anatomic markers occur first, preceding the changes in functional and structural changes that in turn herald the emergence of the clinical manifestation of the disease. As a consequence, it may be difficult to validate changes in molecular signaling as a surrogate end point, being "farther" from the downstream expression of clinical variables (see the article by Keshavan and colleagues elsewhere in this issue). In addition, clinical heterogeneity of overlapping phenotypes and the lack of distinct biomarkers being able to distinguish between major psychiatric disorders compel us still to be overly reliant on symptoms and clinical observation. This drawback has been brought into sharp relief in the conceptualization and configuration of the *Diagnostic and Statistical Manual of Mental Disorders*, Fourth Edition (DSM IV).[106] Finally, replication of findings from biomarker studies is essential.

SUMMARY

- Identification of biomarkers in schizophrenia is still in the early stages of development compared with other areas in medicine.
- Several opportunities are available to develop and validate schizophrenia-specific biomarkers.
- BDNF is a candidate biomarker, although several questions need to be addressed concerning its validity.

REFERENCES

1. Higgins MJ, Baselga J. Targeted therapies for breast cancer. J Clin Invest 2011; 121(10):3797–803.
2. Maitland ML, Schilsky RL. Clinical trials in the era of personalized oncology. CA Cancer J Clin 2011;61(6):365–81.
3. Holmes MV, Perel P, Shah T, et al. CYP2C19 genotype, clopidogrel metabolism, platelet function, and cardiovascular events. JAMA 2011;306(24):2704–14.
4. Snyderman R. Creating meaningful health care reform. J Clin Invest 2009; 119(10):2855–6.
5. Barch DM, Mathalon DH. Using brain imaging measures in studies of precognitive pharmacologic agents in schizophrenia: psychometric and quality assurance considerations. Biol Psychiatry 2011;70(1):13–8.
6. Carter CS, Barch DM, Bullmore E, et al. Cognitive neuroscience treatment research to improve cognition in schizophrenia II: developing imaging biomarkers to enhance treatment development for schizophrenia and related disorders. Biol Psychiatry 2011;70(1):7–12.
7. Luck SJ, Mathalon DH, O'Donnell BF, et al. A roadmap for the development and validation of event-related potential biomarkers in schizophrenia research. Biol Psychiatry 2011;70(1):28–34.
8. Cornblatt BA, Malhotra AK. Impaired attention as an endophenotype for molecular genetic studies of schizophrenia. Am J Med Genet 2001;105(1):11–5.

9. Moritz S, Heeren D, Andresen B, et al. An analysis of the specificity and the syndromal correlates of verbal memory impairments in schizophrenia. Psychiatry Res 2001;101(1):23–31.

10. Glahn DC, Kim J, Cohen MS, et al. Maintenance and manipulation in spatial working memory: dissociations in the prefrontal cortex. Neuroimage 2002;17(1): 201–13.

11. Calkins ME, Gur RC, Ragland JD, et al. Face recognition memory deficits and visual object memory performance in patients with schizophrenia and their relatives. Am J Psychiatry 2005;162(10):1963–6.

12. Conklin HM, Curtis CE, Calkins ME, et al. Working memory functioning in schizophrenia patients and their first-degree relatives: cognitive functioning shedding light on etiology. Neuropsychologia 2005;43(6):930–42.

13. Clementz BA, McDowell JE, Zisook S. Saccadic system functioning among schizophrenia patients and their first-degree biological relatives. J Abnorm Psychol 1994;103(2):277–87.

14. Adler LE, Freedman R, Ross RG, et al. Elementary phenotypes in the neurobiological and genetic study of schizophrenia. Biol Psychiatry 1999;46(1):8–18.

15. Levy DL, Lajonchere CM, Dorogusker B, et al. Quantitative characterization of eye tracking dysfunction in schizophrenia. Schizophr Res 2000;42(3):171–85.

16. Braff DL, Geyer MA, Swerdlow NR. Human studies of prepulse inhibition of startle: normal subjects, patient groups, and pharmacological studies. Psychopharmacology (Berl) 2001;156(2–3):234–58.

17. Baldeweg T, Klugman A, Gruzelier J, et al. Mismatch negativity potentials and cognitive impairment in schizophrenia. Schizophr Res 2004;69(2–3):203–17.

18. Bramon E, McDonald C, Croft RJ, et al. Is the P300 wave an endophenotype for schizophrenia? A meta-analysis and a family study. Neuroimage 2005;27(4):960–8.

19. Davidson LL, Heinrichs RW. Quantification of frontal and temporal lobe brain-imaging findings in schizophrenia: a meta-analysis. Psychiatry Res 2003;122(2): 69–87.

20. Davatzikos C, Shen D, Gur RC, et al. Whole-brain morphometric study of schizophrenia revealing a spatially complex set of focal abnormalities. Arch Gen Psychiatry 2005;62(11):1218–27.

21. Thermenos HW, Goldstein JM, Buka SL, et al. The effect of working memory performance on functional MRI in schizophrenia. Schizophr Res 2005;74(2–3): 179–94.

22. Greenwood TA, Lazzeroni LC, Murray SS, et al. Analysis of 94 candidate genes and 12 endophenotypes for schizophrenia from the Consortium on the Genetics of Schizophrenia. Am J Psychiatry 2011;168(9):930–46.

23. Laruelle M, Abi-Dargham A. Dopamine as the wind of the psychotic fire: new evidence from brain imaging studies. J Psychopharmacol 1999;13(4):358–71.

24. Kim JS, Kornhuber HH, Schmid-Burgk W, et al. Low cerebrospinal fluid glutamate in schizophrenic patients and a new hypothesis on schizophrenia. Neurosci Lett 1980;20(3):379–82.

25. Javitt DC, Sershen H, Hashim A, et al. Inhibition of striatal dopamine release by glycine and glycyldodecylamide. Brain Res Bull 2000;52(3):213–6.

26. Bartha R, Williamson PC, Drost DJ, et al. Measurement of glutamate and glutamine in the medial prefrontal cortex of never-treated schizophrenic patients and healthy controls by proton magnetic resonance spectroscopy. Arch Gen Psychiatry 1997;54(10):959–65.

27. Tuominen HJ, Tiihonen J, Wahlbeck K. Glutamatergic drugs for schizophrenia. Cochrane Database Syst Rev 2006;(2):CD003730.

28. Patil ST, Zhang L, Martenyi F, et al. Activation of mGlu2/3 receptors as a new approach to treat schizophrenia: a randomized Phase 2 clinical trial. Nat Med 2007;13(9):1102–7.

29. Chaki S, Hikichi H. Targeting of metabotropic glutamate receptors for the treatment of schizophrenia. Curr Pharm Des 2011;17(2):94–102.

30. Gonzalez-Burgos G, Hashimoto T, Lewis DA. Alterations of cortical GABA neurons and network oscillations in schizophrenia. Curr Psychiatry Rep 2010; 12(4):335–44.

31. Costa E, Chen Y, Dong E, et al. GABAergic promoter hypermethylation as a model to study the neurochemistry of schizophrenia vulnerability. Expert Rev Neurother 2009;9(1):87–98.

32. Costa E, Chen Y, Davis J, et al. REELIN and schizophrenia: a disease at the interface of the genome and the epigenome. Mol Interv 2002;2(1):47–57.

33. Schurov IL, Handford EJ, Brandon NJ, et al. Expression of disrupted in schizophrenia 1 (DISC1) protein in the adult and developing mouse brain indicates its role in neurodevelopment. Mol Psychiatry 2004;9(12):1100–10.

34. Callicott JH, Straub RE, Pezawas L, et al. Variation in DISC1 affects hippocampal structure and function and increases risk for schizophrenia. Proc Natl Acad Sci U S A 2005;102(24):8627–32.

35. Emamian ES, Hall D, Birnbaum MJ, et al. Convergent evidence for impaired AKT1-GSK3beta signaling in schizophrenia. Nat Genet 2004;36(2):131–7.

36. Freyberg Z, Ferrando SJ, Javitch JA. Roles of the Akt/GSK-3 and Wnt signaling pathways in schizophrenia and antipsychotic drug action. Am J Psychiatry 2010;167(4):388–96.

37. Xu MQ, Xing QH, Zheng YL, et al. Association of AKT1 gene polymorphisms with risk of schizophrenia and with response to antipsychotics in the Chinese population. J Clin Psychiatry 2007;68(9):1358–67.

38. Thiselton DL, Vladimirov VI, Kuo PH, et al. AKT1 is associated with schizophrenia across multiple symptom dimensions in the Irish study of high density schizophrenia families. Biol Psychiatry 2008;63(5):449–57.

39. Benson MA, Newey SE, Martin-Rendon E, et al. Dysbindin, a novel coiled-coil-containing protein that interacts with the dystrobrevins in muscle and brain. J Biol Chem 2001;276(26):24232–41.

40. Li W, Zhang Q, Oiso N, et al. Hermansky-Pudlak syndrome type 7 (HPS-7) results from mutant dysbindin, a member of the biogenesis of lysosome-related organelles complex 1 (BLOC-1). Nat Genet 2003;35(1):84–9.

41. Fanous AH, van den Oord EJ, Riley BP, et al. Relationship between a high-risk haplotype in the DTNBP1 (dysbindin) gene and clinical features of schizophrenia. Am J Psychiatry 2005;162(10):1824–32.

42. Guo AY, Sun J, Riley BP, et al. The dystrobrevin-binding protein 1 gene: features and networks. Mol Psychiatry 2009;14(1):18–29.

43. Talbot K, Eidem WL, Tinsley CL, et al. Dysbindin-1 is reduced in intrinsic, glutamatergic terminals of the hippocampal formation in schizophrenia. J Clin Invest 2004;113(9):1353–63.

44. Tang J, LeGros RP, Louneva N, et al. Dysbindin-1 in dorsolateral prefrontal cortex of schizophrenia cases is reduced in an isoform-specific manner unrelated to dysbindin-1 mRNA expression. Hum Mol Genet 2009;18(20):3851–63.

45. Mei L, Xiong WC. Neuregulin 1 in neural development, synaptic plasticity and schizophrenia. Nat Rev Neurosci 2008;9(6):437–52.

46. Stefansson H, Sigurdsson E, Steinthorsdottir V, et al. Neuregulin 1 and susceptibility to schizophrenia. Am J Hum Genet 2002;71(4):877–92.

47. Hong LE, Wonodi I, Stine OC, et al. Evidence of missense mutations on the neuregulin 1 gene affecting function of prepulse inhibition. Biol Psychiatry 2008; 63(1):17–23.
48. McIntosh AM, Moorhead TW, Job D, et al. The effects of a neuregulin 1 variant on white matter density and integrity. Mol Psychiatry 2008;13(11):1054–9.
49. Winterer G, Konrad A, Vucurevic G, et al. Association of 5' end neuregulin-1 (NRG1) gene variation with subcortical medial frontal microstructure in humans. Neuroimage 2008;40(2):712–8.
50. Lessmann V, Gottmann K, Malcangio M. Neurotrophin secretion: current facts and future prospects [Erratum in: Prog Neurobiol 2004;72(2):165–6]. Prog Neurobiol 2003;69(5):341–74.
51. Murer MG, Yan Q, Raisman-Vozari R. Brain-derived neurotrophic factor in the control human brain, and in Alzheimer's disease and Parkinson's disease. Prog Neurobiol 2001;63(1):71–124.
52. Bramham CR, Messaoudi E. BDNF function in adult synaptic plasticity: the synaptic consolidation hypothesis. Prog Neurobiol 2005;76(2):99–125.
53. Minichiello L, Korte M, Wolfer D, et al. Essential role for TrkB receptors in hippocampus-mediated learning. Neuron 1999;24(2):401–14.
54. Xu B, Gottschalk W, Chow A, et al. The role of brain-derived neurotrophic factor receptors in the mature hippocampus: modulation of long-term potentiation through a presynaptic mechanism involving TrkB. J Neurosci 2000;20(18): 6888–97.
55. Mizuno K, Carnahan J, Nawa H. Brain-derived neurotrophic factor promotes differentiation of striatal GABAergic neurons. Dev Biol 1994;165(1):243–56.
56. Arenas E, Akerud P, Wong V, et al. Effects of BDNF and NT-4/5 on striatonigral neuropeptides or nigral GABA neurons in vivo. Eur J Neurosci 1996;8(8): 1707–17.
57. Brünig I, Penschuck S, Berninger B, et al. BDNF reduces miniature inhibitory postsynaptic currents by rapid downregulation of GABA(A) receptor surface expression. Eur J Neurosci 2001;13(7):1320–8.
58. Elmariah SB, Crumling MA, Parsons TD, et al. Postsynaptic TrkB-mediated signaling modulates excitatory and inhibitory neurotransmitter receptor clustering at hippocampal synapses. J Neurosci 2004;24(10):2380–93.
59. Henneberger C, Kirischuk S, Grantyn R. Brain-derived neurotrophic factor modulates GABAergic synaptic transmission by enhancing presynaptic glutamic acid decarboxylase 65 levels, promoting asynchronous release and reducing the number of activated postsynaptic receptors. Neuroscience 2005; 135(3):749–63.
60. Yamada MK, Nakanishi K, Ohba S, et al. Brain-derived neurotrophic factor promotes the maturation of GABAergic mechanisms in cultured hippocampal neurons. J Neurosci 2002;22(17):7580–5.
61. Vicario-Abejón C, Collin C, McKay RD, et al. Neurotrophins induce formation of functional excitatory and inhibitory synapses between cultured hippocampal neurons. J Neurosci 1998;18(18):7256–71.
62. Linnarsson S, Björklund A, Ernfors P. Learning deficit in BDNF mutant mice. Eur J Neurosci 1997;9(12):2581–7.
63. Tyler WJ, Perrett SP, Pozzo-Miller LD. The role of neurotrophins in neurotransmitter release. Neuroscientist 2002;8(6):524–31.
64. Figurov A, Pozzo-Miller LD, Olafsson P, et al. Regulation of synaptic responses to high-frequency stimulation and LTP by neurotrophins in the hippocampus. Nature 1996;381(6584):706–9.

65. Kang H, Welcher AA, Shelton D, et al. Neurotrophins and time: different roles for TrkB signaling in hippocampal long-term potentiation. Neuron 1997;19(3): 653–64.
66. Ashe PC, Chlan-Fourney J, Juorio AV, et al. Brain-derived neurotrophic factor (BDNF) mRNA in rats with neonatal ibotenic acid lesions of the ventral hippocampus. Brain Res 2002;956(1):126–35.
67. Fiore M, Korf J, Antonelli A, et al. Long-lasting effects of prenatal MAM treatment on water maze performance in rats: associations with altered brain development and neurotrophin levels. Neurotoxicol Teratol 2002;24(2):179–91.
68. Angelucci F, Gruber SH, El Khoury A, et al. Chronic amphetamine treatment reduces NGF and BDNF in the rat brain. Eur Neuropsychopharmacol 2007; 17(12):756–62.
69. Castrén E, da Penha Berzaghi M, Lindholm D, et al. Differential effects of MK-801 on brain-derived neurotrophic factor mRNA levels in different regions of the rat brain. Exp Neurol 1993;122(2):244–52.
70. Angelucci F, Mathé AA, Aloe L. Brain-derived neurotrophic factor and tyrosine kinase receptor TrkB in rat brain are significantly altered after haloperidol and risperidone administration. J Neurosci Res 2000;60(6):783–94.
71. Parikh V, Khan MM, Mahadik SP. Olanzapine counteracts reduction of brain-derived neurotrophic factor and TrkB receptors in rat hippocampus produced by haloperidol. Neurosci Lett 2004;356(2):135–9.
72. Pillai A, Terry AV Jr, Mahadik SP. Differential effects of long-term treatment with typical and atypical antipsychotics on NGF and BDNF levels in rat striatum and hippocampus. Schizophr Res 2006;82(1):95–106.
73. Lipska BK, Khaing ZZ, Weickert CS, et al. BDNF mRNA expression in rat hippocampus and prefrontal cortex: effects of neonatal ventral hippocampal damage and antipsychotic drugs. Eur J Neurosci 2001;14(1):135–44.
74. Bai O, Chlan-Fourney J, Bowen R, et al. Expression of brain-derived neurotrophic factor mRNA in rat hippocampus after treatment with antipsychotic drugs. J Neurosci Res 2003;71(1):127–31.
75. Xu H, Qing H, Lu W, et al. Quetiapine attenuates the immobilization stress-induced decrease of brain-derived neurotrophic factor expression in rat hippocampus. Neurosci Lett 2002;321(1–2):65–8.
76. Thompson Ray M, Weickert CS, Wyatt E, et al. Decreased BDNF, trkB-TK+ and GAD67 mRNA expression in the hippocampus of individuals with schizophrenia and mood disorders. J Psychiatry Neurosci 2011;36(3):195–203.
77. Weickert CS, Hyde TM, Lipska BK, et al. Reduced brain-derived neurotrophic factor in prefrontal cortex of patients with schizophrenia. Mol Psychiatry 2003; 8(6):592–610.
78. Hashimoto T, Bergen SE, Nguyen QL, et al. Relationship of brain-derived neurotrophic factor and its receptor TrkB to altered inhibitory prefrontal circuitry in schizophrenia. J Neurosci 2005;25(2):372–83.
79. Dunham JS, Deakin JF, Miyajima F, et al. Expression of hippocampal brain-derived neurotrophic factor and its receptors in Stanley consortium brains. J Psychiatr Res 2009;43(14):1175–84.
80. Pillai A. Decreased expression of Sprouty2 in the dorsolateral prefrontal cortex in schizophrenia and bipolar disorder: a correlation with BDNF expression. PLoS One 2008;3(3):e1784.
81. Issa G, Wilson C, Terry AV Jr, et al. An inverse relationship between cortisol and BDNF levels in schizophrenia: data from human postmortem and animal studies. Neurobiol Dis 2010;39(3):327–33.

82. Carlino D, Leone E, Di Cola F, et al. Low serum truncated-BDNF isoform correlates with higher cognitive impairment in schizophrenia. J Psychiatr Res 2011; 45(2):273–9.

83. Buckley PF, Pillai A, Evans D, et al. Brain derived neurotropic factor in first-episode psychosis. Schizophr Res 2007;91(1–3):1–5.

84. Pillai A, Kale A, Joshi S, et al. Decreased BDNF levels in CSF of drug-naive first-episode psychotic subjects: correlation with plasma BDNF and psychopathology. Int J Neuropsychopharmacol 2010;13(4):535–9.

85. Jindal RD, Pillai AK, Mahadik SP, et al. Decreased BDNF in patients with antipsychotic naïve first episode schizophrenia. Schizophr Res 2010;119(1–3):47–51.

86. Chen da C, Wang J, Wang B, et al. Decreased levels of serum brain-derived neurotrophic factor in drug-naïve first-episode schizophrenia: relationship to clinical phenotypes. Psychopharmacology (Berl) 2009;207(3):375–80.

87. Xiu MH, Hui L, Dang YF, et al. Decreased serum BDNF levels in chronic institutionalized schizophrenia on long-term treatment with typical and atypical antipsychotics. Prog Neuropsychopharmacol Biol Psychiatry 2009;33(8):1508–12.

88. Reis HJ, Nicolato R, Barbosa IG, et al. Increased serum levels of brain-derived neurotrophic factor in chronic institutionalized patients with schizophrenia. Neurosci Lett 2008;439(2):157–9.

89. Takahashi M, Shirakawa O, Toyooka K, et al. Abnormal expression of brain-derived neurotrophic factor and its receptor in the corticolimbic system of schizophrenic patients. Mol Psychiatry 2000;5(3):293–300.

90. Soontornniyomkij B, Everall IP, Chana G, et al. Tyrosine kinase B protein expression is reduced in the cerebellum of patients with bipolar disorder. J Affect Disord 2011;133(3):646–54.

91. Hori H, Yoshimura R, Yamada Y, et al. Effects of olanzapine on plasma levels of catecholamine metabolites, cytokines, and brain-derived neurotrophic factor in schizophrenic patients. Int Clin Psychopharmacol 2007;22(1):21–7.

92. Yoshimura R, Hori H, Sugita A, et al. Treatment with risperidone for 4 weeks increased plasma 3-methoxy-4-hydroxypnenylglycol (MHPG) levels, but did not alter plasma brain-derived neurotrophic factor (BDNF) levels in schizophrenic patients. Prog Neuropsychopharmacol Biol Psychiatry 2007;31(5):1072–7.

93. Pang PT, Teng HK, Zaitsev E, et al. Cleavage of proBDNF by tPA/plasmin is essential for long-term hippocampal plasticity. Science 2004;306(5695):487–91.

94. Chen ZY, Patel PD, Sant G, et al. Variant brain-derived neurotrophic factor (BDNF) (Met66) alters the intracellular trafficking and activity-dependent secretion of wild-type BDNF in neurosecretory cells and cortical neurons. J Neurosci 2004;24(18):4401–11.

95. Szeszko PR, Lipsky R, Mentschel C, et al. Brain-derived neurotrophic factor val66met polymorphism and volume of the hippocampal formation. Mol Psychiatry 2005;10(7):631–6.

96. Agartz I, Sedvall GC, Terenius L, et al. BDNF gene variants and brain morphology in schizophrenia. Am J Med Genet B Neuropsychiatr Genet 2006; 141B(5):513–23.

97. Chen ZY, Bath K, McEwen B, et al. Impact of genetic variant BDNF (Val66Met) on brain structure and function. Novartis Found Symp 2008;289:180–8 [discussion: 188–95].

98. Dutt A, McDonald C, Dempster E, et al. The effect of COMT, BDNF, 5-HTT, NRG1 and DTNBP1 genes on hippocampal and lateral ventricular volume in psychosis. Psychol Med 2009;39(11):1783–97.

 99. Koolschijn PC, van Haren NE, Bakker SC, et al. Effects of brain-derived neuro-trophic factor Val66Met polymorphism on hippocampal volume change in schizophrenia. Hippocampus 2010;20(9):1010–7.
100. Smith GN, Thornton AE, Lang DJ, et al. Hippocampal volume and the brain-derived neurotrophic factor Val66Met polymorphism in first episode psychosis. Schizophr Res 2012;134(2–3):253–9.
101. Egan MF, Kojima M, Callicott JH, et al. The BDNF val66met polymorphism affects activity-dependent secretion of BDNF and human memory and hippo-campal function. Cell 2003;112(2):257–69.
102. Dempster E, Toulopoulou T, McDonald C, et al. Association between BDNF val66 met genotype and episodic memory. Am J Med Genet B Neuropsychiatr Genet 2005;134B(1):73–5.
103. Ho BC, Milev P, O'Leary DS, et al. Cognitive and magnetic resonance imaging brain morphometric correlates of brain-derived neurotrophic factor Val66Met gene polymorphism in patients with schizophrenia and healthy volunteers. Arch Gen Psychiatry 2006;63(7):731–40.
104. Goldberg TE, Iudicello J, Russo C, et al. BDNF Val66Met polymorphism signif-icantly affects d' in verbal recognition memory at short and long delays. Biol Psychol 2008;77(1):20–4.
105. Mandelman SD, Grigorenko EL. BDNF Val66Met and cognition: all, none, or some? A meta-analysis of the genetic association. Genes Brain Behav 2012; 11(2):127–36.
106. Kraemer HC, Kupfer DJ, Clarke DE, et al. DSM-5: how reliable is reliable enough? Am J Psychiatry 2012;169(1):13–5.

Antipsychotic Polypharmacy
A Comprehensive Evaluation of Relevant Correlates of a Long-Standing Clinical Practice

Christoph U. Correll, MD[a,b,c,d],*, Juan A. Gallego, MD, MS[a,d]

KEYWORDS

- Antipsychotic • Polypharmacy • Combination • Reasons • Rationale • Correlates
- Schizophrenia

KEY POINTS

- Despite insufficient evidence for its safety and effectiveness, antipsychotic polypharmacy (APP) has remained a common treatment strategy in the management of patients with psychotic disorders, especially those with schizophrenia spectrum disorders.
- The risks and uncertainties regarding APP have to be weighed against the well-established risk-benefit ratio of clozapine treatment.
- Concerns with APP include the possibility of higher than necessary total chlorpromazine equivalent dosages, increased acute or long-term side effects, anticipated (or unanticipated) drug-drug interactions, increased rates of noncompliance caused by an increased complexity of drug regimens, difficulties in determining cause and effect of multiple treatments, and substantially higher cost.
- APP is related to patient, illness, and treatment variables that all point toward a greater illness acuity, severity, and chronicity.
- However, some studies suggest that about half of the patients on APP can be successfully converted to antipsychotic monotherapy, indicating that the use of APP may not be required in a relevant number of cases.
- Future randomized controlled studies are needed to understand risks and benefits of APP in comparison with antipsychotic monotherapy and, possibly, high dose antipsychotic monotherapy.

Financial disclosures: Dr Correll has been a consultant or advisor to or has received honoraria from: Actelion, Alexza; American Academy of Child and Adolescent Psychiatry, AstraZeneca, Biotis, Bristol-Myers Squibb, Cephalon, Desitin, Eli Lilly, Gerson Lehrman Group, GSK, IntraCellular Therapies, Lundbeck, Medavante, Medscape, Merck, Novartis, Ortho-McNeill/Janssen/J&J, Otsuka, Pfizer, ProPhase, Sunovion, Takeda and Teva. He has received grant support from BMS, Feinstein Institute for Medical Research, Janssen/J&J, National Institute of Mental Health (NIMH), National Alliance for Research in Schizophrenia and Depression (NARSAD), and Otsuka. Dr Gallego has nothing to disclose. This study was supported in part by the Zucker Hillside Hospital Advanced Center for Intervention and Services Research for the Study of Schizophrenia (MH090590) from the National Institute of Mental Health, Bethesda, MD.

[a] The Zucker Hillside Hospital, Division of Psychiatry Research, North Shore-LIJ Health System, 75-59, 263rd Street, Glen Oaks, NY 11004, USA; [b] Hofstra North Shore-LIJ School of Medicine, Hempstead, NY 11549, USA; [c] Albert Einstein College of Medicine, 1300 Morris Park Avenue, Bronx, NY 10461, USA; [d] The Feinstein Institute for Medical Research, 350 Community Drive, Manhasset, NY 11030, USA
* Corresponding author.
E-mail address: ccorrell@lij.edu

OVERVIEW

The treatment of schizophrenia has remained a challenge despite various pharmacologic advances.[1] Although antipsychotic treatment is the cornerstone of successful treatment of the acute psychotic episode and of relapse prevention, evidence-based therapies are currently still limited to the use of medications with antidopaminergic activity.[2] This restriction to antidopaminergic therapy is caused by absent knowledge about the exact pathopyhysiological mechanisms underlying the exacerbation, persistence, and relapse of psychosis, precluding the development and implementation of rational pharmacologic augmentation and combination strategies in the management of schizophrenia.

One common strategy for the management of refractory and significant residual psychotic signs and symptoms is the use of 2 or more antipsychotics, also called antipsychotic polypharmacy (APP). In a separate article,[3] we undertook a systematic literature review of APP prevalences across 4 decades and geographical regions. Pooling data from 147 studies published between the 1970s and 2009, we found a median APP prevalence of 19.6% (interquartile range [IQR]=12.9%–35.0%). We also found significant differences in pooled APP prevalences across geographical regions, with higher prevalences observed in:

- Asia (median = 32%, IQR = 19.2%–53.0%) and
- Europe (median = 23%, IQR = 15.0%–42.1%)

compared with:

- North America (median = 16%, IQR = 7.2%–24.4%) and
- Oceania (median = 16.4%, IQR = 9.8%–20.0)

Although in North America, global APP prevalences were lower than in Asia and Europe, the median APP prevalence in North America increased steadily from 12.7% in the 1980s to 17.0% in the 2000s. Conversely, the median APP prevalence in Asia markedly decreased monotonously from 55.5% in the 1980s to 19.2% in the 2000s, whereas in Europe an increase from the 1980s (17.6%) to the 1990s (26.3%) was observed, followed by a plateau in the 2000s (25.0%).[3]

Multiple reasons for the use of APP, considered both appropriate and inappropriate, have been discussed (**Table 1**).[4] Justifiable reasons for antipsychotic combinations include active cross-titration and the co-utilization of a different route of administration. Theoretically justifiable reasons include the treatment of different symptom domains (such as cognitive and negative symptoms), or of comorbid conditions (such as anxiety, insomnia, depression); the exploitation of pharmacodynamic or pharmacokinetic drug-drug interactions hoping to augment or speed up the efficacy of the first antipsychotic, especially after insufficient response to clozapine; and the exploitation of pharmacodynamic or pharmacokinetic drug-drug interactions hoping to minimize adverse effects.[5–9] Reasons, which are difficult to justify, include arrested cross-titration caused by intraswitch symptom improvements, miscommunication between services, reliance on unfounded marketing strategies, patients' or family's demand without supportive data for that given individual, and idiosyncratic prescriber habits.[4,7,10]

Over the years, APP has even become a source of debate and strong concern.[4,11–16] Several states have included the reduction of APP as a key performance improvement and quality-of-care target.[17] This situation stems mainly from the fact that robust evidence is lacking for the effectiveness of APP.[18,19] Moreover, although several potential reasons for APP have been discussed, significant concerns exist, fueled by the fact

Table 1 Potential reasons for and concerns about APP	
Potential Reasons	**Potential Concerns**
Active cross-titration	Higher than necessary total dosage
Aborted cross-titration	Increased acute side effects
Enhancement of efficacy	Increased long-term side effects
Speeding up of efficacy	Loss of atypicality
Treatment of different symptom domain (eg, agitation, cognition, negative symptoms)	Drug-drug interactions (known and unforeseen)
Treatment of comorbidity (eg, insomnia, anxiety, depression)	Increased risk of nonadherence
Reduction of dose of first antipsychotic	Difficulty determining cause and effect
Reduction of adverse effects of first antipsychotic	Lack of evidence base
Different route of administration	Increased mortality
Combining complementary pharmacologic and side effects profiles	Cost
Poor communication between services	
Patient's/family's choice/pressure	
Prescriber habit	
Marketing influences	

that most reasons are not justified or not backed up by data, and that there are potential downsides to combining antipsychotics (see **Table 1**).

Concerns include the possibility of higher than necessary total chlorpromazine equivalent dosages, increased acute or long-term side effects, anticipated (or unanticipated) drug-drug interactions, increased noncompliance caused by an increased complexity of drug regimens, difficulties in determining cause and effect of multiple treatments, and substantially higher cost.[4,15,16,20–22]

Although even monotherapy with newer antipsychotics that block multiple receptor systems and subsystems at a lower dose than is required to lead to dopamine blockade that is sufficient for antipsychotic efficacy[23] can already be considered a type of intrinsic polytherapy, the use of antipsychotic cotreatment is generally discouraged by treatment algorithms and is suggested only as a last resort strategy after clozapine (the standard of care for treatment-refractory psychotic illness) has failed.[24–29] Nevertheless, many patients receive APP in clinical practice,[3] despite a general dearth of controlled data on the efficacy and safety of this strategy.[18,19] Because of this critical gap between clinical practice and evidence-based data, APP was recently listed among the 10 areas in schizophrenia research that are in dire need of investigation.[30]

Although debated, discouraged, and defamed, rationales and correlates of APP are unclear. Therefore, in order to provide leads for a better understanding of the motivation for using more than 1 antipsychotic concurrently and to guide initiatives for a reduction of potentially inappropriate use of APP, we reviewed the literature regarding correlates of APP.

METHODS

We conducted an electronic search in PubMed for correlates of APP (last update September 09, 2011), using the following key words: "(antipsychotic OR antipsychotics OR neuroleptic OR neuroleptics) AND (polypharmacy OR combination OR combined OR comedication OR concomitant OR cotreatment OR adjunct OR adjunctive) AND (human) AND (schizophrenia OR schizoaffective OR psychosis OR psychotic OR bipolar OR mania)." In addition, reference lists from retrieved articles and relevant reviews were surveyed to identify additional studies.

Articles were included that reported explicitly on significant or nonsignificant associations between APP and study design, patient, illness, treatment, and prescriber characteristics. We excluded associations between APP and adverse effects, because this was the topic of a separate review, requiring a more fine-grained assessment of individual APP combinations, which can yield different outcomes, including opposing effects of increased or even decreased adverse effects with some combinations.[31] Whenever multiple regression analyses were reported, these results, rather than results from univariate analyses, were included, in order to focus on independent associations whenever possible. Only results that were either explicitly significantly different or explicitly not significantly different between patients treated with APP or antipsychotic monotherapy were included in this review, using descriptive statistics.

RESULTS

Out of 6416 initial hits, 5996 articles were excluded on the abstract level, and 447 full text articles were reviewed. Of these articles, 98 studies provided explicit information on study patient, illness, treatment, prescriber, or study design associations with APP and are included in this review.

STUDY CHARACTERISTICS

The 98 included studies were published between 1977 and 2011, reported on 611,078 patients (range: 38–116,114; median: 534; IQR: 225–3047), and originated from Europe (N = 47, 48.0%), the United States and Canada (N = 37, 37.8%), Asia (N = 11, 11.2%) and Oceania (N = 3, 3.1%). Sixty-seven studies (68.4%) were cross-sectional and 31 (31.6%) were longitudinal. About half of the studies (N = 45, 51.1%) were conducted in inpatients, whereas the rest of the studies were conducted in outpatients (N = 24, 27.2%) or patients treated in both settings (N = 19, n = 21.6%). Among 60 studies that specified the time period of their assessment, most (N = 32, 53.3%) covered the time period between 2000 and 2010. The remaining studies covered the 1990s (N = 16, 26.7%), late 1990s into early 2000s (N = 6, 10.0%), 1980s (N = 3, 5.0%), 1970s (N = 2, 3.3%) or the period spanning the 1970s to 1990s (N = 1, 1.7%). Among 95 studies with information, 88 (92.6%) were conducted in adults and 7 (7.4%) were conducted in children and adolescents. Patients were on average 41.3 years old (66 studies with information), 58.7% were male (83 studies with information) and 60.3% were white (25 studies with information). In 68 studies with diagnostic information, 66.7% had a diagnosis of schizophrenia or schizophrenia spectrum disorders (range: 3%–100%, median 70.5%). APP was defined simply as the use of 2 or more antipsychotics at the study assessment time point in most studies (86, 87.8%). The remaining studies required a minimum duration of APP of at least 3 to 7 days (N = 4, 4.1%), 28 to 30 days (N = 2, 2.0%), 60 days (N = 4, 4.1%), or 90 days (N = 2, 2.0%). Across studies reporting on APP correlates, the mean APP prevalence was 29.9% (range: 3%–95%; IQR: 14.6%–46.0%; median: 26.7%).

PATIENT CHARACTERISTICS

Substantial evidence exists for the association of younger age and APP (**Table 2**).[5,32–41] Only 1 study found older age to be associated with APP,[42] and 1 study reported that

Table 2
Patient variables associated with APP

Variable	Studies	
Younger age	Aparasu et al,[32] 2009 Molina et al,[33] 2009 Lerma-Carrillo et al,[34] 2008 Morrato et al,[35] 2007 Kreyenbuhl et al,[36] 2007 Kogut et al,[37] 2005 Biancosino et al,[5] 2005 Jaffe and Levine 2003[38] Weissman et al,[39] 2002 Leslie et al,[40] 2001 Raschetti et al,[41] 1993	Opposite: Lass et al,[42] 2008 adolescents > children: Constantine et al,[43] 2010
Male sex	Molina et al,[33] 2009 Lerma-Carillo et al,[34] 2008 Morrato et al,[35] 2007 Biancosino et al,[5] 2005 Ganguly et al,[68] 2004 Lelliott et al,[52] 2002 Fourrier et al,[53] 2000	Opposite: Kreyenbuhl et al,[70] 2007
White/non-Latino	Covell et al,[44] 2002 Leslie and Rosenheck,[40] 2001	No differences between Whites and Blacks: Connolly et al,[45] 2007
African American race	Jaffe and Levine,[38] 2003	Opposite: Kreyenbuhl et al,[36] 2007
Unmarried	Santone et al,[46] 2011 Kreyenbuhl et al,[36] 2007 Biancosino et al,[5] 2005 Covell et al,[44] 2002	

APP was more common in adolescents than in children.[43] Moreover, except for 1 study that found females to be treated with more APP,[5] all other studies reported that male sex was associated with higher APP utilization. Data on race and ethnicity were inconclusive. Some studies reported higher APP in White/non-Latino patients,[40,44] others showed either higher[38] or lower[36] APP prevalences in Blacks/African Americans, and 1 study reported no differences between Whites and Blacks.[45] By contrast, 4 studies reported that APP was more common in unmarried patients (see **Table 2**).[5,36,44,46]

ILLNESS CHARACTERISTICS

APP was most prevalent in patients with schizophrenia and schizoaffective disorder and[5,35,39,46–53] psychotic disorders (**Table 3**).[32,43] Moreover, APP was more common in patients with earlier illness onset[47] and longer illness duration,[54–60] with only 1 study finding the opposite.[5] Furthermore, APP was consistently related to greater illness severity or acuity.[5,7,36,40,47,53–55,61–65] Only risk of relapse was not increased in APP patients in 1 2-year study.[47] In addition, patients with APP showed less treatment improvement,[20] had less illness insight,[46,47] greater treatment resistance,[55,66] a history of violence,[60] and more negative symptoms.[35] The effect of comorbidities was assessed. Psychiatric comorbidity,[35] in general, and more comorbid depression[36] and nicotine use[67] were related to APP. Conversely, data on substance use were mixed, showing both higher[40,63] and lower[8,36] APP prevalences (see **Table 3**).

Table 3
Illness variables associated with APP

Variable	Studies	
Schizophrenia/schizoaffective disorder	Millier et al,[47] 2011 Santone et al,[46] 2011 Procyshin et al,[48] 2010 Castberg et al,[49] 2008 Correll et al,[50] 2007 Morrato et al,[35] 2007 Biancosino et al,[5] 2005 Procyshin et al,[51] 2004 Lelliot et al,[52] 2002 Weissman et al,[39] 2002 Fourrier et al,[53] 2000	
Psychotic disorder	Constantine et al,[43] 2010 Aparasu et al,[32] 2009	
Earlier illness onset	Millier et al,[47] 2011	
Longer illness duration	De Hert et al,[54] 2006 Barbui et al,[55,76] 2006 Sim et al,[56] 2004 Janssen et al,[57] 2004 Correll et al,[58] 2003 Chong et al,[59] 2004 Yip et al,[60] 1997	Opposite: Biancosino et al,[5] 2005
Greater illness acuity or severity	Millier et al,[47] 2011 Stroup et al,[61] 2009 Kreyenbuhl et al,[36,70] 2007 De Hert et al,[54] 2006 Barbui et al,[55,76] 2006 Centorrino et al,[62] 2005 Biancosino et al,[5] 2005 Janssen et al,[57] 2004 Weinmann et al,[63] 2004 Schumacher et al 2004 Tapp et al,[7] 2003 Brunot et al,[65] 2002 Leslie and Rosenheck,[40] 2001 Fourrier et al,[53] 2000	Not relapse: Millier et al,[47] 2011
Less improvement	Rupnow et al,[20] 2007	
Less illness insight	Santone et al,[46] 2011 Millier et al,[47] 2011	
Treatment resistance	Tomasi et al,[66] 2006 Barbui et al,[55,76] 2006	
History of violence	Yip et al,[60] 1997	
More negative symptoms	Morrato et al,[35] 2007	
More psychiatric comorbidity	Morrato et al,[35] 2007	
Comorbid depression	Kreyenbuhl et al,[36] 2007	
Comorbid nicotine abuse	Paton et al,[67] 2004	
Comorbid substance abuse	Weinmann et al,[63] 2004 Leslie and Rosenheck,[40] 2001	Opposite: Kreyenbuhl et al,[36] 2007 Ganguly et al,[68] 2004

TREATMENT SETTING AND MEDICATION CHARACTERISTICS

Treatment setting variables associated with APP also point toward greater illness severity (**Table 4**). These variables include involuntary treatment,[52] inpatient treatment,[53,63,65,69–71] longer inpatient stay,[60,69,72,73] except for 1 study,[33] and longer treatment in general.[53,68] In addition, a history of multiple antipsychotic switches[38] and nonadherence or partial medication adherence[74,75] was related to APP. Patients receiving APP at study baseline were also more likely to receive APP at end point in prospective studies (see **Table 4**).[5,64,76]

One of the most consistent and replicated findings is the relationship between APP and greater total antipsychotic dose (see **Table 4**).[18,36,37,48,50,52,56,71–73,77–95] In addition, treatment with quetiapine,[20,38,50,68,73,96–98] depot antipsychotics,[99–101] and first-generation antipsychotics (FGAs)[68,78,85,102] has also been consistently associated with APP. Conversely, results regarding treatment with clozapine and olanzapine have been mixed. Some studies showed greater clozapine[35,68] and olanzapine[96] utilization among APP users, whereas others showed lower clozapine[103] or olanzapine[68] prescribing. In a single study, APP was associated with less treatment discontinuation of aripiprazole.[104]

Not surprisingly, because of the increased total antipsychotic dose, anticholinergic use was significantly higher in patients receiving APP than in those treated with antipsychotic monotherapy.[36,54,56,68,72,84,85,92,100,105–114] In addition, cotreatment with antidepressants,[47,70] anxiolytics,[47,54,70,79] and mood stabilizers[36,68,79] has also been associated with APP (see **Table 4**).

PRESCRIBER CHARACTERISTICS

APP varied substantially by region and provider (**Table 5**).[55,56,59,83,115–118] Higher APP use has been reported for metropolitan location/populations,[32] nonteaching hospital settings and those with less research involvement.[119,120] In addition, higher APP was associated with less physician attendance of local continuous medical education events,[119] but greater attendance at educational programs sponsored by a pharmaceutical company.[70] Furthermore, APP has been associated with (see **Table 5**):

- Treatment by the same doctor for more than 2 years[70]
- Treatment by a more senior staff member as opposed to a trainee[10]
- Having inherited a patient on APP from a previous treatment provider
- Endorsing a specific APP combination preference[10]

STUDY DESIGN AND COST

Shorter observation times and cross-sectional definitions of APP have been associated with higher APP use,[44,68,121] which, in turn, have been related to greater medication cost (see **Table 5**).[20–22,96,122–125]

DISCUSSION

The reviewed literature indicates that APP is related to patient, illness, and treatment variables that are related to greater illness acuity, severity, complexity, and chronicity. This finding seems to validate the notion that APP is prescribed for patients who are difficult to manage with standard antipsychotic monotherapy. In keeping with the association between APP and greater psychiatric comorbidity as well as higher total antipsychotic dose, nonantipsychotic cotreatment, especially anticholinergic use, has also been related to APP. Antipsychotic medication variables suggest that quetiapine, long-acting injectable formulations, and FGAs are consistently related to APP,

Table 4
Treatment setting and medication variables associated with APP

Variable	Studies		
Involuntary treatment	Lelliott et al,[52] 2002		
Hospitalization	Gilmer et al,[69] 2007 Kreyenbuhl et al,[70] 2007 Weinmann et al,[63] 2004	Brunot et al,[65] 2002 Fourrier et al,[53] 2000 Tibaldi et al,[71] 1997	
Longer inpatient stay	Ghio et al,[72] 2011 Gilmer et al,[69] 2007 Centorrino et al,[73] 2004 Yip et al,[60] 1997	Opposite: Molina et al,[33] 2009	
Longer treatment duration	Ganguly et al,[68] 2004 Fourrier et al,[53] 2000		
History of multiple antipsychotic switches	Jaffe and Levine,[38] 2003		
Nonadherence/ partial adherence	Ahn et al,[74] 2008 Simon et al,[75] 2005		
APP at baseline	Barbui et al,[76] 2006 Biancosino et al,[5] 2005 Schumacher et al,[64] 2003		
Higher total dose	Ghio et al,[72] 2011 Procyshyn et al,[48] 2010 Ranceva et al,[77] 2010 Correll et al,[18] 2009 Elie et al,[78] 2010 Centorrino et al,[79] 2008 Hung and Cheung,[80] 2008 Paton et al,[81] 2008 Kreyenbuhl et al,[36] 2007 Correll et al,[50] 2007	Wheeler et al,[82] 2006 Carnahan et al,[84] 2006 Florez Menendez et al,[85] 2004 Centorrino et al,[73] 2004 Kogut et al,[37] 2005 Linden et al,[86] 2004 Humberstone et al,[83] 2004 Sim et al,[56] 2004 Bingefors et al,[87] 2003	Suzuki et al,[88] 2003 Centorrino et al,[89] 2002 Harrington et al,[90] 2002 Lelliott et al,[52] 2002 Chong et al,[91] 2000 Tognoni,[92] 1999 Galletly and Tsourtos 1997[93] Tibaldi et al,[71] 1997 Rosholm et al,[94] 1994 Remington et al,[95] 1993
Quetiapine treatment	Rupnow et al,[20] 2007 Correll et al,[50] 2007 Faries et al,[96] 2005	Ganguly et al,[68] 2004 Centorrino et al,[73] 2004	Ereshefsky,[98] 1999
Depot antipsychotic treatment	Hori et al,[99] 2006 Xiang et al 2008 Chiu et al,[101] 1991		
First-generation antipsychotic treatment	Elie et al,[78] 2010 Divac et al,[102] 2007 Correll et al,[58] 2006		Florez Menendez et al,[85] 2005 Ganguly et al,[68] 2004
Clozapine treatment	Morrato et al,[35] 2007 Ganguly et al,[68] 2004		Opposite: Taylor et al,[103] 2008
Olanzapine treatment	Faries et al,[96] 2005		Opposite: Ganguly et al,[68] 2004
Lower aripiprazole discontinuation	Shahajan et al,[104] 2008		

(continued on next page)

Table 4 (continued)			
Variable		**Studies**	
Anticholinergic treatment	Ghio et al,[72] 2011 Hong and Bishop,[105] 2010 Kreyenbuhl et al,[36] 2007 Xiang et al,[100] 2008 De Hert et al,[54] 2006 Chakos et al,[106] 2006 Florez Menendez et al,[85] 2005	Carnahan et al,[84] 2006 Ganguly et al,[68] 2004 Sim et al 2004[56] Procyshyn et al,[107] 2001 Taylor et al,[108] 2000 Tognoni et al,[92] 1999	Brambilla et al,[109] 1999 Hida et al,[110] 1997 Kivet 1995 Clark and Holden,[112] 1987 Morgan and Gopalaswamy,[113] 1984 Mason et al,[114] 1977
Antidepressant treatment	Millier et al,[47] 2011 Kreyenbuhl et al,[70] 2007		
Anxiolytic treatment	Millier et al,[47] 2011 Centorrino et al,[79] 2008 Kreyenbuhl et al,[70] 2007 De Hert et al,[54] 2006		
Mood stabilizer treatment	Centorrino et al,[79] 2008 Kreyenbuhl et al,[36] 2007 Ganguly et al,[68] 2004		

whereas data on clozapine and olanzapine have been inconsistent. In addition, there was wide provider variability regarding APP use. This finding may be related to variations in regional or national treatment paradigms and cultures as well as to differences in patient populations, but it has also been related to lower academic and education levels, idiosyncratic practices and beliefs, and marketing or time pressure. Longer observation periods that minimize the capturing of temporary, overlapping switches have been related to less APP, whereas APP itself has been associated with greater medication treatment cost.

Patient Variables

The fact that younger age was associated with APP could be because younger age at onset is associated with greater illness severity and poorer outcomes.[126] However, by contrast, it is also possible that younger patients are undergoing more treatment changes and that cross-sectional studies captured overlapping antipsychotic switches as APP. However, arguing against the latter argument is the fact that about half of the studies reporting a significant relationship between younger age and higher APP use required a duration of APP of at least 90 days,[36,37] 60 days,[35] or 28 days,[38] whereas the only study showing that older age was associated with APP required only a 3-day antipsychotic overlap.[42] The finding that adolescents had more APP than children can be explained by the fact that child psychiatrists are more cautious in prescribing medications in prepubertal children, let alone multiple agents from the same class, especially combinations with little evidence in adults and absent evidence in youth. The association of male sex with APP may have to do with greater illness severity, chronicity, or dangerousness in males. The same may be true for unmarried status, which is associated both with younger age and greater illness severity/chronicity. Information on race and ethnicity was mixed and difficult to interpret. Therefore, more data are needed that focus on the relationship between race/ethnicity and APP, taking into account other illness-related and patient-related factors as well.

Table 5
Provider and other variables associated with APP

Variable	Studies	
Provider Characteristics		
Region/country/prescriber	Patrick et al,[115] 2006	Humberstone et al,[83] 2004
	Barbui et al,[55,76] 2006	Muscettola et al,[116] 1987
	Sim et al,[56] 2004	Muijen et al,[117] 1987
	Chong et al,[59] 2004	Edwards and Kumar,[118] 1984
Metropolitan area	Aparasu et al,[32] 2009	
Nonteaching hospital, less research involvement	Baandrup et al,[119] 2010 Johnson and Wright 1990[120]	
Attendance at educational programs sponsored by a pharmaceutical company	Kreyenbuhl et al,[70] 2007	
Less attendance at local continuous medical education activities	Baandrup et al,[119] 2010	
Treatment by same doctor for >2 y	Kreyenbuhl et al,[70] 2007	
More senior staff vs trainees	Correll et al,[10] 2011	
Specific APP preference	Correll et al,[10] 2011	
Inherited APP by previous provider, greater reliance on previous provider's APP recommendation	Correll et al,[10] 2011	
Time pressure, workload	Baandrup et al,[119] 2010	
Other Characteristics		
Shorter study observation periods	Kreyenbuhl et al,[121] 2006 Ganguly et al,[68] 2004 Covell et al,[44] 2002	
Greater medication cost	Baandrup et al,[122] 2011 Zhu and Ascher-Svanum,[21] 2008 Rupnow et al,[20] 2007 Valuck et al,[123] 2007	Stahl et al,[22] 2006 Faries et al,[96] 2005 Loosbrock et al,[124] 2003 Clark et al,[125] 2002

Illness Variables

Illness characteristics also all point toward an association of APP with greater illness severity, acuity, complexity, chronicity, and refractoriness. Although these characteristics could justify APP, most patients receiving APP have not received a trial with clozapine,[127] a step in the treatment algorithm endorsed by most, if not all, treatment guidelines.[24–29] However, it is also possible that at least some of the reported APP frequencies in patients with correlates that point toward greater illness severity and complexity may relate to antipsychotic switching that is under way at the time of the survey. The inconclusive results regarding substance use disorders may be caused by undisclosed differences, whether or not substance use disorders are primary or comorbid with other severe mental disorders, which needs to be pursued in future studies.

Treatment Setting and Medication Variables

Similar to patient and illness variables, treatment setting variables associated with APP also point toward greater illness severity and chronicity of those individuals who are treated with APP. The fact that an increased total antipsychotic dose is the most consistent and replicated correlate of APP raises the important question if prescribers avoid using antipsychotic doses that are significantly higher than doses used in regulatory trials and rather prefer adding a second antipsychotic to increase dopamine blockade in patients with insufficient antipsychotic response. The problem has been raised before that patients enrolled in regulatory trials that help establish the approved medication doses are atypical patients.[128] Only a few eligible patients consent to double-blind randomized trials,[129,130] and treatment responsiveness may be greater in these highly selected populations.[131] Moreover, in order not to increase adverse effect frequencies, drug makers are not interested in studying in the pivotal trials whether a dose increase in patients with insufficient response would improve if the dose were raised.[132] Given this situation, studies should compare continuation of antipsychotic monotherapy with APP and with high-dose antipsychotic treatment, a design that has only rarely been implemented.[133]

Several medication variables were significantly associated with APP. For example, decanoate antipsychotics, FGAs and quetiapine were associated with greater APP. The cotreatment of long-acting injectable formulations with a different antipsychotic is not uncommon, because it may be difficult to perform a fine-grained dose adjustment with injectable antipsychotics alone. The cotreatment of FGAs and second-generation antipsychotics (SGAs) was the most frequent combination in the systematic review of APP frequencies[3] and may be related to clinicians' attempts to add more selective D2 blockade to SGAs, which occupy other receptors.[23] Among individual antipsychotics, quetiapine is particularly often prescribed in combination with other antipsychotics. This situation may be because quetiapine has low extrapyramidal side effects (EPS) rates across the dose range, which can be seen as an advantage when attempting to increase total net dopamine blockade. In addition, quetiapine is also used to treat nonpsychotic comorbid conditions, such as anxiety, depression, and sleep disturbances,[134] which seem to be particularly prominent in more complex and chronically ill patients, who are more likely to receive APP. Greater treatment with antidepressants, anxiolytics, and mood stabilizers was also related to APP, corresponding to the higher comorbidity described earlier. By contrast, mixed results were found in the use of clozapine or olanzapine as part of APP combinations, with some authors reporting higher[35,68,96] and lower utilization.[68,103] These seemingly contradictory findings may be because, on the one hand, more severely ill patients who do not even respond to clozapine and olanzapine are predisposed to APP. On the other hand, effective treatment with clozapine or olanzapine may decrease the need for adding a second antipsychotic. Although APP was associated with greater anticholinergic use, data are missing that determine whether this is predominantly driven by the frequent SGA-FGA combinations and whether and which SGA-SGA combinations may not lead to clinically relevant EPS, necessitating anticholinergic cotreatment. The study showing less treatment discontinuation with aripiprazole when it was combined with a second antipsychotic[104] may be because during the initial treatment with aripiprazole its less sedating properties, coupled with its partial D2 agonism, can lead to increased restlessness or agitation, which can be mitigated by co-use of a more sedating, full D2 antagonist.

Provider and Other Variables

Studies suggest that there are considerable regional and provider differences regarding the frequency of APP use.[55,56,59,83,115–118] Moreover, there is concern that less teaching, research, and independent continuous medical education, as well as greater attendance of programs sponsored by the pharmaceutical industry, are related to higher APP. These findings, together with previously described associations of greater perceived work pressure and less available time for patient care, endorsed also by nursing staff,[119] highlight intervention targets for educational, hospital-based and administrative initiatives aimed at reducing inappropriate APP prescribing. Such initiatives have already shown initial success[115,135] and are backed up by research findings from controlled studies in which 50% to 67% of patients on APP could be successfully converted to antipsychotic monotherapy without decompensation.[136,137]

In keeping with reduced inclusion of patients undergoing active antipsychotic switches, longer observation periods and the related requirement of 1, 2, or 3 months of combined antipsychotic use to establish APP have been associated with lower APP.[44,68,121]

In addition, APP has been associated with greater medication cost.[20–22,96,122–125] For example, in an analysis of an outpatient Medicaid population, APP was the most expensive form of SGA use, costing up to 3 times more per patient than monotherapy.[14] In another study of 836 patients treated in New Hampshire between 1995 and 1999, the increase in the prevalence of APP from 6% to 24% resulted in an average increased medication cost of $400/mo per patient.[125] Likewise, a prospective, naturalistic study of 846 patients started on olanzapine, quetiapine, or risperidone and followed for 1 year found that each dollar spent on the index antipsychotic was accompanied by spending an additional $1.31 on concomitant antipsychotics for patients initiated on quetiapine, $0.64 for risperidone, and $0.38 for olanzapine.[21] Similar results were reported in a randomized, placebo-controlled study of risperidone, quetiapine, or placebo in 382 patients with schizophrenia or schizoaffective disorder, in which patients received clinician's choice psychotropic cotreatment of an additional 28 days after a minimum of 14 days of monotherapy. In this trial, the mean projected cost of additional antipsychotics, making up greater than 95% of the added medications, per randomized patient during the additive-therapy phase was $57.03 in the risperidone group and $101.64 in the quetiapine group.[20]

The substantially higher medication costs associated with APP make this treatment strategy with insufficient evidence base for its efficacy and safety an important target for future research and attempts at reducing irrational APP use. Because patients receiving APP have been shown to have a more complex and severe illness, any studies investigating nonmedication service costs before and after initiation of APP need to use methods that take the illness severity and chronicity into account, either by selecting appropriate comparison groups, using an appropriate mirror image design, or using sophisticated statistical methods, which use propensity score matching methods that take into consideration relevant and directly measured patient and illness attributes that are associated with illness severity, APP, and the investigated targeted outcomes.

LIMITATIONS

The results of this systematic review have to be interpreted within its limitations. First, this was a descriptive review of studies that generally did not focus on correlates of APP, but rather focused on the reporting of APP prevalence. Therefore, the reported associations likely do not capture all of the possible associations because such analyses were either not reported or conducted in a large number of studies reporting on APP. Of 147 studies reporting on APP prevalence until 2009,[3] only 88 (50.3%) included in this review reported on correlates of APP. Moreover, most studies selected specific correlates for analysis, but there has not been a comprehensive screening for potential associations, and most studies collected data on only some of the potential and relevant correlates. Furthermore, many studies were cross-sectional and may have included ongoing antipsychotic switches, correlating variables to both patients undergoing active antipsychotic switches and those with sustained APP. Therefore, future studies should focus on persistent APP (eg, >60 or 90 days) and collect data and screen for associations taking the variables summarized in this article as a guide. However, in order to perform multivariate analyses, such studies also need to be large enough. Furthermore, associations do not prove causality. Therefore, future studies are needed that interview clinicians and patients and ask directly about the reasons for the use of APP and about barriers to convert patients to antipsychotic monotherapy. The latter is particularly relevant because, as mentioned earlier, an emerging body of evidence suggests that 50% to 67% of patients receiving longer-term APP can safely be converted to antipsychotic monotherapy regimes.[136,137]

Nevertheless, despite these limitations, this is the first systematic review summarizing correlates of APP and showing that greater illness severity, chronicity, and complexity are all associated with APP, underscoring the need for the discovery of novel mechanism of antipsychotic treatment, so that rational polypharmacy can be used as a pharmacologic tool to help those patients with limited response to standard antipsychotic monotherapy.

SUMMARY

Despite insufficient evidence for its safety and effectiveness, APP has remained a common treatment strategy in the management of patients with psychotic disorders, especially those with schizophrenia spectrum disorders. APP is related to patient, illness, and treatment variables that all point toward a greater illness acuity, severity, and chronicity. However, there also seem to be provider characteristics at play that suggest that, at least, some APP may be idiosyncratic or unfounded. The latter idea is supported by studies suggesting that more than half of patients on longer-term APP can be safely and successfully converted to antipsychotic monotherapy. Although not a topic of this review, adverse effect patterns seem to be less homogeneous and depend on specific combinations, with some increasing adverse effect burden, some not affecting adverse effects, and others reducing specific adverse effects, even in the absence of lowering the dose of the initial antipsychotic.[31]

However, given the established effectiveness of clozapine for treatment-refractory psychotic and mood symptoms,[138,139] at least when adequately dosed,[139] the risks and uncertainties regarding APP have to be weighed against the well-established risk/benefit ratio of clozapine treatment. Although difficult to design, conduct, and obtain funding for, randomized controlled combination and discontinuation studies are necessary before the role of APP in the management of schizophrenia and other severe psychotic disorders can be determined. In addition to controlled trials, direct investigations should focus on reasons for choosing and continuing APP regimes, and on identifying and comprehensively characterizing patients benefiting from APP who cannot be converted to antipsychotic monotherapy, including that with clozapine. Such studies may help shed light on biological underpinnings of treatment refractoriness and on dysfunctional, nondopaminergic pathways that could help identify novel treatment targets.

REFERENCES

1. Kane JM, Correll CU. Past and present progress in the pharmacologic treatment of schizophrenia. J Clin Psychiatry 2010;71(9):1115–24.
2. Correll CU. What are we looking for in new antipsychotics? J Clin Psychiatry 2011;72(Suppl 1):9–13.

3. Gallego JA, Bonetti J, Zhang JP, et al. Prevalence and correlates of antipsychotic polypharmacy from the 1970s to 2009: a systematic review and metaregression. Schizophr Res 2012;138(1):18–28.

4. Correll CU. Antipsychotic polypharmacy, part 1: shotgun approach or targeted cotreatment? J Clin Psychiatry 2008;69(4):674–5.

5. Biancosino B, Barbui C, Marmai L, et al. Determinants of antipsychotic polypharmacy in psychiatric inpatients: a prospective study. Int Clin Psychopharmacol 2005;20(6):305–9.

6. Sernyak MJ, Rosenheck R. Clinicians' reasons for antipsychotic coprescribing. J Clin Psychiatry 2004;65(12):1597–600.

7. Tapp A, Wood AE, Secrest L, et al. Combination antipsychotic therapy in clinical practice. Psychiatr Serv 2003;54(1):55–9.

8. Pandurangi AK, Dalkilic A. Polypharmacy with second-generation antipsychotics: a review of evidence. J Psychiatr Pract 2008;14(6):345–67.

9. McCue RE, Waheed R, Urcuyo L. Polypharmacy in patients with schizophrenia. J Clin Psychiatry 2003;64(9):984–9.

10. Correll CU, Shaikh L, Gallego JA, et al. Antipsychotic polypharmacy: prescriber attitudes, knowledge and behavior. Schizophr Res 2011;131(1–3):58–62.

11. Stahl SM. Antipsychotic polypharmacy, part 1: therapeutic option or dirty little secret? J Clin Psychiatry 1999;60:425–6.

12. Stahl SM. Antipsychotic polypharmacy: evidence based or eminence based? Acta Psychiatr Scand 2002;106(5):321–2.

13. Stahl SM. Antipsychotic polypharmacy: squandering precious resources? J Clin Psychiatry 2002;63(2):93–4.

14. Stahl SM, Grady MM. A critical review of atypical antipsychotic utilization: comparing monotherapy with polypharmacy and augmentation. Curr Med Chem 2004;11(3):313–27.

15. Meltzer HY, Kostakoglu AE. Combining antipsychotics: is there evidence for efficacy? Psychiatr Times 2000;17:25–34.

16. Weiden PJ, Casey DE. "Polypharmacy": combining antipsychotic medications in the treatment of schizophrenia. J Psychiatr Pract 1999;5:229–33.

17. Goren JL, Parks JJ, Ghinassi FA, et al. When is antipsychotic polypharmacy supported by research evidence? Implications for QI. Jt Comm J Qual Patient Saf 2008;34(10):571–82.

18. Correll CU, Rummel-Kluge C, Corves C, et al. Antipsychotic combinations vs monotherapy in schizophrenia: a meta-analysis of randomized controlled trials. Schizophr Bull 2009;35(2):443–57.

19. Barbui C, Signoretti A, Mulè S, et al. Does the addition of a second antipsychotic drug improve clozapine treatment? Schizophr Bull 2009;35(2):458–68.

20. Rupnow MF, Greenspan A, Gharabawi GM, et al. Incidence and costs of polypharmacy: data from a randomized, double-blind, placebo-controlled study of risperidone and quetiapine in patients with schizophrenia or schizoaffective disorder. Curr Med Res Opin 2007;23(11):2815–22.

21. Zhu B, Ascher-Svanum H, Faries DE, et al. Cost of antipsychotic polypharmacy in the treatment of schizophrenia. BMC Psychiatry 2008;8:19.

22. Stahl SM, Grady MM. High-cost use of second-generation antipsychotics under California's Medicaid program. Psychiatr Serv 2006;57(1):127–9.

23. Correll CU. From receptor pharmacology to improved outcomes: individualizing the selection, dosing, and switching of antipsychotics. Eur Psychiatry 2010; 25(Suppl 2):S12–21.

24. Buchanan RW, Kreyenbuhl J, Kelly DL, et al, Schizophrenia Patient Outcomes Research Team (PORT). The 2009 schizophrenia PORT psychopharmacological treatment recommendations and summary statements. Schizophr Bull 2010; 36(1):71–93.

25. National Institute for Clinical Excellence. Schizophrenia: full national guideline on core interventions in primary and secondary care. Leicester (UK) and London: The British Psychological Society and The Royal College of Psychiatrists; 2003.

26. Moore TA, Buchanan RW, Buckley PF, et al. The Texas Medication Algorithm Project antipsychotic algorithm for schizophrenia: 2006 update. J Clin Psychiatry 2007;68(11):1751–62.

27. McGorry PD. Royal Australian and New Zealand College of Psychiatrists clinical practice guidelines for the treatment of schizophrenia and related disorders. Aust N Z J Psychiatry 2005;39(1–2):1–30.

28. Falkai P, Wobrock T, Lieberman J, et al. World Federation of Societies of Biological Psychiatry (WFSBP)–guidelines for biological treatment of schizophrenia, part 1: acute treatment of schizophrenia. World J Biol Psychiatry 2005;6(3):132–91.

29. Lehman AF, Lieberman JA, Dixon LB, et al. Practice guideline for the treatment of patients with schizophrenia, second edition. Am J Psychiatry 2004;161(Suppl 2): 1–56.

30. Nasrallah HA, Keshavan MS, Benes FM, et al. Proceedings and data from The Schizophrenia Summit: a critical appraisal to improve the management of Schizophrenia. J Clin Psychiatry 2009;70(Suppl 1):4–46.

31. Gallego JA, Nielsen J, DeHert M, et al. Safety and tolerability of antipsychotic polypharmacy. Expert Opinion on Drug Safety 2012;11(4):527–42.

32. Aparasu RR, Jano E, Bhatara V. Concomitant antipsychotic prescribing in US outpatient settings. Res Social Adm Pharm 2009;5(3):234–41.

33. Molina JD, Lerma-Carrillo I, Leonor M, et al. Combined treatment with amisulpride in patients with schizophrenia discharged from a short-term hospitalization unit: a 1-year retrospective study. Clin Neuropharmacol 2009;32(1):10–5.

34. Lerma-Carrillo I, de Pablo Bruhlmann S, del Pozo ML, et al. Antipsychotic polypharmacy in patients with schizophrenia in a brief hospitalization unit. Clin Neuropharmacol 2008;31(6):319–32.

35. Morrato EH, Dodd S, Oderda G, et al. Prevalence, utilization patterns, and predictors of antipsychotic polypharmacy: experience in a multistate Medicaid population, 1998–2003. Clin Ther 2007;29(1):183–95.

36. Kreyenbuhl J, Marcus SC, West JC, et al. Adding or switching antipsychotic medications in treatment-refractory schizophrenia. Psychiatr Serv 2007;58(7): 983–90.

37. Kogut SJ, Yam F, Dufresne R. Prescribing of antipsychotic medication in a medicaid population: use of polytherapy and off-label dosages. J Manag Care Pharm 2005;11(1):17–24.

38. Jaffe AB, Levine J. Antipsychotic medication coprescribing in a large state hospital system. Pharmacoepidemiol Drug Saf 2003;12(1):41–8.

39. Weissman EM. Antipsychotic prescribing practices in the Veterans Healthcare Administration–New York metropolitan region. Schizophr Bull 2002;28(1):31–42.

40. Leslie DL, Rosenheck RA. Use of pharmacy data to assess quality of pharmacotherapy for schizophrenia in a national health care system: individual and facility predictors. Med Care 2001;39(9):923–33.

41. Raschetti R, Spila Alegiani S, Diana G, et al. Antipsychotic drug prescription in general practice in Italy. Acta Psychiatr Scand 1993;87(5):317–21.

42. Lass J, Mannik A, Bell JS. Pharmacotherapy of first episode psychosis in Estonia: comparison with national and international treatment guidelines. J Clin Pharm Ther 2008;33(2):165–73.

43. Constantine RJ, Boaz T, Tandon R. Antipsychotic polypharmacy in the treatment of children and adolescents in the fee-for-service component of a large state Medicaid program. Clin Ther 2010;32(5):949–59.

44. Covell NH, Jackson CT, Evans AC, et al. Antipsychotic prescribing practices in Connecticut's public mental health system: rates of changing medications and prescribing styles. Schizophr Bull 2002;28(1):17–29.

45. Connolly A, Rogers P, Taylor D. Antipsychotic prescribing quality and ethnicity: a study of hospitalized patients in south east London. J Psychopharmacol 2007; 21(2):191–7.

46. Santone G, Bellantuono C, Rucci P, et al. Patient characteristics and process factors associated with antipsychotic polypharmacy in a nationwide sample of psychiatric inpatients in Italy. Pharmacoepidemiol Drug Saf 2011;20(5):441–9.

47. Millier A, Sarlon E, Azorin JM, et al. Relapse according to antipsychotic treatment in schizophrenic patients: a propensity-adjusted analysis. BMC Psychiatry 2011;11:24.

48. Procyshyn RM, Honer WG, Wu TK, et al. Persistent antipsychotic polypharmacy and excessive dosing in the community psychiatric treatment setting: a review of medication profiles in 435 Canadian outpatients. J Clin Psychiatry 2010; 71(5):566–73.

49. Castberg I, Spigset O. Prescribing patterns and the use of therapeutic drug monitoring of psychotropic medication in a psychiatric high-security unit. Ther Drug Monit 2008;30(5):597–603.

50. Correll CU, Frederickson AM, Kane JM, et al. Does antipsychotic polypharmacy increase the risk for metabolic syndrome? Schizophr Res 2007;89(1–3):91–100.

51. Procyshyn RM, Thompson B. Patterns of antipsychotic utilization in a tertiary care psychiatric institution. Pharmacopsychiatry 2004;37(1):12–7.

52. Lelliott P, Paton C, Harrington M, et al. The influence of patient variables on polypharmacy and combined high dose of antipsychotic drugs prescribed for inpatients. The Psychiatrist 2002;26:311–414.

53. Fourrier A, Gasquet I, Allicar MP, et al. Patterns of neuroleptic drug prescription: a national cross-sectional survey of a random sample of French psychiatrists. Br J Clin Pharmacol 2000;49(1):80–6.

54. De Hert M, Wampers M, Peuskens J. Pharmacological treatment of hospitalised schizophrenic patients in Belgium. Int J Psychiatry Clin Pract 2006;10(4):285–90.

55. Barbui C, Nose M, Mazzi MA, et al. Determinants of first- and second-generation antipsychotic drug use in clinically unstable patients with schizophrenia treated in four European countries. Int Clin Psychopharmacol 2006;21(2):73–9.

56. Sim K, Su A, Fujii S, et al. Antipsychotic polypharmacy in patients with schizophrenia: a multicentre comparative study in East Asia [Erratum appears in: Br J Clin Pharmacol 2004;58(5):564]. Br J Clin Pharmacol 2004;58(2):178–83.

57. Janssen B, Weinmann S, Berger M, et al. Validation of polypharmacy process measures in inpatient schizophrenia care. Schizophr Bull 2004;30(4):1023–33.

58. Correll CU, Kane JM, O'Shea D, et al. Antipsychotic polypharmacy in the treatment of schizophrenia. Poster presented at the International Congress on Schizophrenia Research. Colorado Springs (CO); March 29–April 2, 2003.

59. Chong MY, Tan CH, Fujii S, et al. Antipsychotic drug prescription for schizophrenia in East Asia: rationale for change. Psychiatry Clin Neurosci 2004; 58(1):61–7.

60. Yip KC, Ungvari GS, Cheung HK, et al. A survey of antipsychotic treatment for schizophrenia in Hong Kong. Chin Med J (Engl) 1997;110(10):792.
61. Stroup TS, Lieberman JA, McEvoy JP, et al. Results of phase 3 of the CATIE schizophrenia trial. Schizophr Res 2009;107(1):1–12.
62. Centorrino F, Fogarty KV, Sani G, et al. Use of combinations of antipsychotics: McLean Hospital inpatients, 2002. Hum Psychopharmacol 2005;20(7):485–92.
63. Weinmann S, Janssen B, Gaebel W. Switching antipsychotics in inpatient schizophrenia care: predictors and outcomes. J Clin Psychiatry 2004;65(8):1099–105.
64. Schumacher JE, Makela EH, Griffin HR. Multiple antipsychotic medication prescribing patterns. Ann Pharmacother 2003;37(7–8):951–5.
65. Brunot A, Lachaux B, Sontag H, et al. Pharmaco-epidemiological study on antipsychotic drug prescription in French psychiatry: patient characteristics, antipsychotic treatment, and care management for schizophrenia. Encephale 2002;28(2):129–38.
66. Tomasi R, de Girolamo G, Santone G, et al. The prescription of psychotropic drugs in psychiatric residential facilities: a national survey in Italy. Acta Psychiatr Scand 2006;113(3):212–23.
67. Paton C, Esop R, Young C, et al. Obesity, dyslipidaemias and smoking in an inpatient population treated with antipsychotic drugs. Acta Psychiatr Scand 2004;110(4):299–305.
68. Ganguly R, Kotzan JA, Miller LS, et al. Prevalence, trends, and factors associated with antipsychotic polypharmacy among Medicaid-eligible schizophrenia patients, 1998–2000. J Clin Psychiatry 2004;65910:1377–88.
69. Gilmer TP, Dolder CR, Folsom DP, et al. Antipsychotic polypharmacy trends among Medicaid beneficiaries with schizophrenia in San Diego County, 1999–2004. Psychiatr Serv 2007;58(7):1007–10.
70. Kreyenbuhl JA, Valenstein M, McCarthy JF, et al. Long-term antipsychotic polypharmacy in the VA health system: patient characteristics and treatment patterns. Psychiatr Serv 2007;58(4):489–95.
71. Tibaldi G, Munizza C, Bollini P, et al. Utilization of neuroleptic drugs in Italian mental health services: a survey in Piedmont. Psychiatr Serv 1997;48(2):213–7.
72. Ghio L, Natta W, Gotelli S, et al. Antipsychotic utilisation and polypharmacy in Italian residential facilities: a survey. Epidemiol Psychiatr Sci 2011;20(2):171–9.
73. Centorrino F, Goren JL, Hennen J, et al. Multiple versus single antipsychotic agents for hospitalized psychiatric patients: case-control study of risks versus benefits. Am J Psychiatry 2004;161(4):700–6.
74. Ahn J, McCombs JS, Jung C, et al. Classifying patients by antipsychotic adherence patterns using latent class analysis: characteristics of nonadherent groups in the California Medicaid (Medi-Cal) program. Value Health 2008;11(1):48–56.
75. Simon AE, Peter M, Hess L, et al. Antipsychotic use in patients with schizophrenia treated in private psychiatry. Swiss Med Wkly 2005;135(7–8):109–15.
76. Barbui C, Nose M, Mazzi MA, et al. Persistence with polypharmacy and excessive dosing in patients with schizophrenia treated in four European countries. Int Clin Psychopharmacol 2006;21(6):355–62.
77. Ranceva N, Ashraf W, Odelola D. Antipsychotic polypharmacy in outpatients at Birch Hill Hospital: incidence and adherence to guidelines. J Clin Pharmacol 2010;50(6):699–704.
78. Elie D, Poirier M, Chianetta J, et al. Cognitive effects of antipsychotic dosage and polypharmacy: a study with the BACS in patients with schizophrenia and schizoaffective disorder. J Psychopharmacol 2010;24(7):1037–44.

79. Centorrino F, Cincotta SL, Talamo A, et al. Hospital use of antipsychotic drugs: polytherapy. Compr Psychiatry 2008;49(1):65–9.
80. Hung GB, Cheung HK. Predictors of high-dose antipsychotic prescription in psychiatric patients in Hong Kong. Hong Kong Med J 2008;14(1):35–9.
81. Paton C, Barnes TR, Cavanagh MR, et al. High-dose and combination antipsychotic prescribing in acute adult wards in the UK: the challenges posed by p.r.n. prescribing. Br J Psychiatry 2008;192(6):435–9.
82. Wheeler A, Humberstone V, Robinson G. Trends in antipsychotic prescribing in schizophrenia in Auckland. Australas Psychiatry 2006;14(2):169–74.
83. Humberstone V, Wheeler A, Lambert T. An audit of outpatient antipsychotic usage in the three health sectors of Auckland, New Zealand. Aust N Z J Psychiatry 2004;38(4):240–5.
84. Carnahan RM, Lund BC, Perry PJ, et al. Increased risk of extrapyramidal side-effect treatment associated with atypical antipsychotic polytherapy. Acta Psychiatr Scand 2006;113(2):135–41.
85. Florez Menendez G, Blanco Ramos M, Gomez-Reino Rodriguez I, et al. Polypharmacy in the antipsychotic prescribing in practices psychiatric out-patient clinic. Actas Esp Psiquiatr 2004;32(6):333–9.
86. Linden M, Scheel T, Xaver Eich F. Dosage finding and outcome in the treatment of schizophrenic inpatients with amisulpride. Results of a drug utilization observation study. Hum Psychopharmacol 2004;19(2):111–9.
87. Bingefors K, Isacson D, Lindström E. Dosage patterns of antipsychotic drugs for the treatment of schizophrenia in Swedish ambulatory clinical practice–a highly individualized therapy. Nord J Psychiatry 2003;57(4):263–9.
88. Suzuki T, Uchida H, Tanaka KF, et al. Reducing the dose of antipsychotic medications for those who had been treated with high-dose antipsychotic polypharmacy: an open study of dose reduction for chronic schizophrenia. Int Clin Psychopharmacol 2003;18(6):323–9.
89. Centorrino F, Eakin M, Bahk WM, et al. Inpatient antipsychotic drug use in 1998, 1993, and 1989. Am J Psychiatry 2002;159(11):1932–5.
90. Harrington M, Lelliott P, Paton C, et al. The results of a multi-centre audit of the prescribing of antipsychotic drugs for in-patients in the UK. Psychiatr Bull 2002; 26(11):414.
91. Chong SA, Remington GJ, Lee N, et al. Contrasting clozapine prescribing patterns in the east and west? Ann Acad Med Singap 2000;29(1):75–8.
92. Tognoni G. Pharmacoepidemiology of psychotropic drugs in patients with severe mental disorders in Italy. Eur J Clin Pharmacol 1999;55(9):685–90.
93. Galletly CA, Tsourtos G. Antipsychotic drug doses and adjunctive drugs in the outpatient treatment of schizophrenia. Ann Clin Psychiatry 1997;9(2):77–80.
94. Rosholm JU, Hallas J, Gram LF. Concurrent use of more than one major psychotropic drug (polypsychopharmacy) in out-patients–a prescription database study. Br J Clin Pharmacol 1994;37(6):533–8.
95. Remington GJ, Prendergast P, Bezchlibnyk-Butler KZ. Dosaging patterns in schizophrenia with depot, oral and combined neuroleptic therapy. Can J Psychiatry 1993;38(3):159–61.
96. Faries D, Ascher-Svanum H, Zhu B. Antipsychotic monotherapy and polypharmacy in the naturalistic treatment of schizophrenia with atypical antipsychotics. BMC Psychiatry 2005;5:26.
97. Stahl SM. Focus on antipsychotic polypharmacy: evidence-based prescribing or prescribing-based evidence? Int J Neuropsychopharmacol 2004;7(2): 113–6.

98. Ereshefsky L. Pharmacologic and pharmacokinetic considerations in choosing an antipsychotic. J Clin Psychiatry 1999;60(Suppl 10):20–30.

99. Hori H, Noguchi H, Hashimoto R, et al. Antipsychotic medication and cognitive function in schizophrenia. Schizophr Res 2006;86(1–3):138–46.

100. Xiang YT, Weng YZ, Leung CM, et al. Clinical and social correlates with the use of depot antipsychotic drugs in outpatients with schizrenia in China. Int J Clin Pharmacol Ther 2008;46(5):245–51.

101. Chiu HF, Shum PS, Lam CW. Psychotropic drug prescribing to chronic schizophrenics in a Hong Kong hospital. Int J Soc Psychiatry 1991;37(3):187.

102. Divac N, Jasovic-Gasic M, Samardzic R, et al. Antipsychotic polypharmacy at the University Psychiatric Hospital in Serbia. Pharmacoepidemiol Drug Saf 2007;16(11):1250–1.

103. Taylor M, Shajahan P, Lawrie SM. Comparing the use and discontinuation of antipsychotics in clinical practice: an observational study. J Clin Psychiatry 2008;69(2):240–5.

104. Shajahan P, Macrae A, Bashir M, et al. Who responds to aripiprazole in clinical practice? An observational study of combination versus monotherapy. J Psychopharmacol 2008;22(7):778–83.

105. Hong IS, Bishop JR. Anticholinergic use in children and adolescents after initiation of antipsychotic therapy. Ann Pharmacother 2010;44(7–8):1171–80.

106. Chakos MH, Glick ID, Miller AL, et al. Baseline use of concomitant psychotropic medications to treat schizophrenia in the CATIE trial. Psychiatr Serv 2006;57(8):1094–101.

107. Procyshyn RM, Kennedy NB, Tse G, et al. Antipsychotic polypharmacy: a survey of discharge prescriptions from a tertiary care psychiatric institution. Can J Psychiatry 2001;46(4):334–9.

108. Taylor D, Mace S, Mir S, et al. A prescription survey of the use of atypical antipsychotics for hospital inpatients in the United Kingdom. Int J Psychiatry Clin Pract 2000;4(1):41–6.

109. Brambilla P, Monzani E, Alessandri M, et al. Uso di psicofarmaci presso l'ex ospedale psichiatrico di Milano: uno studio di follow-up. Epidemiologia e Psichiatria Sociale 1999;8:262–9 [in Italian].

110. Hida H, Faber M, Alberto-Gondouin M, et al. Analyse des prescriptions de psychotropes dans un Centre Hospitalier Psychiatrique–a survey of psychotropic drugs prescribing in a psychiatric hospital. Thèrapie 1997;52(6):573–8 [in French].

111. Kiivet RA, Llerena A, Dahl ML, et al. Patterns of drug treatment of schizophrenic patients in Estonia, Spain and Sweden. Br J Clin Pharmacol 1995;40(5):467–76.

112. Clark A, Holden N. The persistence of prescribing habits: a survey and follow-up of prescribing to chronic hospital in-patients. Br J Psychiatry 1987;150:88.

113. Morgan R, Gopalaswamy AK. Psychotropic drugs: another survey of prescribing patterns. Br J Psychiatry 1984;144:298–302.

114. Mason AS, Nerviano V, DeBurger RA. Patterns of antipsychotic drug use in four Southeastern state hospitals. Dis Nerv Syst 1977;38(7):541–5.

115. Patrick V, Schleifer SJ, Nurenberg JR, et al. Best practices: an initiative to curtail the use of antipsychotic polypharmacy in a state psychiatric hospital. Psychiatr Serv 2006;57(1):21–3.

116. Muscettola G, Casiello M, Bolline P, et al. Pattern of therapeutic intervention and role of psychiatric settings: a survey in two regions of Italy. Acta Psychiatr Scand 1987;75(1):55–61.

117. Muijen M, Silverstone T. A comparative hospital survey of psychotropic drug prescribing. Br J Psychiatry 1987;150:501–4.

118. Edwards S, Kumar V. A survey of prescribing of psychotropic drugs in a Birmingham psychiatric hospital. Br J Psychiatry 1984;145:502–7.

119. Baandrup L, Allerup P, Nordentoft M, et al. Exploring regional variation in antipsychotic coprescribing practice: a Danish questionnaire survey. J Clin Psychiatry 2010;71(11):1457–64.

120. Johnson DA, Wright NF. Drug prescribing for schizophrenic out-patients on depot injections. Repeat surveys over 18 years. Br J Psychiatry 1990;156:827–34.

121. Kreyenbuhl J, Valenstein M, McCarthy JF, et al. Long-term combination antipsychotic treatment in VA patients with schizophrenia. Schizophr Res 2006;84(1):90–9.

122. Baandrup L, Sørensen J, Lublin H, et al. Association of antipsychotic polypharmacy with health service cost: a register-based cost analysis. Eur J Health Econ 2012;13(3):355–63.

123. Valuck RJ, Morrato EH, Dodd S, et al. How expensive is antipsychotic polypharmacy? Experience from five US state Medicaid programs. Curr Med Res Opin 2007;23(10):2567–76.

124. Loosbrock DL, Zhao Z, Johnstone BM, et al. Antipsychotic medication use patterns and associated costs of care for individuals with schizophrenia. J Ment Health Policy Econ 2003;6(2):67–75.

125. Clark RE, Bartels SJ, Mellman TA, et al. Recent trends in antipsychotic combination therapy of schizophrenia and schizoaffective disorder: implications for state mental health policy. Schizophr Bull 2002;28(1):75–84.

126. Kumra S, Kranzler H, Gerbino-Rosen G, et al. Clozapine versus "high-dose" olanzapine in refractory early-onset schizophrenia: an open-label extension study. J Child Adolesc Psychopharmacol 2008;18(4):307–16.

127. Nielsen J, Dahm M, Lublin H, et al. Psychiatrists' attitude towards and knowledge of clozapine treatment. J Psychopharmacol 2010;24(7):965–71.

128. Correll CU. Real-life dosing with second-generation antipsychotics. J Clin Psychiatry 2005;66(12):1610–1.

129. Robinson D, Woerner MG, Pollack S, et al. Subject selection biases in clinical trials: data from a multicenter schizophrenia treatment study. J Clin Psychopharmacol 1996;16(2):170–6.

130. Hofer A, Hummer M, Huber R, et al. Selection bias in clinical trials with antipsychotics. J Clin Psychopharmacol 2000;20(6):699–702.

131. Correll CU, Kishimoto T, Nielsen J, et al. Clinical relevance of treatments for schizophrenia. Clin Ther 2011;33(12):B16–39.

132. Correll CU, Kishimoto T, Kane JM. Randomized controlled trials in schizophrenia: opportunities, limitations and novel trial designs. Dialogues Clin Neurosci 2011;13(2):155–72.

133. Kinon BJ, Kane JM, Johns C, et al. Treatment of neuroleptic-resistant schizophrenic relapse. Psychopharmacol Bull 1993;29(2):309–14.

134. Baune BT. New developments in the management of major depressive disorder and generalized anxiety disorder: role of quetiapine. Neuropsychiatr Dis Treat 2008;4(6):1181–91.

135. Hazra M, Uchida H, Sproule B, et al. Impact of feedback from pharmacists in reducing antipsychotic polypharmacy in schizophrenia. Psychiatry Clin Neurosci 2011;65(7):676–8.

136. Suzuki T, Uchida H, Tanaka KF, et al. Revising polypharmacy to a single antipsychotic regimen for patients with chronic schizophrenia. Int J Neuropsychopharmacol 2004;7(2):133–42.

137. Essock SM, Schooler NR, Stroup TS, et al. Effectiveness of switching from antipsychotic polypharmacy to monotherapy. Am J Psychiatry 2011;168(7):702–8.

138. Essali A, Al-Haj Haasan N, Li C, et al. Clozapine versus typical neuroleptic medication for schizophrenia. Cochrane Database Syst Rev 2009;(1):CD000059.
139. Leucht S, Komossa K, Rummel-Kluge C, et al. A meta-analysis of head-to-head comparisons of second-generation antipsychotics in the treatment of schizophrenia. Am J Psychiatry 2009;166(2):152–63.

Cognitive Enhancement in Schizophrenia

Pharmacological and Cognitive Remediation Approaches

Philip D. Harvey, PhD[a],*, Christopher R. Bowie, PhD[b]

KEYWORDS

- Schizophrenia • Cognitive enhancement • Pharmacological treatment

KEY POINTS

Practice Recommendations

- Patients with schizophrenia benefit from cognitive remediation, and their everyday functioning has been shown to improve with concurrent psychosocial interventions. Neither treatment alone seems to have similar efficacy.
- Cognitive remediation causes neurobiological changes and has evidence of biological validity. The changes that occur do suggest evidence of activation of brain-repair mechanisms.
- Anticholinergic medications negate the benefit of cognitive remediation and other learning-based interventions. Their use should be kept to a minimum.
- Pharmacological compounds commonly used as off-label add-on therapies for cognitive enhancement (cholinesterase inhibitors; mood stabilizers) have no demonstrated efficacy.
- Modafinil appears to have benefits in reversing the effects of sleep deprivation on cognition, and amphetamine improves cognition. Both have safety concerns, with amphetamine being more risky.

INTRODUCTION

Cognitive impairments in schizophrenia are a major contributor to the inability to function adequately in everyday life that is commonly seen in people with schizophrenia.

Disclosures: Dr Harvey has served as a consultant to Abbott Labs, Genentech, Johnson and Johnson, Novartis, Pharma Neuro Boost, Roche Pharma, Shire, and Sunovion Pharma in the past year. Dr Bowie has served on a scientific advisory board and as a consultant for Abbott Pharmaceuticals in the past year.
[a] Department of Psychiatry and Behavioral Sciences, University of Miami Miller School of Medicine, 1120 North West 14th Street, Suite 1450, Miami, FL 33136, USA; [b] Department of Psychology, Queens University, 62 Arch Street, Kingston, ON K0H 1S0, Canada
* Corresponding author.
E-mail address: philipdharvey1@cs.com

Psychiatr Clin N Am 35 (2012) 683–698
http://dx.doi.org/10.1016/j.psc.2012.06.008
0193-953X/12/$ – see front matter © 2012 Elsevier Inc. All rights reserved.

There has been substantial attention paid to cognitive impairments as a determinant of these functional deficits, and our understanding of the subtleties of the relationships between cognitive impairments and disability has been refined considerably as a result. This article discusses the measurement of cognition in schizophrenia, its role as a determinant of disability, and treatment efforts to date, including both pharmacological and behavioral interventions, and critical components of effective treatments that lead to improvements in everyday outcomes. A detailed discussion is presented on how functioning can and should be measured in the office when patients with schizophrenia are receiving treatment.

There is no need for another detailed review of the nature of deficits in people with schizophrenia. Many such reviews have appeared,[1,2] and there have been no substantial new findings for cognitive functioning assessed with clinical neuropsychological tests. The new developments have been in the area of the creation and adoption of a consensus method for the assessment of cognitive functioning in treatment studies, and in the increased appreciation for the need for the assessment of functional skills in the prediction of everyday outcomes, as well as new developments in the basic neuroscience of cognition. As these developments are not yet ready for use in treatment studies, a detailed review here of such findings is deferred.

COGNITIVE ENHANCEMENT AS A THERAPEUTIC TARGET

Almost 10 years ago the senior leadership at the US National Institute of Mental Health (NIMH), Hyman and Fenton,[3] set the stage for the development of consensus cognitive assessments for clinical treatment studies aimed at cognitive enhancement in schizophrenia. This initiative led to the award of a contract for a project entitled Measurement and Treatment Research for Improving Cognition in Schizophrenia (MATRICS[4]). This MATRICS initiative led to consensus meetings, literature reviews, and the eventual selection of a consensus cognitive assessment battery (ie, the MATRICS consensus cognitive battery: MCCB[5–7]) endorsed by academia and regulatory agencies as the standard performance-based cognitive assessment measure for treatment outcomes studies. This battery is presented in **Box 1**, and the premises on which this battery is based are presented.

In the development process of the MCCB, the initial consensus was that cognitive functioning in general was composed of separable cognitive domains and that schizophrenia was marked by the presence of impairments in most of these domains. Thus, the development process was based on the initial selection of important domains of functioning (eg, verbal memory, processing speed, and so forth) and then selection of representative and psychometrically useful exemplars of these domains. It was further designated that unless otherwise specified by the entity conducting the study, the outcome measure would be the composite, which is an unweighted average of the cognitive domains. Thus, despite the focus on selection of tests from domains, global cognitive functioning is the default treatment target.

Functional Capacity

A concurrent development to the MCCB was the increased interest in the identification of the specific functional skills that underlie everyday functioning. Performance-based assessments have been developed that are targeted at the skills required to engage in community activities, social activities, and vocational activities.[8] While there has been a long-term interest in social competence dating back to behavior therapists in the 1970s, interest in everyday living and vocational skills developed in the 1980s and flowered in the early 2000s. Both comprehensive and abbreviated assessments

---

Box 1
MATRICS consensus cognitive battery

Speed of Processing:

    Category fluency

    Brief Assessment of Cognition in Schizophrenia (BACS)—symbol-coding

    Trail Making A

Attention/Vigilance

    Continuous Performance Test—Identical Pairs (CPT-IP)

Working Memory

    Verbal: University of Maryland—letter-number span

    Nonverbal: Wechsler Memory Scale (WMS) III—spatial span

Verbal Learning

    Hopkins Verbal Learning Test (HVLT)—Revised

Visual Learning

    Brief Visuospatial Memory Test (BVMT)—Revised

Reasoning and Problem Solving

    Neuropsychological Assessment Battery (NAB)—mazes

Social Cognition

Meyer-Solovay-Caruso Emotional Intelligence Test

---

have been developed that examine performance in areas such as shopping, cooking, traveling, and financial management.[9,10] These assessments have been found to be quite strongly related to cognitive performance, and may actually be an intermediate step between neurocognition and everyday functioning.

As reviewed by Leifker and colleagues,[11] the correlation between measures of functional capacity aimed at everyday living skills and performance on a variety of neurocognitive measures is quite high ($r > 0.60$) and extraordinarily consistent. Several studies published since that review have found the same correlations. Further, 3 separate large-scale (N > 200) studies identifying the predictors of real-world functioning as rated by highly knowledgable informants have found that functional capacity measures are more strongly related to everyday outcomes than performance on neuropsychological tests.[12,13,14] These data suggest a model whereby neurocognitive abilities influence the ability to perform the functional skills required to succeed in everyday activities. The real-world outcomes have been shown to be influenced by symptoms and opportunities as well as by cognitive and functional abilities. The amount of variance accounted for in activities such as vocational and residential outcomes has been in the vicinity of 40% to 50%, which means that there are substantial influences yet to be identified.

Social Cognition

This concept refers to the cognitively demanding skills that are required for socially relevant activities.[15] These skills include the perception, processing, and interpretation of emotional displays, and the ability to infer intentions and judge facial and nonfacial gestures. Although there are some methodological limitations to date in the study of social cognition, these are important abilities. Meta-analyses have shown that social cognition and neurocognition are minimally related to each other[16] and that social cognition is more consistently associated with social outcomes than is neurocognition.[17] These findings are consistent with some of the authors' most recent work, in which neurocognition was found to be minimally associated with social outcomes when other factors, such as negative symptoms, were considered.[18]

Social cognition is represented in the MCCB, but with only a single test that is aimed at understanding complex social transactions. Research has suggested that this test, the Meyer-Solovey-Caruso Emotional IntelligenceTest,[19] does not correlate particularly highly with other measures on the MCCB, as would be expected on the basis of the meta-analysis[16] by Ventura and colleagues.[20] Thus, treatment of social cognition would likely not be assured by successful treatment of cognitive impairments, and the information available on the treatment of social cognition is examined separately herein.

COGNITIVE ENHANCEMENT RESEARCH DESIGN

As described later, there are potential interventions for cognition and functional capacity that are delivered through both pharmacological and behavioral methods. As result of the MATRICS process, a consensus research design has been endorsed by the US Food and Drug Administration (FDA). This design would apply to studies of pharmacological cognitive enhancement as well as to software or other computer programs aimed at computerized cognitive remediation. The FDA issues approvals for medications and medical devices for specific uses. The primary criteria for FDA approval of an "indication" for a drug or device are evidence that the drug or device is "safe" and "effective." While psychiatric conditions are primarily defined by their symptoms in the DSM (*Diagnostic and Statistical Manual of Mental Disorders*), other aspects of these illnesses often do not benefit from treatments approved for primary indications. Clear examples of this disconnect are psychosis and agitation in dementia and cognitive impairments in schizophrenia. The FDA has previously allowed attempts to develop a treatment indication for these features, as long as it could be proved that these other features were not improved by standard, previously approved treatments. Referred to as a concern about "pseudospecificity," this means that a treatment cannot be approved for the specific treatment of an illness feature already approved for treatment. An example would be an attempt to seek approval for a treatment for "hallucinations in schizophrenia," when the same treatment is already approved for the treatment of schizophrenia (which includes hallucinations).

Beyond these issues, the FDA has in the past required that treatments aimed at cognitive enhancement be supported by evidence of clinical benefit beyond improvements in performance-based assessments. These so-called coprimary measures in studies of dementia typically have included caregiver assessments of the detectable benefits of cognitive-enhancing treatments, collected in double-blind trials.[21] Although one may ask whether our society might benefit if similar expectations were imposed for approval of treatments such as collagen, botox, and breast implants, similar standards to those of Alzheimer disease have been imposed for the approval of cognitive-enhancement agents in schizophrenia, with the functional capacity measures already described expected to be commonly used. Similarly, the FDA has imposed a 6-month duration requirement for the active phase of "acute" treatment trials for cognitive enhancement in schizophrenia, despite the fact that antipsychotics have been approved in 6-week clinical trials and that an atypical antipsychotic medication (aripiprazole) received approval for treatment-resistant depression on the basis of two 3-week double-blind trials.[22]

As described earlier, the MATRICS initiative realized several critical outcomes from this project. A consensus research design was proposed[23] and then revised after 5 years' experience.[24] At present, therefore, there is a path toward approval for cognitive-enhancing medications and devices in schizophrenia. **Box 2** presents the critical features of this regulatory pathway. Included are patient populations, trial design and duration, and primary and coprimary outcomes measures. There are several critical corollary features of this design. Functional improvements in the real world are not required for approval of a treatment, acknowledging that this seems unlikely in a short-term study. No a priori magnitude of improvement is specified, other than significantly greater improvement than placebo in an add-on design. The typical research design aimed at indications for the treatment of cognitive impairments is an add-on polypharmacy approach. This design would result in interpretable results from a clinical trial, in that active treatment added to standing treatment compared with placebo treatment on 2 separate outcomes measures that would only have to achieve an a priori level of statistical significance of $P<.05$ each.

COGNITIVE REMEDIATION

Behavioral treatments for cognitive impairments in schizophrenia have a long history, originating with behavioral modification techniques and borrowing largely from the drill-and-practice restorative philosophy behind neuropsychological rehabilitation for traumatic brain injury. In recent years the number of published studies has accelerated and reflects not only a refinement in treatment techniques, but an expansion of the outcomes measured. These strategies, variously referred to as cognitive remediation therapy, cognitive enhancement, or cognitive training (among others), have many similarities but have branched out to differ quite substantially with regard to the emphasis on the specific techniques.

Although contemporary approaches differ, a commonality includes the recognition that to be viewed as a successful intervention, the treatment-related changes in cognition should manifest in improved everyday functioning and/or quality of life. Earlier efforts faced criticism that the treatments were simply "teaching the test," and the burden of proof for real cognitive change would be evidence for an underlying change

---

Box 2
NIMH, FDA, academia, and pharmaceutical industry consensus entry criteria for cognitive enhancement interventions

Criteria for Enrollment into Cognitive Enhancement Trials

Diagnosis of schizophrenia

No major change in antipsychotic medications for at least 6 weeks before screening

No medications that can influence cognitive functioning:

Anticholinergics

Amphetamines

L-dopa

No hospitalization for psychiatric illness for at least 8 weeks before screening

Moderately severe or less (<5) severity rating on selected Positive And Negative Syndrome Scale (PANSS) positive scale items at both screening and baseline

No evidence of current major depression

to neurobiological functioning or generalization to change in everyday behavior. In the past 10 years new treatments provide substantial evidence for neurobiological mechanisms of action as well as improvements in functioning.

The variety of treatment procedures for cognitive remediation underscores the excitement in the field but also reveals its developmental stage as refined but still evolving. Some approaches rely heavily on a therapist involvement to modify strategies and facilitate the bridging of cognitive gains to everyday behavior exercises.[25] Drill-and-practice exercises have been used with[26] and without[27] computer software to present and modify the complexity of stimuli. Treatment programs can be quite labor intensive, and may include several noncognitive and social-cognitive aspects.[28,29] Improvements in functioning have also been found with compensatory strategies. These techniques place the point of treatment not on modification of the individual's abilities but on the alteration of the environment and/or adaptive technologies with which an individual's cognitive strengths and weaknesses interact.[30,31] Most recently, neuroplasticity-based treatment has emerged (this term should not confuse the fact that all the aforementioned treatments presuppose that treatments operate on the malleability of the organism's brain) for schizophrenia.[32] The philosophy behind this treatment is that manipulation of early sensory processing is critical in improving the signal-to-noise ratio in schizophrenia. Until very recently there were no direct-comparison studies on the type, duration, or style of therapy, which has perhaps slowed replication and widespread clinical dissemination of cognitive remediation. The only direct comparison published to date found more robust improvements in neurobiological (M50, a measure of sensory gating) and neurocognitive abilities with early sensory training compared with an older and graphically underwhelming computer software package that was not specifically developed for schizophrenia.[33] As the field continues to advance, more studies that examine which strategies work, and for whom, will be a priority.

Evidence for Neurobiological Change with Cognitive Remediation

Although cognitive remediation studies appeared in the literature in the 1960s, it has been only 10 years since Wykes and colleagues[34] first demonstrated changes in brain function for schizophrenia patients who received cognitive remediation. Following 40 hours of paper-and-pencil drill-and-practice techniques coupled with strategic monitoring, patients had increased activation in the frontal cortex during a verbal working memory task. This important study provided evidence to deflect the early criticisms that cognitive impairments in schizophrenia, which were believed to represent a stable or progressive encephalopathy, were not truly modifiable but simply the artifact of teaching a person how to take a test better.

In a series of recent studies by Vinogradov and colleagues, the neuroplasticity-based cognitive remediation strategies that target early auditory processing produced normalization in serum levels of brain-derived neurotrophic factor, which provides an indirect measurement of neuroplasticity,[35] and a normalization in electrophysiological markers of auditory stimuli.[36] Further evidence for the validity of cognitive remediation in producing neurobiological changes comes from the limited gains that are found as a function of genes associated with degradation of dopamine[37] and anticholinergic medication usage, which inhibits new learning.[38] One of the most encouraging findings for long-term prognosis comes from a study by Eack and colleagues.[39] This study used a 2-year social and neurocognitive training program and found that, compared with a placebo group, the treatment effectively staved off structural gray matter loss in brain regions thought to be critical to the neuropathophysiology of schizophrenia. Longer-term outcomes for those treated early in the illness will be a critical further step toward evaluating the cost-effectiveness of the intervention.

The biological mechanisms underpinning cognitive remediation have been an important finding and have occurred alongside another fundamentally important series of studies: the transfer of cognitive gains with cognitive remediation to changes in functioning. Early studies were criticized for failing to demonstrate effectiveness that would be indexed by this generalization of gains to everyday functional behavior changes. As mentioned earlier, concomitant changes in functioning following cognitive improvements might be an unrealistic criterion for many individuals with schizophrenia. This neurodevelopmental disease is associated with cognitive impairments well before the onset of psychosis, often disrupting opportunities for engaging in and learning the complex behavior sets that are required for successful academic achievement, occupational success, social skills, and independent living. Unlike traumatic brain injury, whereby it is hoped that neuropsychological rehabilitation will restore the cognitive functions necessary for the patient to return to his or her level of functioning, people with schizophrenia often have impaired functioning before and throughout the illness Thus, it is difficult to imagine how treatments that focus on cognitive impairments but do not take a skills-training approach would manifest in real-world behavior change. A recent meta-analysis supports this notion. McGurk and colleagues[40] found larger effect-size changes in distal measures such as social functioning when cognitive remediation was used within a larger psychosocial treatment framework. The very small and nonsignificant effects on functioning when cognitive remediation is used in isolation speak to the idea that cognitive improvements occur, and indeed might be quite robust, but the likelihood of these changes transferring to real-world functional behavior is greatly diminished and perhaps not likely if the patient is not engaged in other activities that create an environment where he or she has the opportunity to learn and use new skills.

WHAT ARE THE SOCIETAL AND HEALTH CARE IMPLICATIONS OF TREATING COGNITION?

Schizophrenia is an exceptionally costly disease to the individual and to society. Loss of productivity and disability results in billions of dollars in indirect costs each year.[41] Treatments that enhance cognition could reduce this burden if they result in more independence in living and vocational productivity. Several recent studies suggest that this might be the case. When cognitive remediation is used within the context of vocational rehabilitation services, patients have improved outcomes that include reduced time to employment and greater maintenance of jobs, earning higher wages, and working more hours.[42,43] Future research might further examine the role that cognitive remediation plays with other costs such as independent living and the use of intensive clinical services. With clinically meaningful effects that generalize to improvements in everyday functions, cognitive remediation therapy is poised for widespread use in clinical environments.

Pharmacological Cognitive Enhancement

Target selection for pharmacological cognitive enhancement is complicated and has been reviewed elsewhere.[44,45] Neurotransmission is a complex phenomenon and, despite remarkable advances in neuroscience, is still only partially understood. Developing targets for cognitive enhancement requires the decision as to whether to attempt to increase activity by stimulation of receptors (agonist), reducing activity by blocking receptors (antagonist), modifying the endogenous processes of downregulation of activity, and through either stimulating autoreceptors, blocking reuptake (transport), or reducing degradation of transmitters. Although many of these actions would seem to lead to the same result, the complexities of neurotransmission suggest that the situation is not that simple. For instance, stimulating serotonin receptors directly has no impact on depression, but increasing serotonin activity through blocking transport is a very effective antidepressant strategy (serotonin reuptake inhibition).

There have been multiple recent studies on pharmacological cognitive enhancement, with somewhat disappointing results. **Table 1** presents a list of the studies that have had negative results thus far. These studies are clearly negative, with an occasional minimal signal for cognitive change that would not meet the FDA standard for being meaningful. Some recently promising results are reviewed here, and possible reasons for their lack of effects discussed. See Harvey[45] for a detailed review of those previous treatment failures.

One strategy with some promise for efficacy has been implemented to examine medications that otherwise regulate glutamatergic activity. For instance, lamotrigine, an approved anticonvulsant medication, reduces glutamatergic release and may adjust glutamatergic tone. Lamotrigine pretreatment has been shown[59] to reduce the adverse effects of ketamine administration in healthy individuals. Several studies have reported beneficial effects of lamotrigine on symptoms in people with schizophrenia (eg, Ref.[60]), so an assessment of its cognitive effects seems reasonable.

In 2 highly similar clinical trials reported in a single article, Goff and colleagues[61] found that double-blind placebo-controlled treatment with lamotrigine was possibly associated with cognitive improvements. In the 2 studies the cognitive composite score was improved by $z = 0.58$ and $z = 0.47$ in the lamotrigine group, with corresponding improvements in the placebo group of $z = 0.21$ and $z = 0.20$. The effect of treatment compared with placebo was statistically significant in one study and was not in the other. These data suggest improvements beyond placebo that are

Table 1			
Negative results by mechanism of action[a]			
Mechanism	**Specific Drug**	**Ref.**	**Notes**
Cholinergic			
Muscarinic	Donepezil	46	Worse than placebo
	Rivastigmine	47	Small sample
	Galantamine	48	Some domains improved
Nicotinic	DMX-B	49	Crossover design
	AZD3480	50	—
Glutamatergic			
NMDA	Glycine, D-cycloserine	51	Large-scale study
AMPA	AMPA-Kine	52	—
Noradrenergic	Guanfacine	53	Some domains improved
	Atomoxatine	54	Brain activity changed
GABA	MK0877	55	—
Serotonergic	Tandospirone	56	—
	Buspirone	57	—
Cannabinoid	Rimonabant	58	—

Abbreviations: AMPA, 2-amino-3-(5-methyl-3-oxo-1,2-oxazol-4-yl)propanoic acid; GABA, γ-aminobutyric acid; NMDA, N-methyl-D-aspartic acid.
[a] When multiple studies produced similar results, the study with the largest sample size is presented.

consistent with a small effect size. Improvements of this magnitude may not be clinically significant, but the relative importance of different degrees of cognitive improvements is not well understood at present.

Modafinil

Modafinil is an alertness-promoting medication with a mechanism of action that may be distinct from amphetamine, but likely still involves monoaminergic mechanisms. Multiple studies have provided information regarding modafinil that is partially supportive of cognitive-enhancing properties. As reviewed by Morein-Zamir and colleagues,[62] there are more strong findings in areas of executive functioning and attentional processes than in enhancement of memory functions. Furthermore, evidence of heterogeneity of response is clearly evident, with less severe cognitive impairment and several different genetic polymorphisms predicting better response. Cognitive enhancement in healthy individuals is also reported with modafinil, but these improvements are much more substantial in individuals who are sleep deprived at baseline.[63] A further issue with modafinil is the sporadic case reports of exacerbation of psychosis in patients with schizophrenia who are taking the compound. It is not clear whether these are direct medication effects or if they are associated with misuse of the medication, which could then lead to sleep deprivation and associated adverse events.

GABA-Based Interventions

γ-Aminobutyric acid (GABA)-modulating compounds have been used for years as anxiolytics and these compounds, such as lorazepam, are agonists at the $GABA_A$ benzodiazepine site. In a study[64] that used both cognitive assessments and functional magnetic resonance imaging evaluations, a small sample of schizophrenia patients was compared with a similar-sized sample of healthy controls (n = 11) while receiving lorazepam, placebo, or flumazenil, an antagonist at this same GABA site. The primary cognitive outcomes measure was the n-back working memory test, a commonly used test of working memory with maintenance, manipulation, and updating requirements.

In this study, flumazenil was associated with improved n-back performance under conditions of increased processing load in people with schizophrenia, and simultaneously led to a normalized pattern of cortical activity associated with load response. By contrast, lorazepam led to worsened n-back performance compared with placebo. Healthy individuals performed more poorly than those taking placebo in both active pharmacological conditions. These data, albeit in a small sample and with a single cognitive test, suggest cognitive performance improvements and changes in brain activation compared with placebo and treatments that enhance GABA activity. Furthermore, the effect is not a generalized one, because healthy individuals were adversely affected by both pharmacological manipulations. Convergence of cortical activation changes and cognitive task performance stand in contrast to previous studies of noradrenergic and cholinergic medications wherein brain activation was changed but behavioral performance was unaffected. This study[64] seems quite promising, and requires replication with a larger sample size and a more comprehensive cognitive assessment battery. It must be noted that other GABAergic compounds have not met with much success in large-scale trials.

Nontransmitter Interventions

Neuroscience research has identified pharmacological compounds that have effects other than transmitter manipulation/modulation, including compounds that have other central nervous system (CNS) effects. These agents have been the result of long-term interest in the development of compounds that promote neurogenesis or other brain-growth processes, For example, davunetide is a neuroactive peptide that appears to promote neurite outgrowth in animal models. Because postmortem findings of neurite abnormalities are quite consistent, this appears to be a potentially promising intervention. In a single study examining davunetide in people with schizophrenia, Javitt and colleagues[65] found that intranasal administration of 1 of 2 doses of davunitide led to statistically significant improvements in the University of California San Diego Performance-Based Skills Assessment score (UPSA) compared with placebo treatment. The other, higher dose was not associated with improvements in the UPSA and neither dose improved the MCCB compared with placebo. However, this study had a very small sample size and several of the MCCB domains improved to an extent that would have been significant with even a modestly larger sample (n = 50). The effect size for UPSA change was d = 0.74, which is a large and potentially clinically meaningful effect, and the effect size for changes on the MCCB was d = 0.4, which is moderate, close to statistically significant, and potentially clinically meaningful. As interventions such as davunitide bypass some of the shortcomings of transmitter-based interventions (as described later), this may be a promising compound and even more promising cognitive enhancement strategy.

Why the Negative Results?

As can be seen in this review, with some minor exceptions the pharmacological cognitive-enhancement studies to date have been negative. These results span multiple targets and have used compounds that are known to be effective in treating cognitive impairments in other conditions such as attention-deficit disorders, people with schizotypal personality disorder, and healthy individuals. Several possibilities for these results are reviewed as follows.

- Cognitive Impairment is not modifiable by pharmacological means.
- The use of concurrent medications may interfere with the effects of cognitive enhancers.
- Dosing of add-on compounds may be critically important for their efficacy.
- Delivery and pharmacokinetics may lead to problems in administration.
- Neurotransmitters may not be the viable target for cognitive enhancement.

Cognitive impairment is not modifiable by pharmacological means

There is evidence of progressive cortical volume loss in people with schizophrenia,[66] which include progressive loss of gray matter and reduced growth of white matter, particularly in cases with multiple exacerbations.[67] It could be argued that the progressive volumetric changes constrain the ability of pharmacological treatments to induce a benefit. However, the strongest argument against the notion that progressive brain changes preclude cognitive enhancement is that cognitive remediation has been shown to produce cognitive changes and lead to relevant real-world functional improvements, as already discussed.

The use of concurrent medications may interfere with the effects of cognitive enhancers

Patients with schizophrenia are typically treated with antipsychotic medications. The entire spectrum of effects of these medications is not wholly understood, and it is possible that in some way antipsychotic medications alter the effects of add-on pharmacological cognitive enhancers. This problem is a substantial one, because symptomatic relapse associated with discontinuation of antipsychotic medication poses a considerable clinical problem, so simply suggesting that potential cognitive-enhancing medications be tested or used in patients who are not receiving medications is not practical. There are several ways by which antipsychotic medications could interfere with the effects of add-on pharmacotherapy. The first is through their common mechanism of antipsychotic action: dopamine D_2 receptor blockade. The high levels of reduction of activity required to lead to clinical response following exacerbations[68] might lead to reductions in plasticity of other receptor systems that interact with this receptor subtype, including cholinergic, glutamatergic, and serotonergic systems. A second possibility is through the joint activity of atypical medications at the 5-HT_{2A} receptor system. All of these medications blockade this receptor subtype to a greater or lesser extent, and the serotonergic system is intimately involved in the regulation of multiple other neurotransmitters. A third and even more challenging possibility is the additional pharmacological effects of antipsychotic medications in some way contributing to these negative results. While all atypical antipsychotics share serotonin-dopamine antagonism, they vary markedly in their activity at other receptors, including muscarinic cholinergic, serotonergic (including 2_a, 1_a, 7, and 6_a), adrenergic, and histaminergic receptors, with a mix of agonist and antagonist effects.

Dosing of add-on compounds may be critically important for their efficacy

Although medication doses for treatments that are in current clinical use for other conditions (guanfacine, cholinesterase inhibitors, atomoxetine) are established for the original illnesses, it is not clear whether the same doses would be required to enhance cognition in people with schizophrenia. Many of these treatments have dose-dependent side effects (eg, nausea, hypotension) that limit the potential for dose increases in the original target populations, and concurrent antipsychotic medications may either suppress or exacerbate some of these side effects. As most neurotransmitter activity is regulated by multiple other systems, it is hard to estimate a priori what the potential dose of medications introduced into an already altered biological system should be, because of antipsychotic effects.

Delivery and pharmacokinetics may lead to problems in administration

Some drugs, such as the dopamine D1 agonist SKF-38393 that has been shown to be very effective in studies of animals using direct administration into the CNS (eg, Ref.[69]), may not cross the blood-brain barrier when administered peripherally. The consequence is that it is not currently possible to deliver a definitive, specific D1 agonist directly into the brain, Other potentially effective cognitive enhancers either have short half-lives (α7 nicotinic agonists) or lead to receptor sensitization. As a result, some treatments that have solid basic science support (D1 and α7-agonists) have proved difficult to develop into medications that would be useful for treatments. New innovations, such as identification and development of additional compounds, including specific precursors or prodrugs for D1 agonists that cross the blood-brain barrier or compounds that provide allosteric modulation of cholinergic receptors, may be required.

Neurotransmitters may not be the viable target for cognitive enhancement

Neurotransmitter manipulations have the potential to influence cognition, as shown in multiple previous studies. This intervention strategy, however, is predicated on the idea that neuronal targets are intact and available. This situation has already proved to be problematic in Alzheimer disease, where cholinergic interventions may be handicapped by the widespread loss of cholinergic neurons by the time the intervention is delivered. Similar problems may exist in schizophrenia, where abnormalities in cortical structure, circuit connectivity, and axonal/neuronal integrity could possibly reduce the beneficial effects of receptor stimulation. Behavioral interventions may actually have their effect through altering CNS circuitry or connectivity across multiple linked transmitter systems.[70,71] If this was found to be the case, interventions aimed at neurites, circuits, and white matter may provide a more effective intervention strategy, and these interventions may not be sensitive to the effects of a single transmitter system. The case of davunetide (see earlier discussion) is a perfect example of an intervention that has potentially direct effects on brain structure and function provides a signal of a magnitude not seen in studies of medications with known beneficial effects.

COGNITIVE REMEDIATION AS A PLATFORM FOR PHARMACOLOGIC STUDIES

It is possible that many of the experimental pharmacologic interventions will be of only minimal benefit when patients are evaluated in the context of their habitual low level of cognitive stimulation. Part of the explanation for why clinical trials testing the efficacy of cognitive-enhancing medications have so far been largely unsuccessful may be that patients in these trials are not provided with substantive opportunity to use the cognitive benefit that they may have acquired during the drug-treatment study. Thus, analogous to the need for physical exercise in an individual who takes steroids to increase muscle mass, schizophrenia patients in pharmacological intervention trials may require systematic cognitive training to "exercise" any new-found cognitive potential they may have acquired from drug treatment.[72]

Cognitive remediation may provide an excellent platform for enriching the cognitive environment of patients engaged in pharmacologic trials to improve cognition. As noted earlier, cognitive remediation produces medium to large effect-size improvements in cognitive performance and, when combined with psychiatric rehabilitation, also improves functional outcomes (see Ref.[73] for a review). Patients find these programs to be enjoyable and engaging, and they have been linked with increases in participant self-esteem. Ongoing treatment with cognitive remediation may thus provide schizophrenia patients with the necessary cognitive enrichment and motivation to demonstrate the true potential of effective cognitive enhancement with pharmacologic intervention. Recent work suggests that these methods are feasible in clinical trials even at sites without cognitive remediation experience.[74] These results suggest that clinical delivery of cognitive-enhancement treatments may be feasible in many different clinical service systems.

SUMMARY

Cognitive remediation combined with psychosocial interventions improves everyday functioning in people with schizophrenia. Similar consistent, positive results have not been shown with pharmacological interventions. However, studies of combined pharmacological/psychosocial interventions have not been completed. Although pharmacological cognitive enhancement to date has been largely negative, new compounds and research designs are on the horizon. Combined pharmacological and cognitive enhancement intervention, with concurrent psychosocial interventions, appears to be the therapy of the future.

REFERENCES

1. Gold JM, Harvey PD. Cognitive deficits in schizophrenia. Psychiatr Clin North Am 1993;16:295–312.
2. Bowie CR, Harvey PD. Cognition in schizophrenia: impairment, determinants, and functional importance. Psychiatr Clin North Am 2005;28:613–33.

3. Hyman SE, Fenton WS. Medicine. What are the right targets for psychopharmacology? Science 2003;299:350–1.

4. Marder SR, Fenton W. Measurement and Treatment Research to Improve Cognition in Schizophrenia: NIMH MATRICS initiative to support the development of agents for improving cognition in schizophrenia. Schizophr Res 2004;72:5–9.

5. Nuechterlein KH, Green MF, Kern RS, et al. The MATRICS consensus cognitive battery, part 1: test selection, reliability, and validity. Am J Psychiatry 2008;165:203–13.

6. Kern RS, Nuechterlein KH, Green MF, et al. The MATRICS consensus cognitive battery: part 2. Co-norming and standardization. Am J Psychiatry 2008;165:214–20.

7. Green MF, Nuechterlein KH, Kern RS, et al. Functional co-primary measures for clinical trials in schizophrenia: results from the MATRICS Psychometric and Standardization Study. Am J Psychiatry 2008;165:221–8.

8. Moore DJ, Palmer BW, Patterson TL, et al. A review of performance-based measures of everyday functioning. J Psychiatr Res 2007;41:97–118.

9. Patterson TL, Goldman S, McKibbin CL, et al. UCSD performance-based skills assessment: development of a new measure of everyday functioning for severely mentally ill adults. Schizophr Bull 2001;27:235–45.

10. Heaton RK, Marcotte TD, Mindt MR, et al. The impact of HIV-associated neuropsychological impairment on everyday functioning. J Int Neuropsychol Soc 2004;10:317–31.

11. Leifker FR, Patterson TL, Heaton RK, et al. Validating measures of real-world outcome: the results of the VALERO expert survey and RAND Panel. Schizophr Bull 2011;37:334–43.

12. Bowie CR, Leung WW, Reichenberg A, et al. Predicting schizophrenia patients' real world behavior with specific neuropsychological and functional capacity measures. Biological Psychiatry 2008;63:505–11.

13. Bowie CR, Depp C, McGrath JA, et al. Prediction of real-world functional disability in chronic mental disorders: a comparison of schizophrenia and bipolar disorder. American Journal of Psychiatry 2010;167:1116–24.

14. Sabbag S, Twamley EW, Vella L, et al. Assessing everyday functioning in schizophrenia: not all informants seem equally informative. Schizophrenia Research 2011;131:250–5.

15. Harvey PD, Penn D. Social cognition: the key factor predicting social outcome in people with schizophrenia? Psychiatry (Edgmont) 2010;7:41–4.

16. Eack SM, Pogue-Geile MF, Greeno CG, et al. Evidence of factorial variance of the Mayer-Salovey-Caruso Emotional Intelligence Test across schizophrenia and normative samples. Schizophr Res 2009;114:105–9.

17. Fett AK, Viechtbauer W, Dominguez MD, et al. The relationship between neurocognition and social cognition with functional outcomes in schizophrenia: a meta-analysis. Neurosci Biobehav Rev 2011;35:573–88.

18. Leifker FR, Bowie CR, Harvey PD. The determinants of everyday outcomes in schizophrenia: influences of cognitive impairment, clinical symptoms, and functional capacity. Schizophr Res 2009;115:82–7.

19. Mayer JD, Salovey P, Caruso DR. Mayer-Salovey-Caruso Emotional Intelligence Test (MSCEIT) user's manual. Toronto: MHS Publishers; 2002.

20. Ventura J, Wood RC, Hellemann GS. Symptom domains and neurocognitive functioning can help differentiate social cognitive processes in schizophrenia: a meta-analysis. Schizophr Bull, in press.

21. Laughren T. A regulatory perspective on psychiatric syndromes in Alzheimer's disease. Am J Geriatr Psychiatry 2001;9:340–5.

22. Kahn A. Current evidence for aripiprazole as augmentation therapy in major depressive disorder. Expert Rev Neurother 2008;8:1435–47.

23. Buchanan RW, Davis M, Goff D, et al. A summary of the FDA-NIMH-MATRICS workshop on clinical trial design for neurocognitive drugs for schizophrenia. Schizophr Bull 2005;31:5–19.

24. Buchanan RW, Keefe RS, Umbricht D, et al. The FDA-NIMH-MATRICS guidelines for clinical trial design of cognitive-enhancing drugs: what do we know 5 years later? Schizophr Bull 2011;37:1209–17.

25. Medalia A, Revheim N, Herlands T. Cognitive remediation for psychological disorders, therapist guide. New York: Oxford University Press; 2009.

26. Bell B, Bryson G, Wexler BE. Cognitive remediation of working memory deficits: durability of training effects in severely impaired and less severely impaired schizophrenia. Acta Psychiatr Scand 2003;108:101–9.

27. Wykes T, Reeder C, Comer J, et al. The effects of neurocognitive remediation on executive processing in patients with schizophrenia. Schizophr Bull 1993;25:291–307.

28. Brenner HD, Hodel B, Roder V, et al. Treatment of cognitive dysfunction and behavioral deficits in schizophrenia. Schizophr Bull 1992;18:21–6.

29. Hogarty GE, Flesher S, Ulrich R, et al. Cognitive enhancement therapy for schizophrenia: effects of a 2-year randomized trial on cognition and behavior. Arch Gen Psychiatry 2004;61:866–76.

30. Velligan DI, Diamond PM, Mintz J, et al. The use of individually tailored environmental supports to improve medication adherence and outcomes in schizophrenia. Schizophr Bull 2008;34:483–93.

31. Twamley EW, Savla GN, Zurhellen CH, et al. Development and pilot testing of a novel compensatory cognitive training intervention for people with psychosis. Am J Psychiatr Rehabil 2008;11:144–63.

32. Fisher M, Holland C, Subramaniam K, et al. Neuroplasticity-based cognitive training in schizophrenia: an interim report on effects 6 months later. Schizophr Bull 2010;36:869–79.

33. Popov T, Jordanov T, Rockstroh B, et al. Specific cognitive training normalizes auditory sensory gating in schizophrenia: a randomized trial. Biol Psychiatry 2011;69:465–71.

34. Wykes T, Brammer M, Mellers J, et al. Effects on the brain of psychological treatment: cognitive remediation therapy: functional magnetic resonance imaging in schizophrenia. Br J Psychiatry 2002;181:144–52.

35. Vinogradov S, Fisher M, Holland C, et al. Is serum brain-derived neurotrophic factor a biomarker for cognitive enhancement in schizophrenia? Biol Psychiatry 2009;66:549–53.

36. Adcock RA, Dale C, Fisher M, et al. When top-down meets bottom-up: auditory training enhances verbal memory in schizophrenia. Schizophr Bull 2009;35: 1132–41.

37. Bosia M, Bechi M, Marino E, et al. Influence of catechol-O-methyltransferase Val158Met polymorphism on neuropsychological and functional outcomes of classic rehabilitation and cognitive remediation in schizophrenia. Neurosci Lett 2007;417:271–4.

38. Vinogradov S, Fisher M, Warm H, et al. The cognitive cost of anticholinergic burden: decreased response to cognitive training in schizophrenia. Am J Psychiatry 2009;166:1055–62.

39. Eack SM, Hogarty GE, Cho RY, et al. Neuroprotective effects of cognitive enhancement therapy against gray matter loss in early schizophrenia: results from a 2-year randomized controlled trial. Arch Gen Psychiatry 2010;67:674–82.

40. McGurk SR, Twamley EW, Sitzer DI, et al. A meta-analysis of cognitive remediation in schizophrenia. Am J Psychiatry 2007;164:1791–802.
41. Wu EQ, Birnbaum HG, Shi L, et al. The economic burden of schizophrenia in the United States in 2002. J Clin Psychiatry 2005;66:1122–9.
42. McGurk SR, Mueser KT, DeRosa TJ, et al. Work, recovery, and comorbidity in schizophrenia: a randomized controlled trial of cognitive remediation. Schizophr Bull 2009;35:319–35.
43. Bell MD, Zito W, Greig T, et al. Neurocognitive enhancement therapy with vocational services: work outcomes at two-year follow-up. Schizophr Res 2008;105:18–29.
44. Geyer MA, Tamminga CA. Measurement and treatment research to improve cognition in schizophrenia: neuropharmacological aspects. Psychopharmacology 2004;174:1–2.
45. Harvey PD. Pharmacological cognitive enhancement in schizophrenia. Neuropsychol Rev 2009;19:324–35.
46. Keefe RSE, Malhotra AK, Meltzer HY, et al. Efficacy and safety of donepezil in patients with schizophrenia or schizoaffective disorder: significant placebo/practice effects in a 12-week, randomized, double-blind, placebo-controlled trial. Neuropsychopharmacology 2008;33:1217–28.
47. Sharma TS, Reed C, Aasen I, et al. Cognitive effects of adjunctive 24-week rivastigmine treatment to antipsychotics in schizophrenia: a randomized, placebo-controlled, double-blind investigation. Schizophr Res 2006;85:73–83.
48. Buchanan RW, Conley RR, Dickinson D, et al. Galantamine for the treatment of cognitive impairments in people with schizophrenia. Am J Psychiatry 2007;165:82–9.
49. Freedman R, Olincy A, Buchanan RW, et al. Initial phase 2 trial of a nicotinic agonist in schizophrenia. Am J Psychiatry 2008;165:1040–7.
50. Available at: www.astrazeneca.com/itemid4376018. Accessed December 15, 2011.
51. Buchanan RW, Javitt DC, Marder SR, et al. The cognitive and negative symptoms in schizophrenia trial (CONSIST): the efficacy of glutamatergic agents for negative symptoms and cognitive impairments. Am J Psychiatry 2007;164:1593–602.
52. Goff DC, Lamberti JS, Leon AC, et al. A placebo-controlled add-on trial of the ampakine, CX516, for cognitive deficits in schizophrenia. Neuropsychopharmacology 2008;33:465–72.
53. Friedman JI, Adler DN, Temporini HD, et al. Guanfacine treatment of cognitive impairment in schizophrenia. Neuropsychopharmacology 2001;25:402–9.
54. Friedman JI, Carpenter D, Lu J, et al. A pilot study of adjunctive atomoxetine treatment to second-generation antipsychotics for cognitive impairment in schizophrenia. J Clin Psychopharmacol 2008;28:59–63.
55. Buchanan RW, Keefe RS, Lieberman JA, et al. A randomized clinical trial of MK-0777 for the treatment of cognitive impairments in people with schizophrenia. Biol Psychiatry 2011;69:442–9.
56. Sumiyoshi T, Matsui M, Nohara S, et al. Enhancement of cognitive performance in schizophrenia by addition of tandospirone to neuroleptic treatment. Am J Psychiatry 2001;158:1722–5.
57. Sumiyoshi T, Park S, Jayathilake K, et al. Effect of buspirone, a serotonin1A partial agonist, on cognitive function in schizophrenia: a randomized, double-blind, placebo-controlled study. Schizophr Res 2007;95:158–68.
58. Boggs DL, Kelly DL, McMahon RP, et al. Rimonabant for neurocognition in schizophrenia: a 16-week double blind randomized placebo controlled trial. Schizophr Res 2012;134(2–3):207–10.
59. Anand A, Charney DS, Oren DA, et al. Attenuation of the neuropsychiatric effects of ketamine with lamotrigine. Arch Gen Psychiatry 2000;57:270–6.

60. Zoccali R, Muscatello MR, Bruno A, et al. The effect of lamotrigine augmentation of clozapine in a sample of treatment-resistant schizophrenic patients: a double-blind, placebo-controlled study. Schizophr Res 2007;93:109–16.

61. Goff DC, Keefe RSE, Citrome L, et al. Lamotrigine as add-on therapy in schizophrenia results of 2 placebo-controlled trials. J Clin Psychopharmacol 2007;27:582–9.

62. Morein-Zamir S, Turner DC, Sahakian BJ. A review of the effects of modafinil on cognition in schizophrenia. Schizophr Bull 2007;33:1298–306.

63. Minzenberg MJ, Carter CS. Modafinil: a review of neurochemical actions and effects on cognition. Neuropsychopharmacology 2008;33:1477–502.

64. Menzies L, Ooi C, Kamath S, et al. Effects of gamma-aminobutyric acid modulating drugs on working memory and brain function in patients with schizophrenia. Arch Gen Psychiatry 2007;64:156–67.

65. Javitt DC, Buchanan RW, Keefe RS, et al. Effect of the neuroprotective peptide davunetide (AL-108) on cognition and functional capacity in schizophrenia. Schizophr Res 2012;136(1–3):25–31.

66. DeLisi LE, Szulc KU, Bertisch HC, et al. Understanding structural brain changes in schizophrenia. Dialogues Clin Neurosci 2006;8:71–8.

67. Cahn W, Rais M, Stigter FP, et al. Psychosis and brain volume changes during the first five years of schizophrenia. Eur Neuropsychopharmacol 2009;19:147–51.

68. Laruelle M. Dopamine transmission in the schizophrenic brain. In: Hirsch SR, Weinberger DR, editors. Schizophrenia. Oxford (United Kingdom): Blackwell; 1999. p. 365–87.

69. Arnsten AF, Cai JX, Murphy BL, et al. Dopamine D1 receptor mechanisms in the cognitive performance of young adult and aged monkeys. Psychopharmacology 1994;116:143–51.

70. Akbarian S, Kim JJ, Potkin SG, et al. Maldistribution of interstitial neurons in the prefrontal white matter of brains of schizophrenic patients. Arch Gen Psychiatry 1996;53:425–36.

71. Lim KO, Hedehus M, Moseley M, et al. Compromised white matter tract integrity in schizophrenia inferred from diffusion tensor imaging. Arch Gen Psychiatry 1999;56:367–74.

72. Keefe RS, Vinogradov S, Medalia A, et al. Report from the Working Group Conference on multi-site trial design for cognitive remediation in schizophrenia. Schizophr Bull 2010. http://dx.doi.org/10.1093/schbul/sub010.

73. Wykes T, Huddy V, Cellard C, et al. A meta-analysis of cognitive remediation for schizophrenia: methodology and effect sizes. Am J Psychiatry 2011;168:472–85.

74. Keefe RS, Vinogradov S, Medalia A, et al. Feasibility and pilot efficacy results from the multi-site Cognitive Remediation in the Schizophrenia Trials Network (CRSTN) study. J Clin Psychiatry, in press.

Peers and Peer-Led Interventions for People with Schizophrenia

Anthony O. Ahmed, PhD*, Nancy J. Doane, PhD,
P. Alex Mabe, PhD, Peter F. Buckley, MD, Denis Birgenheir, MS,
Nada M. Goodrum, BS

KEYWORDS

- Schizophrenia • Medical versus consumer model of recovery
- Peer-led interventions • Consumer-operated services • Self-help • Peer Support
- Recovery-based care

KEY POINTS

- Peer-led interventions are innovations emerging in the spirit of the recovery movement.
- Peer-led interventions include mutual support/self-help groups, consumer-operated services, and peer support.
- There is clear impetus for peer-led intervention as these programs have grown in number in the mental health system.
- Studies suggest that peer-led interventions may be beneficial for people with schizophrenia by decreasing hospitalization risk, improving recovery attitudes, fostering engagement in traditional care, and improving social support.
- The evidence base for peer-led interventions is limited by the paucity of studies implementing strong research designs.

INTRODUCTION

Contemporary care for people with schizophrenia has evolved beyond traditional psychopharmacological and psychosocial treatments to include a host of peer-led interventions with origins in the consumer/survivor movement. Guided by the recovery model as their overarching philosophy, these interventions have grown steadily in the last 3 decades and have begun to garner enthusiasm among mental health providers. This article provides a snapshot of the nature, guiding philosophy, and empiric status of these types of interventions for people with schizophrenia.

Department of Psychiatry and Health Behavior, Georgia Health Sciences University, 997 Saint Sebastian Way, Augusta, GA 30912, USA
* Corresponding author.
E-mail address: aahmed@georgiahealth.edu

Psychiatr Clin N Am 35 (2012) 699–715
http://dx.doi.org/10.1016/j.psc.2012.06.009
0193-953X/12/$ – see front matter © 2012 Elsevier Inc. All rights reserved.
psych.theclinics.com

THE RECOVERY MODEL

The development and dissemination of psychopharmacological and psychological interventions have been the mainstays of schizophrenia research and care. Although there has been demonstrable progress in treating schizophrenia through these interventions, the overall outcome can be characterized by Sun Tzu's maxim—"winning the battle but losing the war." That is to say, traditional treatment approaches to caring for individuals with schizophrenia have had some success in the remission of symptoms, but relatively little has been gained in the individual's overall wellness, life goals, strengths, aspirations, preferences, personal growth, quality of life, empowerment, and personhood. Moreover, the focus of traditional practice has been guided primarily by a medical notion of recovery that views recovery as an end state or an outcome characterized by symptom remission, asymptomatic states, cure, and functional improvements.[1]

These criteria are objective and clinician-rated—that is, the clinician determines the individual's level of functioning and if symptoms are below threshold; however, they generally exclude the individual's own subjective experience of improvement, which may be discordant with clinician rating.[2,3] Thus those aspects of life that patients have historically valued have been largely ignored, including the resumption key social roles, responsibilities, and preferences.[4,5] It is therefore not surprising that only about 50% of individuals with severe mental illnesses who need treatment actually seek care.[6] Traditional care is characterized by high rates of nonadherence, no-show, drop-out, and treatment disengagement.[7–9]

Consumer Model Challenges the Medical Model

Within the last 3 decades, former patients, patient advocates, and many progressive practitioners have begun to challenge the medical model, including its view of schizophrenia.

- The consumer movement has encouraged the mental health system to embrace a consumer or experiential notion of recovery that underscores the subjective experience of hope, empowerment, independence, and strengths as key ingredients to adapting to illness and living a full and meaningful life despite the limitations of illness.[10–12]
- It views recovery as a nonlinear process and a journey rather than an end state or outcome that may be characterized by setbacks, but is defined by the individual's desire to continue to pursue overall wellness and a meaningful life despite setbacks.
- It has attempted to reframe psychiatric care for people with schizophrenia and other severe mental illnesses in ways that demonstrate respect for their rights as people and social justice.

Patients and patient advocates have criticized traditional care on grounds that it ignored or devalued the experiences of patients, their needs, and perspectives, and excluded from treatment planning their strengths, coping, suggestions, and interpretations. This has historically led to feelings of disenfranchisement, hopelessness, and disability on the part of patients.[13] In response to the consumer movement, the mental health arena has begun to recognize the need to give patients voices in treatment settings and to incorporate the services of peers (patients and former patients) in the care of people with schizophrenia.[14–16]

WHAT ARE PEER-LED INTERVENTIONS?

With its emphasis on strengths and abilities rather than disability, recovery has led to growing interest in the role that people who have embarked on a journey of recovery can play in enriching the lives of others with psychiatric illnesses. The emergence of peer-led interventions has created opportunities for people living with mental illness to encourage, support, model, empower, and learn from each other in ways that were not possible under the hospice of traditional care. Peer-led interventions can be broadly defined as a collection of mental health practices emerging in the spirit of the consumer/survivor movement in which people dealing with the challenge of psychiatric illness foster the experience of recovery for others with similar challenges.

The essential characteristics of peer-led interventions are that

1. They are dispensed or offered mutually by individuals who have experienced the challenge of mental illness. Individuals further along in recovery offer mentorship and guidance to those at earlier stages of recovery, often drawing lessons from their own personal experience.
2. Providers and consumers are referred to as peers, a terminology that establishes a collaborative, mutual, and equal partnership.
3. Peers self-identify as individuals who have dealt with or are currently living with psychiatric illnesses, an essential characteristic that distinguishes peer-led interventions from traditional care.
4. Relationships among peers are grounded in self-determination, respect, and shared responsibility.

It is conceivable in traditional care that some providers may have themselves dealt with the challenge of mental illness. Their services would not however be considered peer-led, even if such providers have identified publically with the recovery movement, made public declarations about their own mental illness and recovery, or occasionally used examples from their own life experience, because their services are offered in the context of their roles in traditional care.

There has been some confusion about what constitutes the various forms of peer-led interventions. Some authors (eg, Solomon[17]) have used the term "peer support" to describe the entire host of peer-led interventions, whereas Davidson and colleagues[18] have limited the terminology to describe support services provided by peer specialists in traditional care settings to individuals with psychiatric illnesses. In an earlier publication, Davidson and colleagues[19] also used the term "peer support" to describe the universe of peer-led interventions. The current authors have chosen Davidson and colleagues'[18] later taxonomy of peer-led intervention for its parsimony. In this scheme, the family of peer-led interventions comprises mutual support/self-help, consumer-operated services, and peer support services. A discussion of the distinction among these classes of interventions is necessary to evaluate their empiric support.

The historical roots of peer-led interventions have been covered in detail elsewhere.[17–20] There are factions within the consumer/survivor movement with philosophic differences that have contributed to differences in the types of peer-led interventions that have emerged out of the consumer/survivor movement.[20] The perspectives represented among consumers/survivors about traditional care has ranged from consumers, who accept the basic premise of the medical model and seek to reform it, to those who have totally rejected traditional care and view it as fostering disability, stigma, and discrimination and see themselves as survivors of it.[20] The earlier have sought to collaborate with traditional care providers to transform mental health care systems to provide services that are responsive to patient needs, choices, and alternatives. In contrast, survivors/ex-patients have not only rejected the medical model, but they have sought to provide alternative services outside of traditional care systems that focus on helping people with psychiatric illnesses reconnect with valued social, recreational, political, and occupational opportunities. Whereas mutual support and consumer-operated services are often provided in organizations outside of traditional care systems, peer support interventions are usually provided within traditional care systems as adjunctions to traditional interventions. There is evidence that many individuals who use mutual support and consumer-operated services also receive traditional treatments as well such as medication management and psychotherapy.[21]

The Growth of Peer-led Interventions

There is clear impetus for peer-led interventions in the mental health system. The logic of such interventions is self-evident—people with schizophrenia and other severe mental illnesses would clearly benefit from opportunities to interact with others who have successfully dealt with or are currently dealing with the challenges of psychiatric illnesses.[17,19] Such interactions would serve to combat hopelessness and internalized stigma of mental illness as well as provide opportunities for interpersonal learning and growth. Peer-led interventions have increased worldwide in countries where the recovery model has made headway. In the United States, the growth of peer-led interventions has also been fostered by state and federal government initiatives to promote the recovery.

The need for peer providers is highlighted in the New Freedom Commission[22] and the US Substance Abuse and Mental Health Services Administration's (SAMSHA) principles of recovery-based care.[23] The New Freedom Commission final report called for the involvement of patients and their family members in the development of community-based recovery-oriented practices and encouraged the provision of peer-led services with emerging evidence base.

In Canada, key publications outlining the mental health needs and strategy for recovery-based systems transformation in Canadian provinces highlighted the benefits of mutual and peer support services and recommended that the provision of such services be escalated in Canada. Since 2007, the Canadian Mental Health Commission has been embarking on a project to dispense information about the benefits of peer support programs and recommendations for implementing programs in Canadian provinces.[24]

In many states in the United States, peers now provide Medicare/Medicaid reimbursable services within and outside of traditional care systems. As a result, the number of peer-led services has grown significantly in the last decade. Goldstrom and colleagues[25] reported that in 2002, there were 7467 consumer-operated services, self-help organizations, and mutual support groups in the United States. These peer-led interventions provided services to a large number of people, including over 1 million members of self-help organizations and over 500,000 individuals receiving services from consumer-operated services. Most of the peer-led interventions were in the form of mutual support groups (about 44%) and self-help organizations (approximately 40%); about 15% were in the form of consumer-operated services. The survey did not obtain an estimate of the number of people receiving peer support services within traditional clinical and rehabilitative settings, suggesting that the numbers reported may represent underestimates of the actual number of peer-led interventions in 2002. In 2006, Goldstrom and colleagues[26] revisited their classification of peer-led programs and updated the number of programs that were represented in each type of peer-led intervention. They concluded that the numbers of consumer-operated services were underestimated in their original survey and that 29% of peer-led interventions were consumer-operated services. In light of the increasing popularity and acceptance of peer services in mainstream psychiatry, it is likely that peer-led services have substantially grown in the past 5 years.

MUTUAL SUPPORT/SELF-HELP GROUPS

In mutual support, individuals with psychiatric illnesses enroll in groups to support each other in the journey of recovery. Mutual support groups share some similarities with psychotherapy groups offered in traditional care settings.[27]

Social Microcosm

First, the relationships formed among peers in the mutual support group provide a context for role modeling, problem solving, social support, learning, and corrective experiences. Similar to traditional groups, mutual support groups provide a social microcosm in which the individual can receive feedback about current status, improvements, problems, and emerging symptoms from other group members. Mutual support groups provide an opportunity for peers to seek universality in share experiences, which may decrease feelings of isolation and social ambivalence for people with schizophrenia and has potential to increase the size and quality of the social support network. The universality of experiences in mutual support groups also provides an opportunity for peers to assume expert roles that they may experience as empowering and fostering a sense of hope and personal responsibility.[28]

Psychoeducational Information

Mutual support groups may also provide a psychoeducational context for peers to acquire knowledge and information about psychiatric symptoms; gain new perspectives on treatment, wellness, and recovery; and learn skills that may foster improvements such as problem solving and coping skills.

Cognitive and Environmental Antidotes

Davidson and colleagues[19] note that mutual support can also provide cognitive and environmental antidotes to the various difficulties that people with psychiatric illnesses experience. They define cognitive antidotes as a set of beliefs, tenets, and ideologies held by a group that defines the activities of its members, the relationships in the group, skills learned, and group members' perception of their challenges (see also Wituk and colleagues[28]). In the care of people with schizophrenia and other severe mental illnesses, mutual support groups adopt the recovery model as a cognitive antidote that changes their view of psychiatric symptoms by increasing their hope of recovery and encouraging them to embrace a comprehensive view of self as fully human, despite the limitations of placed upon them by psychiatric illness. Environmental antidotes are an asset of mutual support groups in that they provide a source of social networking that may stave off isolation and loneliness.

Patient and Family Education

Since the 1970s, mutual support groups have extended to provide support and education for patients and their family members.[29-31] These family support groups serve as alternatives to traditional provider-led psychoeducational efforts (see Dixon and colleagues[32]). An example in the United States is the National Journey of Hope (JOH) Institute's JOH Program that provides a 12-week educational curriculum and ongoing support for families of patients.[33] The National Alliance on Mental Illness (NAMI) has initiated a set of educational programs that are grounded in mutual support including the NAMI Peer-to-Peer and Family-to-Family[34–36] nationwide initiatives to support the recovery of people with severe mental illnesses.

Empiric studies of mutual/self-help programs

Given the recovery context of mutual support programs, an evaluation of their empiric status should address their benefits for patients and their family members in areas that include yet extend beyond mere symptom reduction. Other dimensions such as recovery orientation (including increased feelings of hope and empowerment), social and interpersonal functioning, continued medication management, educational/vocational functioning, continued medication management, and overall wellness are also relevant to the overall quality of life of people with schizophrenia and other severe psychiatric illnesses.[3] Unfortunately, few studies have simultaneously evaluated the treatment efficacy of any intervention along the aforementioned dimensions.

The earliest empiric studies examined the GROW and Recovery Incorporated programs. These early studies conducted in the 1980s and the 1990s suggested that participation in both programs was associated with decreased symptom severity; improvements in coping skills; reduced risk of relapse, rehospitalization, and length of hospital stay; and increased involvement in traditional treatment.[19] Participants appeared to fare even better the longer they remained in such programs—improving in psychiatric symptoms, social networking, social adjustment, and self-esteem, and increasing pursuit of educational and vocational goals. A few studies were conducted to evaluate the benefits of mutual support groups for families of people with schizophrenia. These studies produced evidence that family support groups had an impact on the clinical course of symptoms experienced by individuals with schizophrenia and improved vocational and overall life outcomes. These improvements were evident even in the absence of significant reductions in expressed emotion—an index of the amount of criticism, emotional overinvolvement, and hostility displayed by families and believed to confer risk for relapse—in such families.[37–40] One randomized control trial suggested that a self-help group initiated by relatives produced benefits that matched outcomes produced by a therapeutic relatives group initiated by psychiatrists, psychologists, and psychotherapists. There were no differences on their impact on rehospitalization rates at 2-year follow-up and other outcome indicators.[39]

A methodological limitation of most of the studies conducted during the 1980s and the 1990s is that very few studies were systematically controlled clinical trials. Studies conducted in the last decade have not improved significantly in methodological rigor, limiting the strength of the inference that can be drawn from their results. In 1 exception, Castelein and colleagues[41] reported on the results of a randomized clinical trial examining the benefits of a minimally Guided Peer Support Group (GPSG) on a set of outcome indicators including social support and networking, self-esteem, self-efficacy, and quality of life. Participants (N = 106) with schizophrenia and other psychotic disorders were assigned to either the GPSG group or a treatment-as-usual condition. The authors found that participants in the GPSG condition improved their social networking and social support, self-esteem, self-efficacy, and quality of life at post-treatment follow-up. The only differences between the GPSP group and the control group on the outcome dimensions, however, were in the areas of social networking and social support (ie, people in the control group receiving traditional care experienced improvements as well). Remarkably, increased connection with group peers did not translate to increased interaction with others outside of the support group such as family members. Although there were no differences in hospitalizations rates, they found that individuals in the GPSG group had fewer negative symptoms and experienced less distress after intervention. They also found that individuals who attended groups more frequently benefited more from the program than low-attendees, suggesting a dose–response effect. Chien and colleagues[42] conducted a randomized clinical trial to examine the benefits of a family-led mutual support group for relatives of people with schizophrenia. They assigned 76 families to either a 12-session mutual support group or a usual psychiatric care condition and compared groups on several outcomes including family burden, functioning, social support, and rehospitalization at the end of the 6-month intervention and at 12-month follow-up. The study found that relatives in the experimental condition experienced significantly higher reductions in family burden, and greater increases in family functioning and social support compared with the treatment-as-usual group. They also found that the mutual support group experienced reductions in their duration of rehospitalization at follow-up, whereas this increased slightly in the control group.

Burti and colleagues[43] conducted a cross-sectional study with 88 subjects diagnosed with serious mental illness participating in either a self-help group (led by consumers) or not, and found that there were no statistically significant differences between groups on any dependent measure (including changes in psychiatric symptoms, disability, quality of life, global assessment of functioning [GAF], and assessment of needs). Hospitalization and costs associated with mental health care were higher at first but went down over time for consumers in self-help groups, whereas they went up for those who were not, although the differences were not statistically significant. Lucksted and colleagues[36] conducted a before and after survey of 550 participants in the NAMI-sponsored Peer-to-Peer program. They found that participating in the program resulted in increased knowledge of psychiatric symptoms and management of symptoms, increased their sense of self-efficacy, and connection with others. Their pilot study suggests that the Peer-to-Peer program is beneficial, but a more rigorous study is clearly needed.

There remains a dearth of tightly controlled systematic studies of mutual support. The studies reported suggest that mutual support interventions may hold promise for people with schizophrenia and their family members, but results have been slightly mixed. Most cross-sectional surveys and qualitative studies suggest that participation in mutual/self-help groups is associated with improvements in wellness, recovery, and decreased relapse.

CONSUMER-OPERATED SERVICES

Consumer-operated services are programs developed, operated, and financed by people who are dealing with or have dealt with the challenge of mental illness in the service of others dealing with similar challenges. Consumer-operated services exist outside of traditional mental health settings as alternatives or adjuncts to traditional care. They hire peers as service providers to offer forms of support to individuals seeking services in such settings, and as educators, administrators, board members, and volunteers. According to Campbell and colleagues,[44] consumer-operated services and programs exist as

1. Drop-in centers, community settings that individuals with psychiatric illnesses can visit as needed that offer a range of services including recreational, vocational, and other support programs

2. Education and advocacy training programs that provide information about psychiatric illnesses, recovery, wellness skills, and advocacy
3. Specialized support services that attend to specific areas of need such as assisting with obtaining housing, education, or employment
4. Multiservice agencies that provide different categories of services including case management, peer counseling, education, and recovery support
5. Warm lines—forms of telephone peer support and crises intervention—are alternatives to traditional crisis hotlines and are run by people in recovery to support others with psychiatric illnesses during crises

Consumer-operated services somewhat overlap and consequently are confused with mutual support programs given that both classes of peer-led interventions provide forms of social and emotional support and may be avenues for modeling and mentorship in recovery.[19] The primary distinguishing factors are that

1. Whereas mutual support often involves a bidirectional provision of support, the nature of support in consumer-operated services may not necessarily be bidirectional. Rather, support provided in consumer-operated services falls somewhere between the support that is provided in mutual support and that provided in traditional care by providers.[18]
2. Second, the nature of support provided in these settings is much more structured, consistent, and defined than that provided in mutual support settings.

In the last 3 decades, consumer-operated services have become better organized and managed and their scope of practice better defined, leading to increased enthusiasm for their services.[15] Although consumer-operated services emerged as a reaction to growing dissatisfaction with traditional care, modern consumer-operated services have evolved to collaborate with traditional providers and offer adjunctive services to individuals receiving care in traditional settings. Modern consumer-operated services also serve to connect patients with community resources, providers, mutual support, and other peer interventions as part of their case management services. Overall, as alternatives and adjuncts to traditional care, consumer-operated services have potential to reduce the burden of heavy caseloads often carried by providers in traditional care, and their proliferation in mental health care may improve the quality of services.[17,45] Some mental health systems have also viewed consumer-operated services as potentially cost saving, as they may allow traditional care settings to focus exclusively on clinical symptoms.[46]

Empiric Studies of Consumer-Operated Services

The empiric evidence offered in support of consumer-operated services is currently limited. Similar to empiric studies of mutual support, few studies have rigorously evaluated the outcomes of consumer-operated services. Most studies conducted during the 1980s and the 1990s focused on using correlational designs to identify the characteristics of participants and their subjective evaluations of the benefits of such programs. Overall, these studies suggest an association between participation in consumer-operated services and improvement in social adjustment, quality of life, life satisfaction, coping and problem-solving skills, treatment engagement, decreased psychiatric symptoms, and reductions in hospitalization.[47–50] It also appeared that the benefits of consumer-operated services were only maintained when participants remained engaged in the peer program.[51] Corrigan[52] conducted a multisite randomized control design examining the impact of participating in peer support programs (offered within a consumer-operated program) on dimensions of recovery and empowerment. Corrigan obtained data from 1824 individuals with schizophrenia and other severe mental illnesses who were receiving services in consumer-operated programs. Participants were assigned to a peer support and no-peer support groups. The author found that participation in peer support had a small association with all but 1 of the subscales generated from measures of recovery and empowerment. That is, the results were generally in the direction of peer support having a benefit when examining measures of recovery and empowerment, although the effect sizes were modest.

Recently, there has been more emphasis on implementing rigorous trials to study the effectiveness of consumer-operated services. In this regard, Campbell and colleagues'[53] initiated the Consumer-Operated Services Project (COSP) Multisite Research Initiative, a collaborative research effort of consumers and providers to evaluate consumer-operated programs. The study recruited 1827 individuals with schizophrenia and other severe mental illnesses, all of whom were receiving services in traditional care settings. Some of the participants, randomly assigned to and designated as members of the experimental group, were offered additional services in consumer-operated services around the country, including 4 drop-in centers, 2 mutual support programs, and 2 advocacy programs. Their outcomes with regard to empowerment and overall wellness were compared with those of individuals randomly assigned to a control group that was comprised individuals who were receiving traditional treatment alone. The researchers found that individuals who participated in consumer-operated services had greater increases in wellness and empowerment scores at 1-year follow-up compared with individuals in the control group receiving only traditional care. They also found that the level of participation in consumer-operated services was associated with increases in empowerment. Nelson and colleagues[51] used a nonequivalent group design to compare people receiving consumer-operated services with people not receiving such services. The study design included 3 groups comprised of a control group and 2 treatment groups. One of the treatment groups received Consumer/Survivor Initiative (CSI) services for 36 months and another group received services for 9 to 18 months. The study outcome indicators, which included social support, community integration, personal empowerment, quality of life, symptom distress, psychiatric hospitalization, emergency services use, and instrumental role involvement, were measured at 9-, 18-, and 36-month follow-up. The authors found that participants receiving CSI services at 36-month follow-up obtained higher scores on community integration, instrumental role involvement, and quality of life (daily activities), and lower scores on symptom distress than individuals in the other 2 groups. The authors did not obtain significant differences on empowerment and housing and safety domains of quality of life. Both studies suggest that consumer-operated services may positively impact recovery attitudes such as empowerment, overall wellness, and community functioning.

Segan and colleagues,[54] however, obtained noncorroborating results when they evaluated the benefit of partnerships between a COSP drop-in center and community mental health agencies (CMHA) for people with schizophrenia and other severe mental illnesses. They recruited 139 individuals seeking services at a CMHA and randomly assigned individuals to either CMHA services alone or combined COSP drop-in and CMHA services. The COSP service offered included only drop-in services. The study outcome measures were severity of psychiatric symptoms and recovery-related outcomes including empowerment, self-efficacy, hopelessness, and social integration. The authors found that change scores in social integration, self-efficacy, and personal empowerment were lower for the combined COSP drop-in and CMHA group compared with the CMHA only group. They also found no differences between groups on symptom severity and hopelessness scores.

Overall, they concluded that the combination of COSP drop-in and CMHA appeared to be less beneficial than CHMA alone. The apparent lower benefit drawn from the combined programs is puzzling and may represent a project-specific anomaly. Most of these studies reported suggest that consumer-operated services confer some benefits in empowerment, wellness, recovery, and social support. However, benefits have not been demonstrated in all studies. In the presence of such negative findings, it would appear that there is a need for additional rigorous studies of the benefits of consumer-operated services.

PEER SUPPORT SERVICES

The third category of peer-led interventions—peer support services—exists within and outside of traditional care settings. Outside of traditional care settings, peer support and mutual/self-help services are offered in consumer-operated programs, but the following section focuses on peer support offered by peers to individuals with schizophrenia and other severe mental illnesses within traditional care systems. Peer support is a category of peer-led intervention that places people with a history of psychiatric illnesses in provider roles to support others with psychiatric disabilities. The responsibilities of peer providers in traditional mental health settings have been defined.[17–19] By virtue of their experience with schizophrenia and other severe mental illnesses and their willingness to disclose their mental illness and experience in treatment, peer providers connect with patients through empathy, acceptance, and shared experiences. As noted by Peebles and colleagues,[55] peer support plays a role in the larger mental health care system beyond the provision of support services to patients. In the context of efforts to transform traditional care systems into recovery-based systems, peer providers serve as advocates for patients in settings that have historically ignored patient voices in treatment planning. Peer specialists receive training and certification from peer programs (eg, Georgia Mental Health Consumer Network) in advocacy and support skills that allow them to advocate for consumers, provide supportive services to consumers and their families, and offer consultation to other members of the treatment team. They are thus in unique roles that allow them to provide insights, education, and perspectives to providers, consumers, and stakeholders about the development and delivery of care from their own lived experience.[56]

System-level changes potentially confer the benefit of improved overall care for people with schizophrenia when the recovery model leads to vital restructuring of funding and reimbursement mechanisms, improvements in the training of practitioners, provision of recovery-based interventions, improved choices, and system-wide policy changes.[55] In a more direct way, peer support and other peer-led interventions provide a source of social support for people with schizophrenia, although relative to mutual support and consumer-operated services, the form of social support is more 1-directional and less reciprocal.[18] Like traditional care, the peer support relationship could provide a context for developing behavior-based coping and problem-solving skills that may contribute to recovery. Whereas skill acquisition in psychotherapy often happens through formal learning, during which the psychotherapist implements techniques such as role playing, peer providers often use self-disclosure and their own life experiences to help patients learn about strategies for dealing with difficulties and maintain wellness. Although peer providers are providers in the traditional sense, the peer provider–consumer relationship departs significantly from the traditional doctor–patient dynamic embraced in traditional care. There is a de-emphasis of power differentials; rather, the relationship is viewed as egalitarian, with shared experiences that foster connection, understanding, and working alliance.[16,57] There is a de-emphasis of psychiatric diagnoses and manualized interventions; rather, the peer relationship is believed to drive the individual's own experiential recovery.[57]

The implementation of peer support in mental health settings has not been without its challenges. Some authors have expressed concerns that peer providers often have poorly defined roles, responsibilities, and job descriptions in certain mental health settings.[58] This potential challenge has also been beneficial in some respects as it allows peer providers to have some flexibility in defining their roles in ways that best meet organizational demands or needs of patients being served in care settings. For example, in some organizations, peer providers play significant roles in crises management, vocational rehabilitation, case management, and program planning.[59] Moreover, the skills, education, and interests of peer providers may be so diverse that having only a few circumscribed roles for peer support may lead to boredom, burnout, and dissatisfaction. Some authors have identified other challenges that peer providers experience in traditional care settings including potential power struggles with traditional care providers; limited resources for peer providers including availability of supervision and community resources; and long-standing stigma and negative attitudes about people with psychiatric diagnoses.[55] These challenges are problems with traditional care rather than peer support; for example, traditional providers may often feel that peer providers are impugning on their professional territories. When the patient's recovery and overall welfare takes precedence, such conflicts should give way to collaboration between traditional providers and peer providers to address the needs of the patient.

Empiric Status of Peer Support

Before 2000, only 2 randomized controlled trials were conducted on the effectiveness of peer support for individuals diagnosed with serious mental illness.[18,60] Other studies conducted at this time suffered serious methodological flaws, including small sample size and low power, or were exploratory and descriptive in nature.[18] Unfortunately, there has been little improvement in the research on the effectiveness of peer support since 2000. In their review of the literature, Davidson and colleagues[18] identified 4 randomized controlled trials on the effectiveness of peer support conducted before 2006. Three of these studies compared case management services provided by peer providers to those provided by traditional providers, and 1 compared peer-provided social support to those of unpaid volunteers. The studies demonstrated that there were no differences on outcome measures, such as in symptom improvement, quality of life, service satisfaction, and employment, based on group assignment, indicating that peer support case management was at least as effective as traditional provider case management services. Remarkably, Clark and colleagues[61] found that consumers who received peer-led case management experienced fewer hospitalizations and remained in the community longer than consumers who received standard case management or treatment as usual.

Research on Vet-to-Vet, a peer initiative for veterans diagnosed with serious mental illness, has produced promising findings.[62,63] Vet-to-Vet is a peer education and support program designed by Moe Armstrong, a decorated veteran who has been diagnosed with schizophrenia, that provides a structured model of peer support and possesses established guidelines for implementation and recommendations for educational material to be used groups. Data suggest that individuals diagnosed with serious mental illness who participate in this program endorse stronger veteran recovery attitudes and empowerment, and more frequent attendance is associated with feeling more involved in daily activities and greater feelings of accomplishment, pride, and growth. Furthermore, those veterans who received services from paid peers, rather than volunteers, exhibited greater veteran recovery attitudes and sense of spirituality and engagement in meaningful activity.

Sell and colleagues'[64] randomized control trial evaluating peer-delivered case management for people with schizophrenia and other severe mental illness (N = 137) demonstrated that that peers were better able to establish a working alliance with service recipients than traditional providers. The alliance was also associated with better engagement in services, which is important given attrition rates in psychiatric settings and associated negative outcomes. Several quasi-experimental cross-sectional or longitudinal studies have demonstrated that individuals with schizophrenia receiving peer support services remained in the community longer and were hospitalized for fewer days.[65,66] This effect has not been demonstrated for internet peer support, however.[67,68] In Kaplan and colleagues'[67] study, individuals who participated in internet peer support exhibited less well-being and endorsed higher levels of distress. Indeed, greater participation was associated with higher levels of distress; but, counterintuitively, greater participation was also associated with higher levels of satisfaction with internet peer support.

These results are promising and suggest that peer support services can lower associated mental health care costs, increase the number of days in the community between hospitalizations, and reduce the likelihood of rehospitalization. Support from peers was associated with attitudes of recovery and empowerment. The limitation of the current empiric base is that there have been few randomized control trials conducted to date, and some trials have obtained negative results. A semi-exhaustive review of the extant literature identified only 3 randomized controlled trials of the benefits of peer support for individuals diagnosed with schizophrenia and other serious mental illness conducted since Davidson and colleagues'[18] review, one of which was unable to tease apart the influence of peer-led interventions due to study design.[69]

IMPLICATIONS AND EMERGING FRONTIERS FOR PEER-LED INTERVENTIONS

Peer-led interventions have potential to increase the accessibility of services to people with schizophrenia. Given that most people in need of services do not seek traditional treatment perhaps due to fears of being labeled mental patients, peer-led interventions represent alternatives that may be acceptable to individuals aversive to traditional care. The responsibilities of peer providers in mental health systems have evolved recently to address emerging needs for educational interventions for consumers and recovery-based training for providers. Peer providers are helping people with psychiatric illnesses manage symptoms, reduce hospitalization risk, and maintain overall wellness. The most prominent of these systems is Mary Ellen Copeland's Wellness Recovery Action Planning (WRAP),[70] which helps people with severe mental illnesses identify triggers, harbingers of symptom exacerbation, and wellness tools for managing such situations while pursuing life goals. In 2 statewide studies conducted in Minnesota and Vermont, Cook and colleagues[71] found that peer providers were able to train people with severe mental illnesses to use the WRAP, and its implementation was associated with increased knowledge of symptoms, improved symptom self-management, and recovery attitudes. Peer-led educational efforts have been extended to educate practitioners and trainees targeted toward improving their attitudes about mental illness and the recovery model. While not directly serving patients with schizophrenia, targeting providers has the potential to confer indirect benefits to service recipients. An example of this endeavor is Project GREAT (Georgia Recovery-based Educational Approach to Treatment), a peer-and-provider collaborative effort to educate practitioners about the recovery model.[56,72]

The Project GREAT curriculum was developed by a team of peers and providers, who teach recovery-based principles using lectures, focus groups, and recovery stories. Peebles and colleagues[72] demonstrated that the Project GREAT curriculum fostered knowledge and attitude change toward a recovery orientation, and was also associated with improved satisfaction among consumers receiving services in a mental health care system. The inclusion of peers as educators for consumers and providers is an emerging frontier for the recovery movement.

Despite growing enthusiasm for peer-led interventions, their limited empiric status is the reason they are not currently included in the Schizophrenia Patient Outcomes Research Team (PORT) guidelines as 1 of the recommended psychosocial interventions for schizophrenia.[73] The specific therapeutic elements of peer-led interventions such as role modeling, social support, recovery stories, and shared experiences should be identified and their relative importance demonstrated through defragmenting studies, so that greater emphasis can be placed on elements that are most beneficial. Notwithstanding, the schizophrenia PORT guidelines noted that peer-led interventions are of growing interest. While empiric studies have focused on the benefits of peer-led interventions for people receiving services, it would be of interest to learn about the impact of assuming a provider role for peer specialists providing peer support in traditional care settings. What impact does supporting another individual's own recovery have on the peer provider's overall wellness and sense of recovery? Does it contribute to mastery or represent a stressor requiring management?

SUMMARY

Peer-led interventions including self-help, consumer-operated services, and peer support are innovations emerging in the spirit of the recovery movement that place patients and ex-patients in position to support the recovery of people with schizophrenia and other severe mental illnesses. There is growing enthusiasm for these interventions in mental health settings, given their cost-saving benefits and usefulness as adjuncts to traditional care. The empiric evidence demonstrating the benefits of peer-led interventions is currently limited, but overall, studies suggest that peer-delivered interventions foster the experience of recovery, decrease the risk of hospitalization, and foster overall wellness. The role of peer providers in the mental health system is evolving and has extended beyond providing support and coping models to patients. Emerging roles include case management, patient-education, and emergency support. Further study of peer-led interventions is warranted, including examining their benefits for improving patient care and their impact at fostering the recovery experiences of peer providers.

REFERENCES

1. Andreasen NC, Carpenter WC, Kane JM, et al. Remission in schizophrenia: proposed criteria and rationale for consensus. Am J Psychiatry 2005;162:441–9.
2. Bellack A. Scientific and consumer models of recovery in schizophrenia: concordance, contrasts, and implications. Schizophr Bull 2006;32:432–42.
3. Nasrallah HA, Targum SD, Tandon R, et al. Defining and measuring clinical effectiveness in the treatment of schizophrenia. Psychiatr Serv 2005;56:273–82.
4. Deegan P. Recovery as a journey of the heart. Psychiatr Rehabil J 1996;19:91–7.
5. Mead S, Copeland ME. What recovery means to us: consumer perspectives. Community Health J 2000;36:315–28.
6. Kessler RC, Berglund PA, Bruce ML, et al. The prevalence and correlates of untreated serious mental illness. Health Serv Res 2001;36:987–1007.

7. O'Brien A, Fahmy IR, Singh SP. Disengagement from mental health services: a literature review. Soc Psychiatry Psychiatr Epidemiol 2009;44(7):558–68.

8. Corry P, Hogman G, Sandamas G. That's just typical. London: National Schizophrenia Fellowship; 2001.

9. Kreyenbuhl J, Nossel IR, Dixon LB. Disengagement from mental health treatment among individuals with schizophrenia and strategies for facilitating connections to care: a review of the literature. Schizophr Bull 2009;35(4):696–703.

10. Deegan PE, Drake RE. Shared decision-making and medication management in the recovery process. Psychiatr Serv 2006;57(11):1636–9.

11. Ahmed AO, Mabe PA, Buckley PF. Recovery in schizophrenia: Perspectives, evidence, and implications. In: Ritsner MS, editor. Handbook of schizophrenia spectrum disorders: therapeutic approaches comorbidity and outcomes. New York: Springer; 2011. p. 1–22.

12. Anthony WA. Recovery from mental illness: the guiding vision of the mental health service system in the 1990s. Psychosoc Rehabil J 1993;16:11–23.

13. Jacobson N, Curtis L. Recovery as policy in mental health services: strategies emerging from the states. Psychiatr Rehabil J 2000;23:333–41.

14. Herbert M, Rosenheck R, Drebing C, et al. Integrating peer support initiatives in a large healthcare organization. Psychol Serv 2008;5(3):216–27.

15. Campbell J. The historical and philosophical development of peer-run support programs. In: Clay S, Schell B, Corrigan P, et al, editors. On our own, together: peer programs for people with mental illness. Nashville (TN): Vanderbilt University Press; 2005. p. 17–64.

16. Mead S, Hilton D, Curtis L. Peer support: a theoretical perspective. Psychiatr Rehabil J 2001;25:134–41.

17. Solomon P. Peer support/peer provided services: underlying processes, benefits, and critical ingredients. Psychiatr Rehabil J 2004;27:392–401.

18. Davidson L, Chinman M, Sells D, et al. Peer support among adults with serious mental illnesses: a report from the field. Schizophr Bull 2006;32(3):443–50.

19. Davidson L, Chinman M, Kloos B, et al. Peer support among individuals with severe mental illness: a review of the evidence. Clin Psychol Sci Prac 1999;6: 165–87.

20. Adame AL, Leitner L. Breaking out of the mainstream: the evolution of peer support alternatives to the mental health system. Ethical Hum Psychol Psychiat 2008;10(3):146–62.

21. Kessler RC, Mickelson KD, Zhao S. Patterns and correlates of self-help group membership in the United States. Soc Policy 1997;27:27–46.

22. New Freedom Commission on Mental Health. Achieving the promise: transforming mental health in America. final report. US Department of Health and Human Services. Pub. number SMA-03-3832. Rockville (MD): Department of Health and Human Services; 2003.

23. Substance Abuse, Mental Health Services Administration. National consensus conference on mental health recovery and systems transformation. Rockville (MD): Department of Health and Human Services; 2005.

24. Kirby MJL, Keon WJ. Out of the shadows at last: transforming mental health, mental illness, and addiction services in Canada (online). Mental Health Commission, 2006. Available at: http://www.parl.gc.ca/39/1/parlbus/commbus/senate/com-e/soci-e/rep-e/pdf/rep02may06part1-e.pdf. Accessed December 28, 2011.

25. Goldstrom ID, Campbell J, Rogers JA, et al. National estimates for mental health mutual support groups, self-help organizations, and consumer-operated services. Adm Policy Ment Health 2006;31(1):92–103.

26. Goldstrom I, Campbell J, Rogers J, et al. Mental health consumer organizations: a national picture. In: Manderscheid RW, Berry JT, editors. Center for Mental Health Services: Mental Health, United States, 2004. DHHS Pub No. (SMA)-4195. Rockville (MD): Substance Abuse and Mental Health Services Administration; 2006. p. 247–55.

27. Yalom I. The theory and practice of group psychotherapy. 4th edition. New York: Basic Books; 1995.

28. Wituk S, Shepherd MD, Slavich S, et al. A topography of self-help groups: an empirical analysis. Soc Work 2000;45(2):157–65.

29. Perkins DD, Zimmerman MA. Empowerment theory, research, and application. Am J Psychol 1995;23(5):569–79.

30. Murray P. Recovery, Inc., as an adjunct to treatment in an era of managed care. Psychiatr Serv 1996;47(12):1378–81.

31. Corrigan P, Slopen N, Garcia G, et al. Some recovery processes in mutual-help groups for persons with mental illness; II: qualitative analysis of participant interviews. Community Ment Health J 2005;41(6):721–35.

32. Dixon L, Adams C, Lucksted A. Update on family psychoeducation for schizophrenia. Schizophr Bull 2000;26(1):5–10.

33. Pickett-Schenk SA, Cook JA, Laris A. Journey of Hope program outcomes. Community Ment Health J 2000;36(4):413–24.

34. Dixon L, Stewart B, Burland J, et al. Pilot study of the effectiveness of the family-to-family education program. Psychiatr Serv 2001;52:965–7.

35. Dixon L, Lucksted A, Stewart B, et al. Outcomes of the peer-taught 12-week family-to-family education program for severe mental illness. Acta Psychiatr Scand 2004;109:207–15.

36. Lucksted A, McNulty K, Brayboy L, et al. Initial evaluation of the peer-to-peer program. Psychiatr Serv 2009;60:250–3.

37. Rappaport J, Seidman E, Toro P, et al. Collaborative research with a mutual help organization. Soc Policy 1985;15:12–24.

38. Schulz M. Self-help groups for families of schizophrenic patients: formation, development, and therapeutic impact. Soc Psychiatry Psychiatr Epidemiol 1994;29(3):149–54.

39. Posner CM, Wilson KG, Kral MJ, et al. Family psychoeducational support groups in schizophrenia. Am J Orthopsychiatry 1992;62(2):206–18.

40. Buchkremer G, Monking HS, Holle R, et al. The impact of therapeutic relatives' groups on the course of illness of schizophrenia patients. Eur Psychiatry 1995; 10:17–27.

41. Castelein S, Bruggeman R, van Busschbach JT, et al. The effectiveness of peer support groups in psychosis: a randomized controlled trial. Acta Psychiatr Scand 2008;118:64–72.

42. Chien W, Thompson DR, Norman I. Evaluation of a peer-led mutual support group for Chinese families of people with schizophrenia. Am J Community Psychol 2008;42:122–34.

43. Burti L, Amaddeo F, Ambrosi M, et al. Does additional care provided by a consumer self-help group improve psychiatric outcome? A study in an Italian community-based psychiatric service. Community Ment Health J 2005;41(6):705–20.

44. Campbell J. Key ingredients of peer programs identified (online). Available at: http://www.power2u.org/downloads/COSP-CommonIngredients.pdf. Accessed December 28, 2011.

45. Hardiman ER. Networks of caring: a qualitative study of social support in consumer-run mental health agencies. Qual Soc Work 2004;3:431–48.

46. Segal SP, Hardiman ER, Hodges JQ. Characteristics of new clients at self-help and community mental health agencies in geographic proximity. Psychiatr Serv 2002;53:1145–52.
47. Mowbray CT, Chamberlain P, Jennings M, et al. Consumer-run mental health services: results from five demonstration projects. Community Ment Health J 1988;24:151–6.
48. Mowbray CT, Wellwood R, Chamberlain P. Project Stay: a consumer-run support service. Psychosoc Rehabil J 1988;12:33–42.
49. Silverman S, Blank M, Taylor L. On our own: preliminary findings from a consumer run service model. Psychiatr Rehabil J 1997;21(2):151–9.
50. Mowbray C, Tan C. Consumer-operated drop-in centers: evaluation of operations and impact. J Ment Health Adm 1993;20:8–19.
51. Nelson G, Ochocka J, Janzen R, et al. A longitudinal study of mental health consumer/survivor initiatives: part V—outcomes at three-year follow-up. J Community Psychol 2007;35:655–65.
52. Corrigan PW. Impact of consumer-operated services on empowerment and recovery of people with psychiatric disabilities. Psychiatr Serv 2006;57:1493–6.
53. Campbell J, Lichtenstein C, Teague G, et al. The Consumer-Operated Services Program (COSP) multisite research initiative: final report. Saint Louis (MO): Coordinating Center at the Missouri Institute of Mental Health; 2006.
54. Segal S, Silverman CJ, Temkin TL. Outcomes from consumer-operated and community mental health services: a randomized control trial. Psychiatr Serv 2011;62(8):915–21.
55. Peebles SA, Mabe PA, Davidson L, et al. Recovery and systems transformation for schizophrenia. Psychiatr Clin North Am 2007;30:567–83.
56. Ahmed AO, Mabe PA, Buckley PF. Peer specialists as educators for recovery-based systems transformation: the Project GREAT experience. Psychiatr Times 2012;29:1–7.
57. Mead S, Hilton D. Crisis and connection. Psychiatr Rehab J 2003;27:87–95.
58. Mowbray C, Moxley D, Colins M. Consumers as mental health providers: first person accounts of benefits and limitations. J Behav Health Serv Res 1998;25: 397–411.
59. Schwenk EB, Brusilovskiy E, Salzer MS. Results from a national survey of certified peer specialist job titles and job descriptions: evidence of a versatile behavioral health workforce. Philadelphia: The University of Pennsylvania Collaborative on Community Integration; 2009.
60. Chinman MJ, Rosenheck R, Lam JA, et al. Comparing consumer and nonconsumer provided case management services for homeless persons with serious mental illness. J Nerv Ment Dis 2000;188(7):446–53.
61. Clarke GN, Herincks HA, Kinney RF, et al. Psychiatric hospitalizations, arrests, emergency room visits, and homelessness of clients with serious and persistent mental illness: findings from a randomized trial of two ACT programs vs. usual care. Ment Health Serv Res 2000;2(3):155–64.
62. Barber JA, Rosenheck RA, Armstrong M, et al. Monitoring the dissemination of peer support in the VA healthcare system. Community Ment Health J 2008;44:433–41.
63. Resnick SG, Rosenheck RA. Integrating peer-provided services: a quasi-experimental study of recovery orientation, confidence, and empowerment. Psychiatr Serv 2008;59(11):1307–14.
64. Sells D, Davidson L, Jewell C, et al. The treatment relationship in peer-based and regular case management for clients with severe mental illness. Psychiatr Serv 2006;57(8):1179–84.

65. Min S, Whitecraft J, Rothband AB, et al. Peer support for persons with co-occurring disorders and community tenure: a survival analysis. Psychiatr Rehab J 2007;30(3):207–13.
66. Lawn S, Smith A, Hunter K. Mental health peer support for the hospital avoidance and early discharge: an Australian example of consumer driven and operated service. J Ment Health 2008;17(5):498–508.
67. Kaplan K, Salzer MS, Solomon P, et al. Internet peer support for individuals with psychiatric disabilities: a randomized controlled trial. Soc Sci Med 2011;72: 54–62.
68. Salzer M, Palmer S, Kaplan K, et al. A randomized, controlled study of Internet peer-to-peer interactions among women newly diagnosed with breast cancer. Psychooncology 2010;19:441–6.
69. Rowe M, Bellamy C, Baranoski M, et al. A peer support, group intervention to reduce substance use and criminality among persons with severe mental illness. Psychiatr Serv 2007;58(7):955–61.
70. Copeland ME. Wellness recovery action plan. Dummerston (VT): Peach Press; 1997.
71. Cook JA, Copeland ME, Corey L, et al. Developing the evidence-base for peer-led services: challenges among participants following Wellness Recovery Action Planning (WRAP) education in two statewide initiatives. Psychiatr Rehab J 2010; 34:113–20.
72. Peebles SA, Mabe PA, Fenley G,, et al. Immersing practitioners in the Recovery model: an educational program evaluation. Community Ment Health J 2009;45: 239–45.
73. Dixon LB, Dickerson F, Bellack AS, et al. The 2009 schizophrenia PORT psycho-social treatment recommendations and summary statements. Schizophr Bull 2010;36(1):48–70.

Homelessness in Schizophrenia

Adriana Foster, MD*, James Gable, PharmD, John Buckley

KEYWORDS

- Homeless • Schizophrenia • Outreach • Assertive community treatment • Housing
- Shelter

HOMELESSNESS IN THE UNITED STATES AND WORLDWIDE
How Big Is the Problem?

A single point-in-time count in January 2010 found 649,917 homeless people in the United States, of whom 109,812 were chronically homeless and 246,374 were unsheltered. Throughout the year, 1.59 million people in the United States spent at least one night in a shelter.[1] There were 26,248 homeless people in New York City's Department of Homeless Services records in 2006, 2525 of whom were veterans.[2] The 2006 Australian census estimated 104,676 homeless individuals.[3] In 2007 in the United Kingdom there were a total of 98,744 homeless households in temporary accommodation.[4] A 2003 report estimated that there were 410,000 homeless people in Germany and the same number in France.[5] Exact homeless counts are difficult to estimate because homelessness is most often transient and a multitude of settings need to be included in the assessment (shelters, hospitals, and jails as well as streets, parks, abandoned buildings, and other areas not meant for human habitation).

Challenges in Homelessness Research

The definition of homelessness varies and may include individuals who lack a fixed, regular, and adequate nighttime residence[1]; may be more restrictive, including only unsheltered or street homeless; or may be broader, including those who double up in housing or reside in single-room occupancy hotels, jails, residential substance abuse programs, and transitional housing for people with mental illness (see **Box 1** for definitions).

Sampling sites influence the prevalence of mental disorders found in the homeless population. In a sample of homeless people from streets and shelters, the rates of

Disclosures: All authors work as volunteers performing mental health screenings of homeless persons at shelters in Augusta, Georgia, as part of the Helping Hands program, sponsored by a grant from American Psychiatric Foundation. Adriana Foster, has received grant support from National Institute of Mental Health and Sunovion on topics unrelated to this article. James Gable and John Buckley do not have any conflicts of interest to report.
Department of Psychiatry and Health Behavior, Medical College of Georgia, Georgia Health Sciences University, 997 Saint Sebastian Way, Augusta, GA 30912, USA
* Corresponding author.
E-mail address: afoster@georgiahealth.edu

Box 1
Terms used in this article

Unsheltered homeless

Persons who reside in a place not meant for human habitation, such as cars, parks, sidewalks, abandoned buildings, or on the street.

Rough sleepers[a]

Individuals who sleep in the open air, such as in the streets, tents, doorways, parks, or bus shelters, and people in buildings or other places not designed for habitation, such as stairwells, sheds, cars, derelict boats, or stations.

Sheltered homeless

Persons who reside in an emergency shelter, which is transitional housing for homeless persons who originally came from the streets or other shelters.

Precariously housed

People on the edge of becoming literally homeless who may be staying with friends or relatives or who may be paying an extremely high percentage of their income on rent. They are often characterized as at imminent risk of becoming homeless.

Chronically homeless

Unaccompanied homeless individuals with a disabling condition who have been continuously homeless for a year or more or who have had at least 4 separate, distinct, and sustained periods of homelessness in the past 3 years.

Homeless household[a]

A single homeless individual or a family of homeless individuals.

[a] Term used in United Kingdom.

---

alcohol and drug use are high (70%–86% and 48%–61%, respectively) and mental illness can be found in up to 90%. The prevalence of these disorders is lower in temporary housing facilities and tends to be high in hospital samples of homeless.[6]

The sampling method may affect research outcomes; for example a cross-sectional sample may overestimate the prevalence of mental illness because people with mental illness are homeless longer than those without it and thus have a higher probability to be selected in such a sample. Alternatively, studying people who enter homelessness during a specific period or selecting a sample that is stratified based on the duration of homelessness has been proposed.[7]

The diagnostic methods used to determine mental illness in homeless research vary broadly. Tools that have been used include psychiatric evaluation; clinical assessment with diagnostic instruments, such as the Diagnostic Interview Schedule[8] or the Structured Clinical Interview for DSM Disorders[9]; or screening instruments (for example, the Addiction Severity Index, which was validated in a homeless sample[10]), intended to detect the probable cases that can be confirmed with further evaluation.[6]

Outcome measures for interventions used for homeless with mental illness include housing, mental health, severity of psychiatric symptoms, recovery from substance use, employment, social support, victimization, and overall quality of life, used alone or in combination. Instruments used to assess quality of life include the Lehman Quality of Life Interview[11] and the Colorado Symptoms index[12] or multidimensional assessments, such as the Colorado Client Assessment Record,[13] which includes symptoms, cognition, behavioral domains, level of function, and the global severity of impairment. Illness severity is measured with various instruments, such as the Global Severity Index of the Brief Symptom Inventory of the Symptom Checklist-90.[14]

Attrition is common in homeless studies. Sample retention rates reported are 74.8% to 81%[15,16] and become lower as the follow-up period extends; for example, in a sample of homeless veterans, 57% completed follow-up interviews at 3 months whereas only 37% were still available at 12 months.[14]

Morbidity and Mortality in the Homeless

Physical illness, injury, and mortality in the homeless

Vazquez and colleagues[17] compared the prevalence of physical illness among home-less persons in Madrid, Spain (N = 289), and Washington, DC (N = 908), and found that in both samples, 70% of the persons reported at least one significant health problem in the year before the study with respiratory and cardiovascular illnesses leading in both samples. The Spanish homeless people were older, became homeless later in life, and remained homeless for longer time than the group in Washington, DC. The Spanish sample had significantly higher 12-months prevalence rates of hepatitis and jaundice, other digestive system problems, AIDS, and HIV. The American sample had signifi-cantly more sexual and respiratory diseases. Spanish homeless women had poorer health and a significantly higher prevalence of tuberculosis than American homeless women. In an analysis of illness and injury that led to hospitalization in 326,073 home-less versus 1,202,622 housed low-income residents in New York City in 2000 to 2002, Frencher and colleagues[18] found that unintentional injury rates, including falls, were higher in the young children, adults, and elderly homeless compared with the low-income housed group. Homeless adults and elderly were more likely to be hospitalized for injury related to cold temperature and homeless elderly were admitted for heat-related problems more than the low-income group. Injury due to assault was higher in homeless adolescents, adults, and elderly than the low-income group. More than 5% of all injury-related hospitalizations were due to self-inflicted injury, most of which occurred in homeless adolescents and adults. The age of death in homeless people was found to be 46-years old to 50 years old in men,[19-21] much like the life expectancy in schizophrenia, which is lower than in the general population (**Fig. 1**).[22] Babidge and colleagues[19] described the cause of death among 708 homeless people (506 with schizophrenia) at 10-year follow-up after referral to mental health clinics established

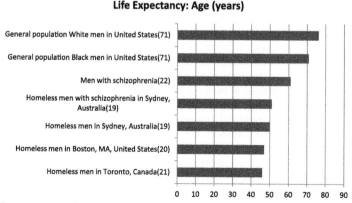

Fig. 1. Life expectancy for men who are homeless, men with schizophrenia, and men in general population (reference numbers in parentheses). *Data from* Refs.[19-22,71]

at shelters in Sydney, Australia. Standardized mortality ratios (SMRs) were obtained by dividing the observed deaths in the homeless by the expected deaths in the general population of New South Wales, Australia. Homeless men and women died 3 to 4 times more frequently than general population. Younger groups of homeless men had highest mortality (SMR 4.54 in the 20–29-year-old group with schizophrenia and 11.59 in the 30–39-year-old group with other mental disorders). Suicide was a leading cause of death, with overdose of prescription medication the most common reason of death, and peaked in the 30-year-old to 39-year-old group with schizophrenia (SMR 11.76) and the 40-year-old to 49-year-old group with other psychiatric disorders (SMR 50). Hwang[21] studied mortality rate ratios by dividing the mortality rate in homeless male shelter users by mortality in a general male population in Toronto, Canada, in 8933 homeless men who used shelters in the city in 1995 through 1997. Similar to the findings in Sydney, Australia, in Toronto, the highest mortality rate ratio was found in younger adults, with 8.3 in 18-year-olds to 24-year-olds, 3.7 in 25-year-olds to 44-year-olds, and 2.3 in 45-year-olds to 64-year-olds. Suicide was among the top causes of death in 18-year-olds to 24-year-olds and in 25-year-olds to 44-year-olds along with poisonings, AIDS, and accidents, whereas in the older group, cancer and cardiovascular disease became the leading causes of death, along with accidents. In the same study, the investigators found that the mortality rates in Toronto were lower than those in Boston and New York City for men in the 25-year-old to 44 year-old group. Hwang[20] also found that the homeless may be underutilizing the health care system because 27% of a sample of 558 homeless people in Boston who died between 1988 and 1993 had no contact with the inner city homeless health care system within 1 year from death. People with HIV and injection drug use were significantly more likely to have made health care contacts in the year before death.

Mental illness in the homeless

Perhaps due to variable methodology, including sample selection and assessment tools, the proportion of mental illness found in the homeless, although higher than in general population, varies in studies from around the world. In a sample of 96 homeless adolescents from Los Angeles (mean age 16.1 years old), 32% endorsed 1 to 3 psychotic symptoms on the Diagnostic Interview Schedule after the responses potentially associated with medications, drug use, or physical conditions were eliminated. Presence of psychotic symptoms was correlated in this sample with mood symptoms, drug use, and abusive life experiences.[23] Fichter and Quadflieg[24] studied a representative sample of 265 single homeless men and an aged-matched general population sample in Munich, Germany, with the Structured Clinical Interview for DSM Disorders,[9] and noted a lifetime prevalence of mental disorders that was 2.4 times more frequent among homeless individuals compared with the community sample; 72.7% of the homeless had alcohol dependence, 32.8% had mood disorders, 15.9% had anxiety disorders, and 9.8% had psychotic disorders. Herrman and colleagues[25] found that 50% of 346 homeless people in Melbourne, Australia (predominantly men), received a *Diagnostic and Statistical Manual of Mental Disorders* (Third Edition Revised)[26] diagnosis of current mental disorder (mood, psychosis, and substance use). In this sample, 9.4% had exclusively mood disorders, 8.5% had only psychotic disorders, and 32.9% had only substance-related disorders whereas 22.8% had comorbid disorders. The studies of mental illness and substance use disorders in the homeless in the 1980s focused on large urban areas, including New York, Boston, St Louis, Baltimore, and Los Angeles.[6] The prevalence of alcohol use disorders in these studies ranged from 12.2% to 68% and drug use prevalence ranged from 1% to 37.1%. In comparison, the prevalence of alcohol use and drug use disorders was found to be 13.3% and

5.9%, respectively, in the US Epidemiologic Catchment Area (ECA) study.[27] Schizophrenia was found in 1.4% to 30.3% of the population studied, whereas 15.1% to 29.5% reported mood disorders. The US ECA study found, in comparison, 1.3% and 8.3% prevalence of schizophrenia and mood disorders, respectively.[27] In a sample of 110 homeless people in rural Pennsylvania, Kales and colleagues[28] found a prevalence of 26.6% for major depressive disorder of which 71% also reported substance use disorder and 6.4% reported psychotic thinking. Among the homeless people surveyed, 30% had a history of hospitalization for psychiatric issues and same percentage reported a past suicide attempt, whereas the sample had an estimated lifetime prevalence of alcohol, drug, or combined abuse or dependence of 57.2%. Haughland and colleagues[29] reported on the prevalence of mental illness in 201 individuals from a suburban county in New York State and found that 21% of their sample had a mental illness, of whom 10% had schizophrenia-spectrum disorders and 4% mood disorders. Drug use history was not included in mental illness; 51% of the sample reported alcohol, 72% reported drug use, and 46% of the sample had evidence of drug metabolites at urinalysis. The subgroup with mental illness were most likely to be in their 30s, had been homeless for significantly longer time, and spent twice as many weeks literally homeless than those without mental illness. A meta-analysis of studies measuring the prevalence of mental disorders, including 5684 homeless persons in 7 countries from 1966 to 2007,[30] found a pooled prevalence of psychotic illness of 12.7%, major depression 11.4%, personality disorders 23.1%, alcohol dependence 37.9%, and drug dependence 24.4%. Caton and colleagues[31] found that a of group of 445 newly homeless single adults (median age 36 years old, 62% black) who entered shelters in New York City, 51% had a lifetime diagnosis of *Diagnostic and Statistical Manual of Mental Disorders* (Fourth Edition) axis I disorder and 53% of substance use disorder, and 44% had received treatment for substance use disorder. Only 377 (85%) of these individuals were available for follow-up at 6 months, 12 months, and 18 months, and 81% of those became housed during the follow-up period, either with family, in supportive housing, or in their own apartments. Younger age, employment, coping skills, family support, absence of substance abuse treatment, and arrest history, all protected against long-term homelessness. Key predictors of duration of homelessness were only older age group (>44 years old) and arrest history but not a diagnosis of mental disability or substance use disorder, as hypothesized at study onset.

Key Points

- Homeless persons have a high prevalence of morbidity of all causes, but especially mental illness, including drug and alcohol use disorders.

- Prevalence of alcohol use is estimated to be between 38% and 68%, drug use 24.4% and 37%, and mood disorders 12% to 30% in various homeless samples.

- Mortality is high among the homeless compared with general population, especially in young men.

- Homelessness seems to increase the risk of suicide, especially in the young male population.

Schizophrenia in the homeless

Folsom and Jeste[32] summarized studies about schizophrenia in the homeless from 1966 to 2001 and found a prevalence range of schizophrenia from 1% to 45%. The studies, which used representative samples and standardized diagnostic instruments, yielded a weighted average of 11% for the prevalence of schizophrenia in the homeless (compared with the ECA findings of 1.3% lifetime prevalence of schizophrenia), with a higher prevalence found in women and in younger and chronically homeless people; 31% to 68% of homeless persons with schizophrenia received mental health treatment in the year before participating in the study.[32]

Geddes et al[33] found a lower prevalence of schizophrenia in 1992 (9%) in a carefully sampled population of homeless from shelters in Edinburgh, Scotland, compared with the prevalence found (25%) in 1966 in a homeless population in Edinburgh. In a sample of 885 homeless persons followed by a psychiatric outreach team in Ottawa, Canada, 16% had symptoms of schizophrenia and 15% had symptoms of psychosis other than schizophrenia. People with schizophrenia and other psychoses were more likely to be foreign born (odds ratios 2.92 for schizophrenia and 4.79 for symptoms of psychosis). Birth in Europe was associated with significantly higher risk for psychosis whereas birth in Asia led to marginally higher risk, and birth in the Caribbean led to no significant risk.[34] These findings mirror those of Cantor-Graae and Selten,[35] who found a relative risk for schizophrenia in migrant populations of 2.9 with a higher relative risk for blacks and second-generation immigrants in a meta-analysis of schizophrenia and migration.

Homelessness in Schizophrenia

Risk factors

Schizophrenia is a risk factor for homelessness: 15% of a population (10,340 people) who had at least one service encounter between 1999 and 2000 for schizophrenia, bipolar disorder, or major depressive disorder at a mental health center in San Diego County were recorded to be homelessness at the time of the encounter[36]; 20% of patients with schizophrenia, compared with 17% with bipolar disorder and 9% with depression, were homeless. African Americans were more likely to be homeless compared with whites, Asians, or Latinos, and men (particularly younger) were more likely to be homeless than women. Odds ratios for homelessness were 2.4 in people with schizophrenia and 1.6 in bipolar disorder compared with major depression, and people who were homeless had a lower global assessment of function score. Substance use disorders and lack of Medi-Cal insurance also increased the risk of homelessness in this population. Among 263 patients with schizophrenia and schizoaffective disorder discharged from hospitals in New York City, those with a higher risk of homelessness at 3 months' follow-up had a combination of severe psychiatric symptoms, a global assessment of function less than 43 (scores between 41 to 50 represent serious psychiatric symptoms or serious impairment in social, occupational, or school functioning), and drug abuse or dependence.[37] One hundred homeless women, 18 years old to 64 years old, with schizophrenia and schizoaffective disorder from shelters, drop-in centers, transitional housing, and psychiatric inpatient units in New York City, were compared with 100 never-homeless women from inpatient and outpatient psychiatric settings. Comorbidity with alcohol and drug abuse and antisocial personality and lack of family support were risk factors for homelessness in women with schizophrenia.[38] In a sample of 500 people with schizophrenia from Xinjin County, Chengdu, in rural China, followed for 10 years, 7.8% became homeless for at least one night. Being separated or never married, living in poor and unstable conditions, lack of income, and family history of mental disorder were identified as independent risk factors for homelessness.[39]

The cost of homelessness in schizophrenia

The cost of homelessness is an integral part of the $9.3 billion annual non–health care expenditures in schizophrenia and was estimated at $6397 million in 2002.[40] Salit and colleagues[41] studied the admissions to public hospitals in New York City in a sample of 18,864 homeless persons versus admissions of a sample of low-income adults who were not homeless: 51% of the homeless admissions were for substance abuse and mental health treatment compared with only 22.8% of the admissions in the other low-income adults; homeless persons spent an average of 4.1 days longer in the hospital than the group of low-income adults who were not homeless, translating to more than $4000 excess cost per patient if the admission was for mental illness— $3370 for AIDS patients and $2414 for other types of admissions. Rosenheck[14] reported on the costs of specific treatment components in the US Homeless Chronically Mentally Ill Veterans Program, calculated from a group of 406 people of whom 48.4% had alcohol use disorders, 32.7% had drug abuse or dependence, 12.9% had depression, 11.5% had schizophrenia, and 9.6% had posttraumatic stress disorder. In this group of homeless veterans, the program led to improvement in most of the outcomes measures (psychiatric symptoms, drug and alcohol use, days worked, frequency of social contacts, and homelessness) 1 year after enrollment. Residential treatment was the most expensive treatment component, with 0.25 SD improvement in days housed (9.9 days) estimated at $3553 and 0.25 SD in days worked (2.6 days) estimated at $5,692, 3 to 5 times higher than the case management costs leading to the same improvement.

Service use by homeless people with schizophrenia

Deinstitutionalization, poor access to mental health services, and housing and support services are all thought to contribute to homelessness in people with severe mental illness. Inability of the mentally ill homeless to navigate the mental health system due to disorganization and severity of illness and their lack of or limited income was also implicated in homelessness. Of 10,340 people with schizophrenia, bipolar disorder, or major depression who accessed mental health services in San Diego County in 1999 to 2000, 15% were homelessness at the time of the encounter.[36] Homeless people in this sample used crisis residential services 10 times and inpatient psychiatric services 4 times more than people who were not homeless. Caton[42] compared the demographic characteristics and mental health service use in a sample of 100 homeless men with schizophrenia from a shelter in Upper Manhattan, New York City, with 100 inpatients or outpatients with schizophrenia from Columbia University– affiliated facilities who have never been homeless. The homeless group was 66% black and the never-homeless group was 54% Hispanic. The homeless spent approximately half of the 3 years before the interview without a residence. The pattern of emergency room, inpatient, and outpatient treatment was not significantly different between the homeless and never-homeless groups. The homeless group had significantly poorer discharge planning in regards to living arrangements, aftercare, and finances planning and was also significantly more likely to leave the hospital against medical advice than the never-homeless group. In a sample of homeless people from a shelter in San Diego, California, with access to on-site free medical and psychiatric clinic, Folsom and colleagues[43] identified 47 people with schizophrenia and 47 with major depression who were older than 45. Homeless people with schizophrenia had fewer medical visits, cholesterol and colon cancer screenings, and documented chronic conditions, including diabetes, hypertension and arthritis. A level-of-care approach was proposed for the homeless with mental illness by Stergiopoulos and colleagues,[44] who administered the Colorado Client Assessment Record to 356 men in a shelter in Ontario, Canada. This validated scale assesses an individual's symptoms, risk behaviors, and social and community functioning; appreciates the overall severity; and assesses the individual's strengths for the month before the interview on a scale from 1 (no problems) to 9 (extreme problems, low functioning). In this sample, according with Colorado Client Assessment Record, 25% of individuals were able to care for themselves, one-third needed moderate community support, 38% needed extensive support and rehabilitation through assertive community treatment (ACT) or intensive case management, and 9% required residential care. The investigators found that only 34% of the homeless group received the recommended level of care, whereas 48% were underserved and 19% were overserved. The homeless people who were underserved were significantly more impaired cognitively and due to medical illness. They were also more resistive, had more severe interpersonal problems, and had lesser supports and resources than the group who was not underserved.

Key Points

- Prevalence of schizophrenia in homeless samples is estimated at approximately 11% compared with 1% in general population.

- Homelessness worsens prognosis in schizophrenia and adds a large cost to the health care system.

- Service planning and use by homeless people with schizophrenia is poorer than in never-homeless samples.

- Life expectancy for homeless men with schizophrenia is approximately 50 years, 25 years lower than in US general population.

OBSTACLES IN TREATING HOMELESS PEOPLE WITH SCHIZOPHRENIA

Treating schizophrenia in the homeless has proved challenging in several aspects. Many patients with schizophrenia experience great difficulty accessing the health care system. Many studies have shown great stigma attached to the treatment of the mentally ill, especially toward those with more obvious characteristics of schizophrenia. Lack of coordinated programs and disparities within the health care system create obstacles for treatment of homeless people with schizophrenia.

Cognitive Dysfunction

Patients with severe persistent mental illness, including schizophrenia, display cognitive dysfunction. A systematic review of studies assessing cognitive function in the homeless found that 4% to 7% of all homeless people exhibit global cognitive deficits with focal deficits in verbal and visual memory, attention, cognitive processing speed, and executive function found in multiple studies, such as seen in Burra et al.[45] The cognitive deficits inherent to schizophrenia necessitate the need for intense case management. Coldwell and Bender,[46] in their meta-analysis of ACT effectiveness in the rehabilitation of homeless with severe mental illness, showed that ACT leads to a 37% greater reduction in homelessness and a 26% greater improvement in psychiatric symptom severity compared with standard case management treatment. Even with the most effective treatment models, however, some people with schizophrenia remain homeless and symptomatic for long-term. Burns and colleagues[47] examined this issue in a retrospective study of an Australian male homeless population. The investigators established domains that could contribute to the failure to function of some homeless people with schizophrenia, despite intensive outreach treatment: limited social contact, poor self-care, poor collaboration, persistent psychotic symptoms, and accommodation instability. The case files of homeless men with schizophrenia and schizoaffective disorder (158 in 2000 and 159 in 2005) with previous intensive outreach treatment were reviewed: 17% of the homeless men met criteria for all 5 domains in 2000 and 23% in 2005 had all 5 criteria (not a statistically significant difference), pointing to the fact that several homeless people with schizophrenia may not obtain basic levels of function despite access to intensive outreach programs. There is evidence[48,49] that IQ drops in homeless people, particularly in those with psychosis. Bremner and colleagues[47] assessed IQ and cognitive speed in 62 homeless men in a shelter and found that both premorbid IQ (mean 95.9) and current IQ (mean 83.5) were lower than general population mean of 100. The men with largest decline in cognitive function from premorbid IQ were most likely to homeless for longer periods and to have schizophrenia (mean IQ drop from 98.1 to 74.8, $P<.01$) or alcohol abuse (mean IQ drop from 95.6 to 78.3, $P<.02$). Adams and colleagues[49] assessed cognitive function in 64 homeless women and found that those with significant mental illness demonstrated significant decline in cognitive function, more so than the cognitive decline in homeless women without mental illness. Mentally ill women in this study also exhibited high rates of psychotic symptoms. Spence and colleagues'[50] review of studies assessing cognitive dysfunction in homeless adults determined that the homeless demonstrate a considerable cognitive dysfunction, which must be taken into consideration when designing policies and programs to help this group. It can be concluded that evaluation of cognitive function of all homeless persons, especially those with mental illness, should be included in the initial assessment of the homeless for services. Furthermore, consideration of cognitive dysfunction must be taken when attempting to reintegrate homeless persons back into the community.

Imprisonment

Homeless people, particularly those with severe mental illness, including schizophrenia, are more likely to be incarcerated than the general population. Release from imprisonment is more likely to lead to homelessness and homelessness is more likely to lead to incarceration. This cycle of imprisonment and homelessness creates more difficulty for homeless individuals with schizophrenia to access services and obtain housing. Imprisonment was shown by Kushel and colleagues[51] to lead to both increased rates of homelessness and increased high-risk health behavior. In a sample of 1426 homeless and marginally housed individuals in San Francisco, 25.8% had a prior psychiatric hospitalization and 23.1% had been to prison in their lifetime (compared with 6.6% of US general population in 2001); 84.4% of this population reported lifetime drug use, 50% used cocaine, and 23.9% reported having had an alcohol problem in the past year. In this group of homeless, cocaine and heroin use, mental illness, HIV infection, and having had more than 100 sexual partners and selling drugs at the time of the study were associated with lifetime imprisonment. History of incarceration in the homeless, however, has not been shown to decrease the success rate of housing programs. Malone demonstrated[52] that a criminal background was not predictive of failure to remain in supportive housing: 332 homeless people who lived in supportive housing, of whom 51% had a criminal history, 72% had mental illness, and 68% abused substances and were followed for attainment of housing—72% of all participants obtained consistent housing for 2 years; 70% of those with a criminal history obtained housing whereas 74% without criminal history obtained housing, not a statistically significant difference. These findings lend support to the idea that regulations governing past criminal history in programs benefiting the mentally ill homeless may be unnecessary and are potentially detrimental to a majority of homeless persons with schizophrenia.

Substance Use Disorders

It has been widely documented that patients with schizophrenia are more likely to abuse substances that the general population and this is also true for homeless persons with schizophrenia. The previously mentioned study by Kushel and colleagues[51] also demonstrated that drug abuse and imprisonment were strongly correlated among the homeless: 93% of homeless persons with a history of imprisonment also had a history of drug abuse compared with 81.7% of those with no history of incarceration ($P<.01$). In a study on the effects of substance use disorders on housing stability in homeless mentally ill persons,[53] drug and alcohol abuse was a major mediator of success in obtaining independent housing. In this study of a McKinney Act supported housing project, 361 people with severe mentally illness (schizophrenia, bipolar disorder, or major depression) were randomly assigned to receive traditional case management or intensive case management, and they were randomized to either receive subsidized housing or not. Although this study found no difference in outcomes between the types of case management, those who received rent subsidy were 4.87 times more likely to obtain housing than those without subsidized housing. Those participants who reported no substance use disorders at the beginning of the study were 2.66 times more likely to maintain stable independent housing over 2 years than those who reported a history of substance use. Women were 2.14 times more likely to achieve consistent housing than men. Mental illness diagnosis was not related to the housing outcome in this study, which supports the notion that supported housing should be seriously considered for people with severe mental illness, including schizophrenia.

Stigma

Stigma and bias have long surrounded mental illness, especially schizophrenia. Public attitudes have an impact on the care of homeless people with schizophrenia in several respects. Discrimination against individuals with schizophrenia as hopeless or useless leads to marginalization, which further increases stigma and social isolation. Public support is also vital to outreach programs' continued survival because funding for such programs comes through the government. Several studies have shown that the public does exhibit many biased attitudes toward people with schizophrenia. Link and colleagues[54] demonstrated that significant fears of violence by the mentally ill exist within the general population; 1444 respondents of the 1996 General Social Survey, representing non–health care professionals from across the United States, were presented with randomly assigned clinical vignettes describing individuals with various mental illness or substance abuse. Respondents were then asked about the potential causes of the situations described in the vignettes. Recognition of mental illness, as represented by a response of very likely or somewhat likely to be caused by mental illness, were found to be 88.1% for schizophrenia, 48.7% for alcohol abuse, 43.5% for cocaine dependence, 69.1% for major depressive disorder, and 21.5% for a subclinical "troubled" person. Respondents were also asked if they believed the person represented in the vignette was dangerous; 61% reported to believe that vignette representing a patient with schizophrenia was very likely or somewhat likely to commit violence, and 63% of respondents desired social distance from the individual with schizophrenia. Pescosolido and colleagues[55] compared the 1996 General Social Survey (described previously) to the 2006 General Social Survey, using the same vignettes, and showed that although public perception of the causes of schizophrenia improved from 1996 to 2006, stigma associated with the perceived risk of violence and desire for social distance did not significantly improve. The same clinical vignettes and response rating system were used in both 1996 and 2006. The identification of schizophrenia as a neurobiologic illness significantly increased from 76% in 1996 to 86% in 2006. Stigma associated with schizophrenia also declined but not at a statistically significant rate. These results demonstrate that antistigma efforts in recent years have been successful in educating the population but that significant bias persists despite these efforts.

In 1995 Link and colleagues[56] explored the phenomenon of "compassion fatigue" toward the homeless, using a nationwide telephone survey to assess individuals' compassion as expressed in their willingness to help, empathy and stigma toward the homeless, and whether or not contact with the homeless makes people less compassionate toward the homeless: 86% of people agreed that they feel "sad and compassionate" when thinking of homeless people and great public support was found for programs to support the homeless; 64% of respondents disagreed or strongly disagreed that programs for the homeless cost too much money; and 77% disagreed or strongly disagreed that they felt less compassion than they once did. Lack of empathy was noted of respondents, however; 72% believed that homelessness was often brought on by irresponsible behavior and 64% believed that homelessness was often precipitated by laziness, showing the respondents' limited understanding of how homelessness occurs. This study also found that those with the most contact with the homeless also had the highest levels of compassion for the homeless in most domains assessed. Although bias within the public is somewhat expected, substantial bias also exists within health care professionals toward both the homeless and the mentally ill. There is evidence that physicians' bias and their belief that their work is not respected by peers are among the 4 top obstacles preventing them from working with homeless.[57] Evidence shows,[58] however, that spending time in homeless clinics encourages resident physicians to continue to volunteer in such clinics and that the same applies to medical students. Residents and students who volunteer to work with the homeless have previous experience with volunteering and show caring attitudes for indigent population.

The authors' team surveyed 2 classes of medical students at Georgia Health Sciences University in Augusta for their attitudes toward the homeless. The class of 2014 was surveyed in the first month of medical school, before they had had an opportunity to volunteer with student-led volunteer programs for the homeless, and the class of 2013 after 2 semesters, when they had the opportunity to volunteer with these groups with a tool adapted from the 1995 Link and colleagues[56] survey of attitudes toward the homeless. Although the number of students who completed the survey was small (56 of the 2013 class and 66 of 2014 class), there was a statistically significant improvement in the class' empathy and a decrease in stigma toward the homeless after having volunteered in homeless clinics.[59]

This suggests that medical schools and residency programs have an opportunity to have a positive impact on the future care of homeless persons by exposing their students and residents to the homeless population.

Key Points

- Cognitive decline and substance use disorders should be assessed as part of the mental health evaluation of the homeless, and treatment planning should address these aspects of illness.

- A history of imprisonment does not prevent homeless people from maintaining housing and thus should not be used to limit their access to a residence.

- Stigma against the homeless still exists in medical students, residents, and practicing physicians but can be reduced by direct exposure to this vulnerable population.

INTERVENTIONS FOR MENTAL ILLNESS IN THE HOMELESS
Outreach

In late 1980s, the Homeless Emergency Liaison Project (HELP)[15] aimed to offer treatment to seriously mentally ill homeless people living on the streets in New York City. The psychiatrist in the project team was empowered to order police to transport homeless people who met program criteria of mental illness and risk of harm to an inpatient unit. Of 298 individuals served by the program, 80% had schizophrenia, 73% had comorbid medical conditions—vascular disease, anemia, tuberculosis, infestations, and 38% had abused substances. People in this program were hospitalized for an average of 61 days and one-half were transferred to a state hospital. At 2 years' follow-up, 30% of patients lived in the community whereas 24.5% were still in a state psychiatric hospital. This program's outcome sheds light on a subset of severely ill homeless who were at the time in need of long-term psychiatric care. The Access to Community Care and Effective Services and Supports (ACCESS) study[60] was able to describe the same subset of individuals further. The study explored how awarding funds to support outreach and ACT for 100 homeless people at 9 intervention sites and in addition providing funds and technical support to promote system services integration worked to improve outcomes of homeless mentally ill compared with awarding just funds for outreach and ACT to 9 comparison sites. Of 11,857 individuals approached, 2260 were contacted through street outreach rather than approached in shelters or other agencies. Of those, 79.2% of were male; they were 42 years old on average; 46.2% were black; 5.4% were Hispanic; 58% were psychotic; 41.9% had alcohol abuse or dependence; 22.9% had drug abuse or dependence; and 15.4% had a serious medical condition. Although the street-outreach individuals were older, more severely ill, and took longer to engage in outreach compared with the homeless engaged in the program from shelters and other institutions, once enrolled in case management and controlling for baseline differences, at 3 months' follow-up, they showed equivalent improvement on housing, mental health, substance use, employment, social support, victimization, and quality of life (**Fig. 2**). Although the

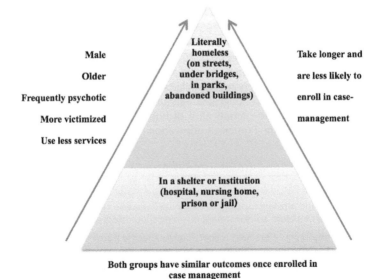

Fig. 2. Characteristics of unsheltered homeless in the United States in the 1990s.

study showed that providing technical support and funds to integrate systems did not improve subject outcomes over the 4 years beyond the improvement owed to outreach and ACT, it offered evidence that the latter 2 strategies are effective in improving a wide array of outcomes. All 18 ACCESS sites showed improvement in all subject outcomes, including mental health, alcohol and substance use, independent housing, public and social support, employment, and quality of life at 1 year after study enrollment for the 7055 study subjects.[61] Women across all sites in the ACCESS sample (2727, followed at 18 months) had significantly better outcomes than men in family relationships, victimization, and social support but being accompanied by children was associated with less change in drug use among women compared with men.[62]

Assertive Community Treatment

ACT uses enrollment criteria and provides a full range of medical, psychosocial, and rehabilitation services by a community-based team that operates around the clock[63] with the goals of stabilizing symptoms, preventing relapse, meeting basic needs, and increasing quality of life and social functioning of its participants. ACT was adapted early after its first implementation to serve the homeless by assigning the individuals to miniteams within ACT and structuring the treatment in engagement, stabilization, and maintenance phases, leading to discharge to a less-intensive program once individuals achieved their program goals.[64] The Critical Time Intervention (CTI) study[65] focused on the transition between the shelter-based psychiatric services and community housing and assigned 96 men with severe mental illness (67% with schizophrenia), substance abuse, and medical comorbidities to CTI or usual services. CTI workers provided up to 9-months of assistance with strengthening of individuals' long-term ties to services, family, and friends and offered emotional and practical support in the transition. The homeless group who received CTI spent an average of 30 days homeless whereas the usual care group spent 90 days homeless during the 18 months' follow-up period.

Morse and colleagues[16] randomly assigned a group of 165 homeless individuals with mental illness to 3 interventions—broker case management, ACT with support from community workers, and ACT only—and followed them for up to 18 months from 1990 to 1993; 81% of these individuals had a diagnosis of schizophrenia (66%), atypical psychosis (12%), and delusional disorder (3%). People assigned to the 2 types of ACT had better contacts with the program and other agencies, lower severity of thought disorder, and higher activity level and satisfaction with the program. People assigned to ACT-only remained in stable housing longer than those in the other treatment conditions. The 3 types of intervention did not generate significantly different effects on income, self-esteem, or substance abuse. In a meta-analysis on the effectiveness of ACT in severely mentally ill homeless, Coldwell and Bender[46] identified 10 studies with a total of 5775 subjects, including 4631 subjects in ACCESS, of which 6 were randomized controlled trials. ACT led to a 37% greater reduction of homelessness and a 26% greater reduction in psychiatric symptoms severity compared with standard case management.

Housing First

Tsemberis and Eisenberg[66–68] advocate Housing First, a concept based on the view that housing is a basic human right of all individuals, including those with disabilities. This concept emphasizes consumer choice and provides housing to the homeless with severe mental illness regardless of their engagement in mental health or substance and alcohol recovery services. Mental and physical health, vocational, and social work services are provided through a modified ACT team, which allows the individuals to determine the type and intensity of services they pursue. This concept requires only that individuals meet with the ACT team regularly and engage in a money management plan. Tsemberis explored whether people with mental illness can maintain independent housing without prior treatment and how the housing retention rate in the Housing First program compares with that of programs that require people to participate in psychiatric and substance abuse treatment and maintain sobriety before providing housing (continuum of care approach). A sample of 206 homeless individuals, 79% men, and 51% homeless, of whom 53% had schizophrenia, were assigned to the Housing First with modified ACT or a continuum of care approach and followed for 24 months between December 1997 and January 2001.[68] Individuals in the Housing First group perceived their consumer choices as significantly more numerous and more stable over time. The Housing First participants were housed sooner and more stably and spent less time homeless than the continuum of care group. There were no differences in the alcohol and substance use between the 2 groups, although people in the Continuum of Care group used substance abuse recovery services significantly more and the groups did not significantly differ in psychiatric symptoms. Tsemberis and colleagues[68] emphasized the 80% housing retention rate for the Housing First group compared with less than 40% for the continuum of care group.

Key Points

- ACT is more effective than other interventions in improving housing rates and psychiatric symptoms in the homeless.
- Providing housing and case management for homeless individuals with chronic mental illness increases their likelihood of retaining a residence. Even if not required by the housing program, they use mental health and substance abuse treatment services.

FUTURE DIRECTIONS FOR THE MENTALLY ILL HOMELESS

Homeless people with mental illness, in particular those with schizophrenia, are a vulnerable yet underserved population who deserve special attention from the policy makers and health care providers. Their particular characteristics, for example, cognitive dysfunction and comorbid substance use, should be acknowledged, evaluated, and addressed in treatment plans. Doing so without amplifying the stigma already existing in society and even among care providers, however, is difficult. ACT is the best-studied and most-effective intervention for homeless with severe mental illness, including schizophrenia. Adding a treatment that addresses cognition in the transition to housing—for example, cognitive adaptive therapy,[69] a manual-driven treatment that uses environmental supports and compensatory strategies to enhance function—and strengthening services for alcohol and substance use disorders may further enhance ACT. Housing availability, although expensive and scarce in the current socioeconomic context, may decrease the societal burden of caring for this population. Health professions' education to address the specific characteristics of the homeless and provide exposure to this population early in professional training is a promising approach to dispel the societal stigma that may extend to doctors, nurses, and other health care providers. In urban centers with a high concentration of homeless people, access to dedicated comprehensive, integrated programs, such as the Boston Health Care for the Homeless Program,[70] can ensure continuity of care from street and shelter to hospital and clinics and eventually may help form a relationship between clinician and patient. Despite increased awareness due to ongoing research and of existing resources to support homeless persons, in particular those with chronic severe mental illness, they remain a vulnerable and underserved population.

REFERENCES

1. HUD's 2010 annual homeless assessment report to congress. 2011. Available at: http://www.hudhre.info/documents/2010HomelessAssessmentReport.pdf. Accessed November 23, 2011.
2. Henderson C, Bainbridge J, Keaton K, et al. The use of data to assist in the design of a new service system for homeless veterans in New York City. Psychiatr Q 2008;79:3–17.
3. Chamberlain C, Mackenzie D. Australian Census Analytic Program "Counting the Homeless". 2008. Available at: http://www.ausstats.abs.gov.au/Ausstats/subscriber. nsf/0/57393A13387C425DCA2574B900162DF0/$File/20500-2008Reissue.pdf. Accessed January 12, 2012.
4. UK Housing Review 2007/2008. Available at: http://www.york.ac.uk/res/ukhr/ ukhr0708/compendium.htm. Accessed January 12, 2012.
5. Edgar B, Doherty J, Meert H. Review of statistics on homeless in europe, FEANTSA European Federation of National Organizations working with the homeless. 2003. Available at: http://www.elsevier.com/framework_products/promis_misc/clinics_ sample_ref.pdf. Accessed January 12, 2012.
6. Fischer PJ, Breakey WR. The epidemiology of alcohol, drug and mental disorders among homeless persons. Am Psychol 1991;46:1115–28.
7. Hwang S. Mental illness and mortality among homeless people. Acta Psychiatr Scand 2001;103:81–2.
8. Robins LN, Helzer JE, Croughan J, et al. National institute of mental health diagnostic interview schedule: its history, characteristics, and validity. Arch Gen Psychiatry 1981;38(4):381–9.
9. Spitzer RL, Williams JB, Gibbon M, et al. The structured clinical interview for DSM-III-R (SCID), I: history, rationale, and description. Arch Gen Psychiatry 1992;49(8): 624–9.
10. Zanis DA, McLellan AT, Cnaan RA, et al. Reliability and validity of the addiction severity index with a homeless sample. J Subst Abuse Treat 1994;11(6):641–8.
11. Lehman AF. A Quality of Life Interview for the chronically mentally ill. Eval Program Plann 1988;11:51–62.
12. Shern DL, Wilson NZ, Coen AS, et al. Client outcomes II: longitudinal client data from the Colorado treatment outcome study. Milbank Q 1994;72:123–48.
13. Ellis RH, Wilson NZ, Foster FM. Statewide treatment outcome assessment in Colorado: the Colorado Client Assessment Record (CCAR). Community Ment Health J 1984;20(1):72–89.
14. Rosenheck RA, Frisman L, Gallup P. Effectiveness and cost of specific treatment elements in a program for homeless mentally ill veterans. Psychiatr Serv 1995; 46(11):1131–9.
15. Marcos LR, Cohen NL, Nardacci D, et al. Psychiatry takes to the streets, the New York City initiative for the homeless mentally ill. Am J Psychiatry 1990;147(11):1557–61.
16. Morse GA, Calsyn RJ, Klinkenberg WD, et al. An experimental comparison of three types of case management for homeless mentally ill persons. Psychiatr Serv 1997;48:497–503.
17. Vazquez C, Munoz M, Crespo M, et al. A comparative Study of the 12-Months Prevalence of physical health problems among homeless people in Madrid and Washington, DC. Int J Ment Health 2006;34(3):35–56.

18. Frencher SK, Benedicto CM, Kendig TD, et al. A comparative analysis of serious injury and illness among homeless and housed low income residents of New York City. J Trauma 2010;69:S191–9.
19. Babidge NC, Buhrich N, Butler T. Mortality among homeless people with schizophrenia in Sidney, Australia: a 10-year follow-up. Acta Psychiatr Scand 2001;103: 105–10.
20. Hwang SW, O"Connell JJ, Lebow JM, et al. Health care utilization among homeless adults prior to death. J Health Care Poor Underserved 2001;12(1):50–8.
21. Hwang SW. Mortality among men using homeless shelters in Toronto, Ontario. JAMA 2000;283(16):2152–7.
22. Hennekens CH, Hennekens AR, Hollar D, et al. Schizophrenia and increased risks of cardiovascular disease. Am Heart J 2005;150:1115–21.
23. Mundy P, Robertson M, Robertson J, et al. The prevalence of psychotic symptoms in homeless adolescents. J Am Acad Child Adolesc Psychiatry 1990;29(5):724–31.
24. Fichter MM, Quadflieg N. Prevalence of mental illness in homeless men in Munich, Germany: results from a representative sample. Acta Psychiatr Scand 2001;103(2):94–104.
25. Herrman HE, McGorry PD, Bennett PA, et al. Age and severe mental disorders in homeless and disaffiliated people in inner Melbourne. Med J Aust 1990;153: 197–205.
26. American Psychiatric Association, Diagnostic and statistical manual of mental disorders, 3rd edition, Revision (DSM-III-R), American Psychiatric Association, 1000 Wilson Boulevard, Arlington, VA 22209-3901, 1987.
27. Regier DA, Boyd JH, Burke JD, et al. One-month prevalence of mental disorders in the United States based on five epidemiologic catchment area sites. Arch Gen Psychiatry 1988;45(11):977–86.
28. Kales JP, Barone MA, Bixler EO, et al. Mental illness and substance use among sheltered homeless persons in lower density population areas. Psychiatr Serv 1995;46(6):592–5.
29. Haughland G, Siegel C, Hopper K, et al. Mental illness among homeless individuals in a suburban county. Psychaitr Serv 1997;48(4):504–9.
30. Fazel S, Khosla V, Doll H, et al. The prevalence of mental disorders among the homeless in western countries: systematic review and meta-regression analysis. PLoS Med 2008;5(12):e225.
31. Caton CL, Dominguez B, Schanzer S, et al. Risk factors for long term homelessness: findings from a longitudinal study of first time homeless single adults. Am J Public Health 2005;95(10):1753–9.
32. Folsom D, Jeste DV. Schizophrenia in homeless persons: a systematic review of literature. Acta Psychiatr Scand 2002;105:404–13.
33. Geddes J, Young G, Bailey S, et al. Comparison of prevalence of schizophrenia among residents of hostels for homeless people in 1966 and 1992. BMJ 1994; 308(6932):814.
34. Dealberto MC, Middlebro A, Farrell S. Symptoms of schizophrenia and psychosis according to foreign birth in a Canadian sample of homeless persons. Psychiatr Serv 2011;62(10):1187–93.
35. Cantor-Graae E, Selten JP. Schizophrenia and migration: a meta-analysis and review. Am J Psychiatry 2005;162:12–24.
36. Folsom DP, Hawthorne W, Lindamer LG, et al. Prevalence and risk factors for homelessness and utilization of mental health services among 10,340 patients with serious mental illness in a large public mental health system. Am J Psychiatry 2005;162(2):370–6.

37. Olfson M, Mechanic D, Hansell S, et al. Prediction of homelessness within three months of discharge among inpatients with schizophrenia. Psychiatr Serv 1999; 50(5):667–73.

38. Caton CL, Shrout PE, Dominguez B, et al. Risk factors for homelessness among women with schizophrenia. Am J Public Health 1995;85:1153–6.

39. Ran MS, Chan CL, Chen EY, et al. Homelessness among patients with schizophrenia in rural China: a 10-year cohort study. Acta Psychiatr Scand 2006;114:118–23.

40. Wu EQ, Birnbaum HG, Shi L, et al. The economic burden of schizophrenia in the United States in 2002. J Clin Psychiatry 2005;66:1122–9.

41. Salit SA, Kuhn EM, Hartz AJ. Hospitalization costs associated with homelessness in New York City. N Engl J Med 1998;338:1734–40.

42. Caton CL. Mental Health Service use among homeless and never-homeless men with schizophrenia. Psychiatr Serv 1995;46(11):1139–43.

43. Folsom DP, McCahill M, Bartels SJ, et al. Medical comorbidity and receipt of medical care by older homeless people with schizophrenia or depression. Psychiatr Serv 2002;53(11):1456–60.

44. Stergiopuolos V, Dewa C, Durbin J, et al. Assessing the mental health service needs of the homeless: a level of care approach. J Health Care Poor Underserved 2010;21:1031–45.

45. Burra TA, Stergiopoulos V, Rourke SB. A systematic review of cognitive deficits in homeless adults: implications for service delivery. Can J Psychiatry 2009;54(2): 123–33.

46. Coldwell CM, Bender WS. The effectiveness of assertive community treatment for homeless populations with severe mental illness: a meta-analysis. Am J Psychiatry 2007;164(3):393–9.

47. Burns A, Robins A, Hodge M, et al. Long-term homelessness in men with a psychosis: limitation of services. Int J Ment Health Nurs 2009;18(2):126–32.

48. Bremner AJ, Duke PJ, Nelson HE, et al. Cognitive function and duration of rooflessness in entrants to a hostel for homeless men. Br J Psychiatry 1996;169(4):434–9.

49. Adams CE, Pantelis C, Duke PJ, et al. Psychopathology, social and cognitive functioning in a hostel for homeless women. Br J Psychiatry 1996;168(1):82–6.

50. Spence S, Stevens R, Parks R. Cognitive dysfunction in homeless adults: a systematic review. J R Soc Med 2004;97(8):375–9.

51. Kushel MB, Hahn JA, Evans JL, et al. Revolving doors: imprisonment among the homeless and marginally housed population. Am J Public Health 2005;95(10): 1747–52.

52. Malone DK. Assessing criminal history as a predictor of future housing success for homeless adults with behavioral health disorders. Psychiatr Serv 2009;60(2): 224–30.

53. Hurlburt MS, Hough RL, Wood PA. Effects of substance abuse on housing stability of homeless mentally ill persons in supported housing. Psychiatr Serv 1996;47(7):731–6.

54. Link BG, Phelan JC, Bresnahan M, et al. Public conceptions of mental illness: labels, causes, dangerousness, and social distance. Am J Public Health 1999; 89(9):1328–33.

55. Pescosolido BA, Martin JK, Long JS, et al. "A disease like any other"? A decade of change in public reactions to schizophrenia, depression, and alcohol dependence. Am J Psychiatry 2010;167(11):1321–30.

56. Link BG, Schwartz S, Moore R, et al. Public knowledge, attitudes, and beliefs about homeless people: evidence for compassion fatigue. Am J Community Psychol 1995;23(4):533–55.

57. Doblin BH, Gelberg L, Freeman HE. Patient care and professional staffing patterns in McKinney Act clinics providing primary care to the homeless. JAMA 1992;267(5):698–701.

58. O'toole TP, Hanusa BH, Gibbon JL, et al. Experiences and attitudes of residents and students influence voluntary service with homeless populations. J Gen Intern Med 1999;14(4):211–6.

59. Murro D, Gable J, Smith L, et al. Students partner with the community to screen homeless mentally ill. Poster presented at the National Outreach Scholarship Conference. Raleigh, 2010.

60. Lam JA, Rosenheck RA. Street outreach for persons with serious mental illness: is it effective? Med Care 1999;37(9):894–907.

61. Rosenheck RA, Lam J, Morrissey JP, et al. Service systems integration and outcomes for mentally ill homeless persons in the ACCESS program. Psychiatr Serv 2002;53(8):958–66.

62. Cheng A, Kelly P. Impact of an integrated service system on client outcomes by gender in a national sample of a mentally ill homeless population. Gend Med 2008;5(4):395–404.

63. Burns BJ, Santos AB. Assertive community treatment: an update of randomized trials. Psychiatr Serv 1995;46(7):660–75.

64. Dixon LB, Krauss N, Kernan E, et al. Modifying the PACT model to serve homeless persons with severe mental illness. Psychiatr Serv 1995;46(7):684–8.

65. Susser E, Valencia E, Conover S, et al. Preventing recurrent homelessness among mentally ill men: a "critical time" intervention after discharge from a shelter. Am J Public Health 1997;87(2):256–62.

66. Tsemberis S, Eisenberg RF. Pathways to housing: supported housing for street-dwelling homeless individuals with psychaitric disabilities. Psychiatr Serv 2000; 51(4):487–93.

67. Tsemberis S, Moran L, Shinn M, et al. Consumer preference programs for individuals who are homeless and have psychiatric disabilities: a drop-in center and a supported housing program. Am J Community Psychol 2003;32(3–4):305–17.

68. Tsemberis S, Gulcur L, Nakae M. Housing first, consumer choice and harm reduction for homeless individuals with a dual diagnosis. Am J Public Health 2004;94(4):651–6.

69. Draper ML, Stutes D, Maples N, et al. Cognitive adaptive training for outpatients with schizophrenia. J Clin Psychol 2009;65(8):842–53.

70. O'Connell JJ, Oppenheimer SC, Judge CM, et al. The Boston health care for the homeless program: a public health framework. Am J Public Health 2010;100(8): 1400–8.

71. Centers for Disease Control. Morbidity and mortality weekly report, quickstats: life expectancy at birth, by race and sex, United States, 2000—2009. 2011;60(18):588. Available at: http://www.cdc.gov/mmwr/preview/mmwrhtml/mm6018a5.htm?s_cid=mm6018a5_w. Accessed January 12, 2012.

Internet-Based Interventions for Psychosis: A Sneak-Peek into the Future

Mario Álvarez-Jiménez, PhD, DClinPsy[a,b],*,
John F. Gleeson, PhD, MClinPsych[c], Sarah Bendall, PhD, MClinPsych[a,b],
R. Lederman, PhD[d], G. Wadley, PhD[d], E. Killackey, DClinPsy[a,b],
Patrick D. McGorry, PhD, MD[a,b]

KEYWORDS

- Psychiatric interventions • Peer support • Family interventions
- Internet interventions • Psychosis • Mental health access

KEY POINTS

- People suffering from psychosis use the Internet regularly and online-based interventions have been well-received by people with psychosis and their carers.
- The use of the Internet in psychosis treatment has been neglected and is overdue.
- Online-based interventions for psychosis should be designed to supplement existing models of care and augment social inclusion, rather than replacing available resources.
- Innovative and flexible interventions that integrate different technologies, evidence-based therapy, and peer and professional support are likely to be more acceptable and effective.
- Internet-based interventions may begin to overcome major challenges in the field of early intervention including engagement with specialised services and maintenance of treatment effects.

INTRODUCTION

Psychotic disorders are among the most costly mental health disorders in terms of human suffering and societal expenditure.[1] Their onset, typically in the critical development period of adolescence and early adulthood, has severe effects on individuals, families, and society.[2] Although advances in antipsychotic medication have led to a better prognosis in relation to psychotic symptoms,[3] this has not translated into

[a] Orygen Youth Health Research Centre, Victoria, Melbourne, Australia; [b] Centre for Youth Mental Health, The University of Melbourne, Victoria, Melbourne, Australia; [c] Department of Psychology, Australian Catholic University, Melbourne, Australia; [d] The Department of Computing and Information Systems, The University of Melbourne, Victoria, Melbourne, Australia
* Corresponding author. Orygen Youth Health Research Centre, Centre for Youth Mental Health, The University of Melbourne, 35 Poplar Road, Parkville 3054, Melbourne, Victoria, Australia.
E-mail address: malvarez@unimelb.edu.au

Psychiatr Clin N Am 35 (2012) 735–747
http://dx.doi.org/10.1016/j.psc.2012.06.011
0193-953X/12/$ – see front matter © 2012 Elsevier Inc. All rights reserved.

improved functional or social outcomes.[4] Compared with the general population, people with psychosis are disproportionally undereducated, unemployed, living in unstable accommodation, or homeless.[5] People living with psychosis experience extreme social isolation, with most experiencing difficulties in maintaining close relationships, and more than half reporting significant unmet needs in relation to their treatment.[5]

Psychosis continues to be one of the most stigmatized conditions, with nearly half of patients experiencing frequent discrimination or victimisation.[6] The diagnosis of psychosis is commonly associated with a perception of a catastrophic loss of social status that often results in self-stigma, shame, and social avoidance.[7] Many medical treatments exacerbate this by disempowering people with psychotic illness, for example through the use of compulsory treatment orders or compulsory commitment to inpatient treatment.[8] Stigma further diminishes self-esteem and self-efficacy[9] and adversely affects help seeking and treatment engagement among many patients.[8]

Family members are as much victims of psychosis as the patients themselves.[10] Caring for a young person with psychosis is demanding, often isolating, and leads to high levels of distress and burden.[11] Moreover, the stigma associated with having a family member with psychosis often leads to social isolation, avoidance, and shame, causing many families to lose their own support network.[11]

The Development and Challenges of Psychosocial Interventions for Psychosis

In recent decades, there has been a growing interest in the development and evaluation of psychosocial interventions focused on improving functional and social outcomes in psychosis. Novel interventions such as cognitive behavioral therapy,[3,12,13] vocational support,[14] peer-support services,[15] psychoeducation,[16] and family interventions[17,18] have been shown to be effective in improving clinical symptoms, relapse rates, vocational outcomes, and quality of life, and reducing the burden of carers. However, despite mounting evidence supporting their effectiveness, studies uniformly point to unacceptably low penetration rates, with less than 10% of patients having access to evidence-based psychosocial interventions.[19,20] Reasons for poor accessibility include costly delivery and dissemination of specialized interventions, geographic barriers and transportation costs, and the stigma associated with mental health treatment, which limits help seeking and treatment attendance among people with severe mental disorders.[8]

The previous decade has witnessed the increasing use of the Internet, which has become more than a simple information and communication tool.[21] With increasing access to novel information and communication technologies in developed countries, a growing number of users resort to the Internet for information on, and support for, mental health disorders.[22] A wide array of different resources exists, ranging from psychoeducation and peer-to-peer support forums to e-counseling and self-help therapy.[23] Given the acceptability and accessibility of novel information and communication technologies, Internet-based interventions have the potential to overcome existing barriers by providing cost-effective, nonstigmatizing, and ongoing support to people with psychosis. However, although research has investigated the use of Web-based and mobile-based applications to support depression[24,25] and anxiety,[26] such approaches have rarely been applied to the treatment of psychotic disorders.

This article provides a critical review of the potential for Internet-based applications to improve clinical and psychosocial outcomes in people with psychosis. Current evidence on Internet-based interventions, potential benefits or harms, and current challenges are reviewed and recommendations are proposed for future interventions for psychosis using these technologies.

IS INTERNET-BASED SUPPORT ACCEPTABLE TO PEOPLE WITH PSYCHOSIS?

The extant research indicates that the Internet is a powerful source of information and support for patients with psychosis, with the potential to significantly influence health-related behaviors and decisions as well as the clinician-patient relationship.[27] Although more studies are needed, preliminary evidence suggests that the use of the Internet by people with psychosis resembles that of individuals not affected by mental illness.[27] In addition to the general advantages such as accessibility and the capacity to access a wide array of resources,[28] people with psychosis resort to the Internet because of the anonymity and absence of a hierarchy on the Web and its potential to assist in overcoming difficulties with social interaction.[27] A reported advantage of Internet-based support is the disinhibiting effect of online communication as well as the potential for such communication to overcome the fear of stigma by removing the face-to-face aspect.[29] In the context of online therapy, disinhibition can encourage therapeutic expression and self-reflection, helping patients to be more open about their illness.[30,31] In this sense, some online therapists report anecdotally that relating through text-based self-disclosure can induce a high degree of intimacy and honesty from early in the therapy process.[32]

Information and communication technologies can be particularly useful for young people, including those with psychosis. Individuals less than 25 years of age are the greatest users of Internet resources[33] and the adolescent population is particularly comfortable interacting within the computer environment.[29] Recent surveys have shown that young people are more likely than their older counterparts to trust mental health information Web sites and perceive them as likely to be helpful.[21] In addition, some young people, particularly teenagers, would sometimes rather interact with a computer than talk to a therapist.[34] Parental attitudes toward the Internet, belief in help seeking, and greater willingness to relate with peers with mental disorders seem to predict whether young people consider the Internet to be helpful in dealing with mental illness.[21] Although there is little evidence on the acceptability and feasibility of online interventions for young people with psychosis, preliminary qualitative research suggests that this population shows positive attitudes toward Internet-based interventions and, in particular, toward online social networking.[29]

WHAT TYPE OF INTERNET-BASED INTERVENTIONS ARE EFFECTIVE IN THE TREATMENT OF PSYCHOSIS?

Until recently, despite their clinical and social potential, online interventions had not been used and tested for the treatment of psychosis. Only a few recent studies have investigated the effectiveness of Internet-based interventions such us online peer-support groups,[30] family interventions,[35,36] psychoeducation,[37] and mobile interventions[38] in the treatment of psychosis, with no studies specifically focused on patients with first-episode psychosis (FEP). However, taken together, the preliminary research provides useful insights into the potential, challenges, and future directions of such interventions.

Online Peer-Support Groups

The development of peer support or user-led services for people with mental disorders has rapidly increased worldwide. The enthusiasm for these services is based on solid theory as well as promising research findings.[15] Peer support rests on the assumption that people who have overcome adversity can provide valuable support, guidance, and hope to others facing similar difficulties.[15] Moreover, consistent with the helper-therapy principle,[39] being able to be of assistance to others can improve self-esteem and reduce experiences of self-stigma.[40] Research on user-led services has found robust associations between peer support, empowerment, and recovery in people with psychosis.[40] Likewise, interactions with peers in settings that respect empowerment and self-determination have been postulated to reduce self-stigma through enhancing group identification and, in turn, increasing self-esteem and self-efficacy.[41] In addition to these benefits, the potential of peer support to enhance social support networks and improve quality of life is widely recognized.[30]

With the widespread use and access to the Internet, online peer-support groups have proliferated, many of which are specifically mental health support groups.[30] However, despite their prevalence and likely benefits, little is known about the effectiveness or risks of such groups in people with psychosis.

The limited existing research suggests that online mental health groups for depression can improve depressive symptoms and increase the use of health services as a result of the information accessed through the Internet.[42] In addition, some people prefer online peer support rather than face-to-face interventions because of the stigma associated with mental illness,[31] making online interventions a valid alternative for those unlikely to engage in traditional treatment.

Research on the effects of these groups for people with psychosis is even more sparse. A recent study that involved patients with depression and psychotic disorders found that participation in an unmoderated, unstructured peer-support group was not associated with clinical or psychological benefits.[30] This finding is in contrast with previous studies examining structured or moderated support groups,[31,43] suggesting that group facilitation and the structure in which peer support occurs may be important elements to bringing about positive results.[30] It has been argued that the lack of moderation and structure may adversely affect the group's ability to attain a sense of community, a pivotal element of peer support.[30] An alternative is that unmoderated and unstructured forums may lead to an excess of expressions of fear and anxiety, which have been associated with increased levels of depression and lower quality of life.[44] In addition, although participants may feel positive about helping others, the absence of formal supervision or guidance may generate higher levels of distress in some peer supporters.

Online Family Interventions

Family intervention is a recommended and evidence-based treatment in schizophrenia.[45] The effectiveness of family interventions in reducing relapse rates and hospital admissions, and improving compliance with medication in schizophrenia, is well documented.[46] Family interventions have shown effectiveness in improving the experience of caregiving and reducing the burden of the caring role.[18] However, despite their widely recognized benefits, only a small proportion of those caring for a family member with schizophrenia have access to such interventions,[19,20] mainly because of high dissemination costs. Online interventions have the potential to overcome some of these barriers and, therefore, to improve the accessibility of evidence-based support for carers.

To date, only 2 studies have investigated the effectiveness of online family interventions in schizophrenia.[35,36] Rotondi and colleagues[35] assessed the effectiveness of an online family psychoeducation program focused on promoting self-efficacy, self-management, and problem-solving strategies, in tandem with professionally moderated patient and carer discussion forums. This study showed a high level of engagement in and usage of the online intervention by patients with schizophrenia and their carers. In addition, the online intervention significantly improved positive psychotic symptoms and knowledge about schizophrenia in both patients and their supporters. However, the intervention showed no effect on other clinical or social variables.[35] Glynn and colleagues[36] evaluated the effectiveness of an online multi-family intervention for relatives of people with schizophrenia. The intervention comprised a real-time, professionally moderated chat program for anonymous groups of 5 to 6 relatives, a discussion board, and educational material on behavioral family interventions. Consistent with the results of Rotondi and colleagues,[35] this study showed a good level of participation and engagement in the online groups, although the intervention did not have a significant effect on clinical status, relatives' distress, or perceived social support.[36]

When taken together, these findings indicate that it may be necessary to involve patients in the online family intervention to realize positive clinical results.[36] In addition, real-time chats for relatives may not be required to obtain clinical benefits, with asynchronous interventions possibly being more acceptable and convenient for carers. In contrast with the study by Glynn and colleagues,[36] Rotondi and colleagues[35] provided an initial 4-hour workshop for participants, which may account for the increased intervention uptake seen in the latter study. Thus, it may be that social networking that is not anonymous fosters a sense of belonging to the virtual community and the motivation to participate in online forums.

Online Psychoeducation

Psychoeducational interventions for schizophrenia seek to enhance patients' knowledge of, and insight into, their illness to assist them in coping more effectively with their condition, thereby improving prognosis.[16] A substantial body of research has provided evidence that psychoeducation improves medication compliance, reduces relapse rates, promotes social functioning, and increases satisfaction with mental health services.[16] Preliminary research suggests that computer-based psychoeducation can be acceptable, as effective as face-to-face or paper-based methods, and preferred by some.[37,47] Although more research is needed to ascertain their effectiveness, useful elements, type of content, and format, novel technologies are likely to provide a cost-effective and acceptable medium to deliver psychoeducation, which may appeal to younger patients and those more familiar with Internet-based technologies. In the meantime, online interventions that provide clear and engaging information and cater for cognitive deficits and levels of insight are likely to produce better outcomes.[13,48,49]

Mobile-Based Interventions

Mobile devices, including microcomputers, tablets, mobile phones, and smart phones, are developing at a rapid rate, and hold great promise for influencing and even transforming treatment delivery in psychosis.[50] Recent evidence shows that mobile technology is helping to bridge the gap between socioeconomic layers through far-reaching access to such devices in relation to computer-based Internet connection or home-serviced Internet packages.[50] With mobile phone subscriptions having reached almost 6 billion worldwide,[51] emerging evidence shows that homeless and socially disadvantaged people use mobile phones regularly.[50,52] US studies suggest that some minority groups such as African American and Latino people have become leading users of mobile Internet devices.[53] Coupled with their widespread accessibility, the portability, online connectivity, and ease of use of current mobile devices provide an unprecedented opportunity to deliver evidence-based interventions, enable real-time support, and gather ecologically valid information in psychosis treatment.

Preliminary evidence shows that mobile devices are both acceptable to, and efficiently used by, people with schizophrenia.[38,50,54,55] In addition, preliminary research shows that mobile interventions can bring about improved outcomes in schizophrenia.

Spaniel and colleagues[56] conducted a 1-year open trial with patients with schizophrenia and their carers in which early warning signs of relapse were assessed weekly by a 10-item questionnaire delivered via a mobile phone. Responses were collected using SMS (short message service), and, if the total score exceeded a given threshold, an alert was declared and the treating psychiatrist notified by an e-mail message. Phone contact with the patient and prompt evaluation of the patient's current status was then recommended. Compared with the year before the intervention, there was a 60% reduction in the number of hospital admissions.[56]

In contrast, Granholm and colleagues[55] recently used mobile devices to administer cognitive behavioral interventions in a therapeutic context. In their study, 55 participants with schizophrenia received 840 text messages over a 12 week-period targeting medication adherence, socialization, and auditory hallucinations. The text-messaging intervention incorporated principles of cognitive behavior therapy, with 4 types of messages sent for each outcome of interest: outcome and cognition assessment, pre-elicited thought-challenging messages, and personalized behavioral coping strategies. The intervention was acceptable to most users and was associated with a significant improvement in auditory hallucinations and number of social interactions.[55] Medication adherence improved for those living independently, suggesting that the intervention was effective in assisting participants with higher functioning and/or lower support in taking medications.[55] However, those with lower functioning and more negative symptoms were less likely to complete the intervention, although newer generations of smart, easier-to-use phones may enable mobile interventions to be effectively used in these patients.[55]

Oorschot and colleagues[57] deployed an experienced sampling method (ESM)[58] to elucidate individual patterns of symptoms, social interaction, contextual factors, and their longitudinal interaction, with the purpose of delivering tailored psychoeducation. This innovative approach may augment face-to-face interventions by improving insight, promoting the therapeutic alliance between clinician and patient, and personalizing treatment strategies.[57]

Internet and FEP

In the preceding 2 decades, early intervention for psychosis has emerged as a major international focus of clinical service delivery.[59] The enthusiasm for early intervention is bolstered by findings that treatment delay leads to symptomatic and psychosocial deterioration[60] and worse clinical response.[61] In addition, the early course of psychosis is thought to be a critical period after which the level of disability sustained,[62] or recovery attained,[4] is likely to endure into the longer term.[63] As a result, it has been argued that there is a window of opportunity to minimize or even prevent disability in this group by providing prompt psychosocial interventions as part of their rehabilitation.[14]

Novel information and communication technologies provide an unprecedented opportunity for enhancing, and even revolutionizing, early intervention for psychosis. Given the general enthusiasm of young people for novel technologies, Internet-based interventions may be particularly effective for, and appealing to, patients with FEP. Innovative interventions using these technologies may play a pivotal role in addressing significant challenges, including access to and engagement with specialized early intervention services, and provision of extended support to maintain the clinical and functional gains of specialized early intervention services.

To our knowledge, despite their theoretic potential, no study has investigated the feasibility or effects of Internet-based interventions for patients with FEP. We therefore conducted a focus group with young people with psychosis with the aim of examining their views on technology-based tools. Qualitative analysis showed that patients with FEP were enthusiastic about the use of Internet-based strategies as part of their treatment program. They preferred a system characterized by connectivity (ie, users should be able to contact peers, share personal experiences, support each other, and contact clinicians if required). In addition, the system should resemble regular social networking programs (ie, asynchronous, ongoing communication), but be separate from them, and expert moderators should guide, but not censor, the interaction to ensure a safe and supportive network. Patients also indicated that the system should provide useful and updated information relevant to their needs, and optional therapeutic interventions (ie, cognitive behavioral strategies).

In contrast, there was little enthusiasm for SMS-based systems, particularly if the messages were automated rather than of human origin. Concerns were also raised about the potential risks of Internet-based strategies when experiencing active psychotic symptoms (ie, acute phase).Patients were also negative about systems that required them to fill out numerous questionnaires, and, on the whole, about content that made them feel worse and focus negatively on their condition.

CHALLENGES, RISKS, AND ETHICAL ISSUES OF INTERNET-BASED INTERVENTIONS IN PSYCHOSIS

In addition to their potential to bring about significant clinical benefits, Internet-based interventions for psychosis pose both familiar and new clinical risks and ethical issues. Some of these challenges and suggested solutions are discussed later.

It has been argued that participation in Internet peer-support forums may cause harm by increasing participants' social isolation, exposing participants to harmful or misleading advice, or reducing engagement with health care providers.[30] Research specifically assessing the potential risk or harm of online forums for schizophrenia is limited, and the evidence coming from mental heath forums and the general community is mixed. Initial research on the general community suggested that Internet use may increase social isolation and reduce well-being, indicating that online ties were displacing strong, face-to-face relationships.[64] In contrast, more recent evidence has challenged these earlier findings by showing an association between Internet usage, decreased loneliness and depression, and increased perceived social support, self-esteem, and well-being.[65,66] There is also evidence that Internet use does not interfere with face-to-face relationships and may serve as a tool to create or augment relationships or enhance users' connection with the community.[67] These mixed results may be partly accounted for by user personal characteristics and social context, with more extroverted and socially connected users benefiting more from Internet usage.[66] It is also likely that Internet content mediates the relationship between Internet use, personal characteristics, and outcomes, with less socially connected users engaging in less beneficial or even harmful online activity. For example, excessive expressions of fear and anxiety have been shown to induce increased stress and reduce quality of life,[44] whereas Internet interventions focused on self-efficacy have produced improved clinical outcomes in patients with schizophrenia.[35]

Concerns about misleading advice or reduced access to health care providers are not supported by the literature. Recent studies have shown that advice provided by peers is generally appropriate, and inaccurate advice is corrected by others in a timely manner.[68] Furthermore, participation in online peer-support groups has been shown to encourage members to seek professional advice[69] and to empower participants to become more involved in their own treatment,[31] indicating that Internet-based support is unlikely to interfere with face-to-face mental health care.

In our view, Internet-based interventions for psychosis that are specifically designed to supplement existing mental health services and augment traditional relationships through online interaction (either enhancing existing relationships or encouraging new ones that carry over to the off-line world) are likely to be most beneficial. In addition, professionally moderated forums focused on positive constructs such as self-efficacy, problem solving, and social recovery may enhance their clinical effectiveness and minimize risks related to negative content or misuse of the online tool.

Internet-based interventions may expose vulnerable participants to hostile interactions or to others who may take advantage of them as a result of disclosing private information, because anonymity reduces accountability for one's actions.[30] One solution to this problem is to develop anonymous forums that ensure users' safety and reduce the risk of sensitive information being disclosed beyond the confines of the online group. However, anonymity may induce a lack of connection to other group members by reducing the sense of trust and, as a result, the likelihood of developing positive relationships, an essential element of peer support and online interventions. An alternative and potentially more cost-beneficial strategy may be to develop closed, secure online forums, in which users are clients of existing clinical services and/or identities are verified by the researchers.[70] Moreover, appropriate screening procedures, with exclusion of high-risk individuals (eg, participants with significant paranoid ideation or antisocial personality traits), regular moderation of online content, a report button for users, clear forum guidelines and usernames specific to the online group[70] (but identities possibly known to other users) may enhance the benefits of online interactions for patients with schizophrenia, the risk of participation being lessened.

In addition, patients with schizophrenia are at risk of experiencing a psychotic relapse, self-harm, and other psychiatric emergencies and Internet and mobile-based interventions typically include assessments of clinical symptoms that extend beyond the traditional model of care. Although around-the-clock monitoring provides a unique opportunity for relapse and suicide prevention, it also introduces significant practical and ethical dilemmas. To address this issue, rigorous protocols for safety need to be carefully devised. Although further work is warranted to optimize online safety in patients with psychosis, general recommendations include visible emergency guidelines and contact information for users,[36] regular monitoring of online interactions,[71] computerized monitoring of self-harm–related terms,[72,73] and a detailed emergency response protocol.[38]

DEVELOPMENT OF INTERNET-BASED INTERVENTIONS FOR PSYCHOSIS: IMPLICATIONS FOR PRACTICE

Although the procedure for devising Internet-based interventions for psychosis is underinvestigated, a systematic and phased development is likely to increase the likelihood of acceptance and the effectiveness of such interventions.[70] To this end, several recommendations have been put forward, including careful analysis of users' needs and preferences before development,[70] active involvement of stakeholders throughout all phases of development,[70] and regular consultations with potential users in all aspects of the protocols (ie, emergency responding, therapy/psychoeducation content and wording, graphic design, and specific features).[38] In addition, the relevance of multimodal and carefully planned induction and training procedures and extensive pilot testing has been highlighted.[38]

SUMMARY AND RECOMMENDATIONS FOR FUTURE RESEARCH

Preliminary research suggests that people with psychosis use the Internet in a similar manner to those not affected by mental illness. Likewise, Internet-based or mobile-based interventions developed to support people with psychosis and their families have been consistently well received by users. Such interventions may be particularly acceptable to, and beneficial for, young people with early psychosis. However, despite their potential, the use of innovative Internet-based technologies in psychosis treatment has been neglected and is overdue.

In the meantime, future interventions for psychosis should be systematically developed in accordance with user needs and in regular consultation with stakeholders. Careful attention should be paid to ethical issues, clinical safety, and emergency procedures. Innovative and flexible interventions that integrate different technologies (eg, mobile phones, chat rooms), evidence-based therapy, and peer and professional support are likely to be both more acceptable and more effective. Online-based interventions should be designed to supplement existing models of care and augment social inclusion, rather than replacing available resources.

Internet-based interventions hold great promise to revolutionize psychosis treatment and early intervention through increasing the accessibility of evidence-based interventions, reducing the stigma and anxiety associated with face-to-face care, and providing around-the-clock peer and professional support to patients and their families. These novel interventions may begin to overcome some major challenges, including engagement with mental health services and maintenance of treatment effects. The Internet has the potential to foster global recovery in people with psychosis beyond what is possible in traditional interventions. Internet-based support can be empowering, enabling consumers to link up, and even shape the nature of the services, support, and care they are receiving in line with the main principles of the recovery framework.[40]

REFERENCES

1. van Os J, Kapur S. Schizophrenia. Lancet 2009;374:635–45.
2. McGorry PD, Killackey E, Yung A. Early intervention in psychosis: concepts, evidence and future directions. World Psychiatry 2008;7:148–56.
3. Alvarez-Jimenez M, Parker AG, Hetrick SE, et al. Preventing the second episode: a systematic review and meta-analysis of psychosocial and pharmacological trials in first-episode psychosis. Schizophr Bull 2011;37:619–30.
4. Alvarez-Jimenez M, Gleeson JF, Henry LP, et al. Road to full recovery: longitudinal relationship between symptomatic remission and psychosocial recovery in first-episode psychosis over 7.5 years. Psychol Med 2012;42(3): 595–606.
5. Morgan VA, Waterreus A, Jablensky A, et al. People living with psychotic illness 2010. Canberra (Australia): Department of Health and Ageing; 2011.
6. Albrecht GL, Walker VG, Levy JA. Social distance from the stigmatized. A test of two theories. Soc Sci Med 1982;16:1319–27.
7. Birchwood M, Trower P, Brunet K, et al. Social anxiety and the shame of psychosis: a study in first episode psychosis. Behav Res Ther 2007;45: 1025–37.
8. Corrigan P. How stigma interferes with mental health care. Am Psychol 2004;59: 614–25.
9. Corrigan PW, Watson AC, Barr L. The self-stigma of mental illness: implications for self-esteem and self-efficacy. J Soc Clin Psychol 2006;25:875–84.
10. McFarlane WR, Cook WL. Family expressed emotion prior to onset of psychosis. Fam Process 2007;46:185–97.
11. Kuipers E, Onwumere J, Bebbington P. Cognitive model of caregiving in psychosis. Br J Psychiatry 2010;196:259–65.

12. Gleeson JF, Cotton SM, Alvarez-Jimenez M, et al. A randomized controlled trial of relapse prevention therapy for first-episode psychosis patients: outcome at 30-month follow-up. Schizophr Bull 2011. [Epub ahead of print].

13. Alvarez-Jimenez M, Gleeson JF, Cotton S, et al. Predictors of adherence to cognitive-behavioural therapy in first-episode psychosis. Can J Psychiatry 2009;54:710–8.

14. Killackey E, Jackson HJ, McGorry PD. Vocational intervention in first-episode psychosis: individual placement and support v. treatment as usual. Br J Psychiatry 2008;193:114–20.

15. Davidson L, Chinman M, Sells D, et al. Peer support among adults with serious mental illness: a report from the field. Schizophr Bull 2006;32:443–50.

16. Xia J, Merinder LB, Belgamwar MR. Psychoeducation for schizophrenia. Cochrane Database Syst Rev 2011;(6):CD002831.

17. Pharoah F, Mari J, Rathbone J, et al. Family intervention for schizophrenia. Cochrane Database Syst Rev 2006;(4):CD000088.

18. Gleeson JF, Cotton SM, Alvarez-Jimenez M, et al. Family outcomes from a randomized control trial of relapse prevention therapy in first-episode psychosis. J Clin Psychiatry 2010;71:475–83.

19. Lehman AF, Steinwachs DM. Patterns of usual care for schizophrenia: initial results from the Schizophrenia Patient Outcomes Research Team (PORT) client survey. Schizophr Bull 1998;24:11–20 [discussion: 20–32].

20. Lehman AF, Kreyenbuhl J, Buchanan RW, et al. The Schizophrenia Patient Outcomes Research Team (PORT): updated treatment recommendations 2003. Schizophr Bull 2004;30:193–217.

21. Oh E, Jorm AF, Wright A. Perceived helpfulness of websites for mental health information: a national survey of young Australians. Soc Psychiatry Psychiatr Epidemiol 2009;44:293–9.

22. Eysenbach G, Kohler C. Health-related searches on the Internet. JAMA 2004; 291:2946.

23. Van't Hof E, Cuijpers P, Stein DJ. Self-help and Internet-guided interventions in depression and anxiety disorders: a systematic review of meta-analyses. CNS Spectr 2009;14:34–40.

24. Christensen H, Griffiths KM, Jorm AF. Delivering interventions for depression by using the internet: randomised controlled trial. BMJ 2004;328:265.

25. Cuijpers P, Smit F, Bohlmeijer E, et al. Efficacy of cognitive-behavioural therapy and other psychological treatments for adult depression: meta-analytic study of publication bias. Br J Psychiatry 2010;196:173–8.

26. Cuijpers P, Marks IM, van Straten A, et al. Computer-aided psychotherapy for anxiety disorders: a meta-analytic review. Cogn Behav Ther 2009;38:66–82.

27. Schrank B, Sibitz I, Unger A, et al. How patients with schizophrenia use the internet: qualitative study. J Med Internet Res 2010;12:e70.

28. Fox S, Rainie L. The online health care revolution. Pew Internet & American Life Project; 2000. Available at: http://www.pewinternet.org/Reports/2000/The-Online-Health-Care-Revolution.aspx. Accessed January 15, 2012.

29. Lederman R, Wadley G, Gleeson JF, et al. Supporting young people with psychosis in the community: an ICT-enabled relapse prevention tool. Paper presented at: Proceedings of the Pacific Asia Conference on Information Systems (PACIS). Brisbane (Australia): PACIS; 2011.

30. Kaplan K, Salzer MS, Solomon P, et al. Internet peer support for individuals with psychiatric disabilities: a randomized controlled trial. Soc Sci Med 2010;72: 54–62.

31. Houston TK, Cooper LA, Ford DE. Internet support groups for depression: a 1-year prospective cohort study. Am J Psychiatry 2002;159:2062–8.
32. Rochlen AB, Zack JS, Speyer C. Online therapy: review of relevant definitions, debates, and current empirical support. J Clin Psychol 2004;60:269–83.
33. Lloyd R, Bill A. Australia online: how Australians are using computers and the internet. 2001 Australian Census Analytic Program. Publication 2056.0. Canberra (Australia): Australian Bureau of Statistics; 2004.
34. Abeles P, Verduyn C, Robinson A, et al. Computerized CBT for adolescent depression ("Stressbusters") and its initial evaluation through an extended case series. Behav Cogn Psychother 2009;37:151–65.
35. Rotondi AJ, Anderson CM, Haas GL, et al. Web-based psychoeducational intervention for persons with schizophrenia and their supporters: one-year outcomes. Psychiatr Serv 2010;61:1099–105.
36. Glynn SM, Randolph ET, Garrick T, et al. A proof of concept trial of an online psychoeducational program for relatives of both veterans and civilians living with schizophrenia. Psychiatr Rehabil J 2010;33:278–87.
37. Jones RB, Atkinson JM, Coia DA, et al. Randomised trial of personalised computer based information for patients with schizophrenia. BMJ 2001;322:835–40.
38. Depp CA, Mausbach B, Granholm E, et al. Mobile interventions for severe mental illness: design and preliminary data from three approaches. J Nerv Ment Dis 2010;198:715–21.
39. Riessman F. The 'helper-therapy' principle. Soc Work 1965;10:27–32.
40. Corrigan PW. Impact of consumer-operated services on empowerment and recovery of people with psychiatric disabilities. Psychiatr Serv 2006;57:1493–6.
41. Watson AC, Corrigan P, Larson JE, et al. Self-stigma in people with mental illness. Schizophr Bull 2007;33:1312–8.
42. Ritterband LM, Gonder-Frederick LA, Cox DJ, et al. Internet interventions: in review, in use, and into the future. Prof Psychol Res Pr 2003;34:527–34.
43. Dunham PJ, Hurshman A, Litwin E, et al. Computer-mediated social support: single young mothers as a model system. Am J Community Psychol 1998;26:281–306.
44. Lieberman MA, Goldstein BA. Not all negative emotions are equal: the role of emotional expression in online support groups for women with breast cancer. Psychooncology 2006;15:160–8.
45. Onwumere J, Bebbington P, Kuipers E. Family interventions in early psychosis: specificity and effectiveness. Epidemiol Psychiatr Sci 2011;20:113–9.
46. Pharoah F, Mari J, Rathbone J, et al. Family intervention for schizophrenia. Cochrane Database Syst Rev 2010;(12):CD000088.
47. Walker H. Computer-based education for patients with psychosis. Nurs Stand 2006;20:49–56.
48. Gonzalez-Blanch C, Crespo-Facorro B, Alvarez-Jimenez M, et al. Cognitive dimensions in first-episode schizophrenia spectrum disorders. J Psychiatr Res 2007;41:968–77.
49. Williams C, Whitfield G. Written and computer-based self-help treatments for depression. Br Med Bull 2001;57:133–44.
50. Ben-Zeev D. Mobile technologies in the study, assessment, and treatment of schizophrenia. Schizophr Bull 2012;38(3):384–5.
51. The World in 2011: ICT Facts and Figures. International Telecommunication Union; 2010. Available at: http://www.itu.int/ITU-D/ict/facts/2011/material/ICTFacts. Accessed January 22, 2012.

52. Le Dantec CA. Exploring mobile technologies for the Urban Homeless. ACM Conference on Computer Supported Cooperative Work (CSCW 2010). Savannah (GA): CSCW; 2010.

53. Smith A. Mobile access 2010. Pew internet & American Life Project; 2010. Available at: http://www.pewinternet.org/Reports/2010/Mobile-Access-2010.aspx. Accessed January 15, 2012.

54. Granholm E, Loh C, Swendsen J. Feasibility and validity of computerized ecological momentary assessment in schizophrenia. Schizophr Bull 2008;34:507–14.

55. Granholm E, Ben-Zeev D, Link PC, et al. Mobile Assessment and Treatment for Schizophrenia (MATS): a pilot trial of an interactive text-messaging intervention for medication adherence, socialization, and auditory hallucinations. Schizophr Bull 2012;38(3):414–25.

56. Spaniel F, Vohlidka P, Hrdlicka J, et al. ITAREPS: information technology aided relapse prevention programme in schizophrenia. Schizophr Res 2008;98:312–7.

57. Oorschot M, Lataster T, Thewissen V, et al. Mobile assessment in Schizophrenia: a data-driven momentary approach. Schizophr Bull 2012;38(3):405–13.

58. Palmier-Claus JE, Myin-Germeys I, Barkus E, et al. Experience sampling research in individuals with mental illness: reflections and guidance. Acta Psychiatr Scand 2011;123(1):12–20.

59. McGorry PD, Yung AR. Early intervention in psychosis: an overdue reform. Aust N Z J Psychiatry 2003;37:393–8.

60. Melle I, Larsen TK, Haahr U, et al. Reducing the duration of untreated first-episode psychosis: effects on clinical presentation. Arch Gen Psychiatry 2004;61:143–50.

61. Alvarez-Jimenez M, Gleeson JF, Henry LP, et al. Prediction of a single psychotic episode: a 7.5-year, prospective study in first-episode psychosis. Schizophr Res 2011;125:236–46.

62. Birchwood M, Todd P, Jackson C. Early intervention in psychosis. The critical period hypothesis. Br J Psychiatry Suppl 1998;172:53–9.

63. Crumlish N, Whitty P, Clarke M, et al. Beyond the critical period: longitudinal study of 8-year outcome in first-episode non-affective psychosis. Br J Psychiatry 2009; 194:18–24.

64. Kraut R, Patterson M, Lundmark V, et al. Internet paradox. A social technology that reduces social involvement and psychological well-being? Am Psychol 1998;53:1017–31.

65. Shaw LH, Gant LM. In defense of the internet: the relationship between Internet communication and depression, loneliness, self-esteem, and perceived social support. Cyberpsychol Behav 2002;5:157–71.

66. Kraut R, Kiesler S, Boneva B, et al. Internet paradox revisited. J Soc Issues 2002; 58:49–74.

67. Katz JE, Aspden P. A nation of strangers? Commun ACM 1997;40:81–6.

68. Esquivel A, Meric-Bernstam F, Bernstam EV. Accuracy and self correction of information received from an internet breast cancer list: content analysis. BMJ 2006; 332:939–42.

69. Mendelson C. Gentle hugs: internet listservs as sources of support for women with lupus. ANS Adv Nurs Sci 2003;26:299–306.

70. Valimaki M, Anttila M, Hatonen H, et al. Design and development process of patient-centered computer-based support system for patients with schizophrenia spectrum psychosis. Inform Health Soc Care 2008;33:113–23.

71. Sharkey S, Jones R, Smithson J, et al. Ethical practice in internet research involving vulnerable people: lessons from a self-harm discussion forum study (SharpTalk). J Med Ethics 2011;37:752–8.

72. Huang YP, Goh T, Liew CL. Hunting Suicide Notes in Web 2.0- Preliminary Findings. Paper presented at Ninth IEEE International Symposium on Multimedia Workshops. Washington, DC: IEEE Computer Society; 2007.
73. Goh TT. Monitoring youth depression risk in Web 2.0. VINE 2009;39:192.

Index

Note: Page numbers of article titles are in **boldface** type

A

Antipsychotic polypharmacy, **661–681**
    concerns with, 663
    electronic search for correlates of, 663–664
        exclusion of adverse effect associations, 663
    prevalences of, geographical, 662
    reasons for, 662–663
Antipsychotic polypharmacy studies, characteristics of, 664
    illness characteristics in, 665–666
    illness variables in, 670
    limitations of, 672–673
    medication costs in, 672
    medication variables in, 670–671
    patient variables in, 664–665, 669
    prescriber characteristics in, 667, 670
    provider variables in, 670–671
    treatment setting in, 667–671
Attention and vigilance, in neurocognitive manifestations of psychosis risk, 601

B

Biomarkers and predictors, **645–659**
    BDNF as putative marker, described, 649
        in chronic schizophrenia, 651–652
        in first-episode psychosis, 650–651
        preclinical studies of, 650
    BDNF Val/Met polymorphism studies, 652
    challenges, lack of validation, 652–653
    classification of, 645
    for schizophrenia, biological markers, 647
        dopamine, 647–648
        endophenotypes, 647
        GABA, 648
        glutamate, 648
        neuronal signaling molecules, 648–649
        opportunities for, 646–649
    of disease, 646

C

Cognitive enhancement, **683–698**
    as therapeutic target, functional capacity in, 684–685

Psychiatr Clin N Am 35 (2012) 749–755
http://dx.doi.org/10.1016/S0193-953X(12)00069-X
0193-953X/12/$ – see front matter © 2012 Elsevier Inc. All rights reserved.

Moving?

Make sure your subscription moves with you!

To notify us of your new address, find your **Clinics Account Number** (located on your mailing label above your name), and contact customer service at:

Email: journalscustomerservice-usa@elsevier.com

800-654-2452 (subscribers in the U.S. & Canada)
314-447-8871 (subscribers outside of the U.S. & Canada)

Fax number: 314-447-8029

Elsevier Health Sciences Division
Subscription Customer Service
3251 Riverport Lane
Maryland Heights, MO 63043

*To ensure uninterrupted delivery of your subscription, please notify us at least 4 weeks in advance of move.

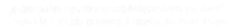

Printed and bound by CPI Group (UK) Ltd, Croydon, CR0 4YY

03/10/2024

01040456-0002